Wearable Bioelectronics

Wearable Bioelectronics

Edited By

Onur Parlak
*Postdoctoral Research Fellow, Materials Science and Engineering,
Stanford University, Stanford, CA, United States*

Alberto Salleo
*Associate Professor of Materials Science, Stanford University,
Stanford, CA, United States*

Anthony Turner
*Emeritus Professor of Biotechnology, SATM, Cranfield University,
Cranfield, Bedfordshire, United Kingdom*

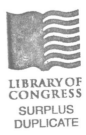

ELSEVIER

Elsevier
Radarweg 29, PO Box 211, 1000 AE Amsterdam, Netherlands
The Boulevard, Langford Lane, Kidlington, Oxford OX5 1GB, United Kingdom
50 Hampshire Street, 5th Floor, Cambridge, MA 02139, United States

Notices
Knowledge and best practice in this field are constantly changing. As new research and experience broaden
our understanding, changes in research methods, professional practices, or medical treatment may become
necessary.

Practitioners and researchers must always rely on their own experience and knowledge in evaluating and
using any information, methods, compounds, or experiments described herein. In using such information or
methods they should be mindful of their own safety and the safety of others, including parties for whom they
have a professional responsibility.

To the fullest extent of the law, neither the Publisher nor the authors, contributors, or editors, assume any
liability for any injury and/or damage to persons or property as a matter of products liability, negligence or
otherwise, or from any use or operation of any methods, products, instructions, or ideas contained in the
material herein.

Library of Congress Cataloging-in-Publication Data
A catalog record for this book is available from the Library of Congress

British Library Cataloguing-in-Publication Data
A catalogue record for this book is available from the British Library

ISBN: 978-0-08-102407-2

For information on all Elsevier publications
visit our website at https://www.elsevier.com/books-and-journals

Publisher: Matthew Deans
Acquisition Editor: Kayla Dos Santos
Editorial Project Manager: Joshua Mearns
Production Project Manager: Maria Bernard
Cover Designer: Christian J. Bilbow

Typeset by SPi Global, India

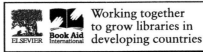

Contents

Chapter 6: Wearable device for thermotherapies *179*

Minyoung Suh, Sergio Curto, Punit Prakash, Gerard van Rhoon

Chapter 7: Soft actuator materials for textile muscles and wearable bioelectronics..*201*

Edwin W.H. Jager, Jose G. Martinez, Yong Zhong, Nils-Krister Persson

Contributors

Yuanyuan Bai   Suzhou Institute of Nano-tech and Nano-bionics, Chinese Academy of Sciences, Beijing, China

Lourdes Basabe-Desmonts   BIOMICs Research Group, Lascaray Ikergunea, Research Center, University of the Basque Country, Vitoria-Gasteiz; Ikerbasque, Basque Foundation for Science, Bilbao, Spain

Fernando Benito-Lopez   Analytical Microsystems & Materials for Lab-on-a-Chip (AMMa-LOAC) Group, Microfluidics Cluster UPV/EHU, Analytical Chemistry Department, University of the Basque Country UPV/EHU, Vitoria-Gasteiz, Spain

Vincenzo F. Curto   Electrical Engineering Division, Department of Engineering, University of Cambridge, Cambridge, United Kingdom

Sergio Curto   Radiation Oncology, Erasmus MC Cancer Institute, Rotterdam, The Netherlands

Ravinder Dahiya   School of Engineering, University of Glasgow, Glasgow, United Kingdom

Sam Emaminejad   Interconnected and Integrated Bioelectronics Lab, Department of Electrical and Computer Engineering, University of California, Los Angeles, CA, United States

Edwin W.H. Jager   Division of Sensor and Actuator Systems, Department of Physics, Chemistry and Biology (IFM), Linköping University, Linköping, Sweden

Jose G. Martinez   Division of Sensor and Actuator Systems, Department of Physics, Chemistry and Biology (IFM), Linköping University, Linköping, Sweden

Sina Moshfeghi   Interconnected and Integrated Bioelectronics Lab, Department of Electrical and Computer Engineering, University of California, Los Angeles, CA, United States

William Navaraj   School of Engineering, University of Glasgow, Glasgow, United Kingdom

Edilberto Ojeda   Analytical Microsystems & Materials for Lab-on-a-Chip (AMMa-LOAC) Group, Microfluidics Cluster UPV/EHU, Analytical Chemistry Department, University of the Basque Country UPV/EHU; BIOMICs Research Group, Lascaray Ikergunea, Research Center, University of the Basque Country, Vitoria-Gasteiz, Spain

Onur Parlak   Department of Materials Science and Engineering, Stanford University, Stanford, CA, United States

Nils-Krister Persson   Smart Textiles, Swedish School of Textiles (THS), University of Borås, Borås, Sweden

Sanaz Pilehvar   Interconnected and Integrated Bioelectronics Lab, Department of Electrical and Computer Engineering, University of California, Los Angeles, CA, United States

Punit Prakash   Electrical and Computer Engineering, Kansas State University, Manhattan, KS, United States

Kamyar Salahi   Interconnected and Integrated Bioelectronics Lab, Department of Electrical and Computer Engineering, University of California, Los Angeles, CA, United States

Alberto Salleo   Department of Materials Science and Engineering, Stanford University, Stanford, CA, United States

Alina Sekretaryova   Department of Chemistry, Uppsala University, Uppsala, Sweden

Clara Smith   School of Engineering, University of Glasgow, Glasgow, United Kingdom

Phoenix Stout   Interconnected and Integrated Bioelectronics Lab, Department of Electrical and Computer Engineering, University of California, Los Angeles, CA, United States

Minyoung Suh   Textile and Apparel, Technology and Management, North Carolina State University, Raleigh, NC, United States

Gerard van Rhoon   Radiation Oncology, Erasmus MC Cancer Institute, Rotterdam, The Netherlands

Shuqi Wang   Suzhou Institute of Nano-tech and Nano-bionics, Chinese Academy of Sciences, Beijing, China

Bo Wang   Interconnected and Integrated Bioelectronics Lab, Department of Electrical and Computer Engineering, University of California, Los Angeles, CA, United States

Andrew Wilhelm   Interconnected and Integrated Bioelectronics Lab, Department of Electrical and Computer Engineering, University of California, Los Angeles, CA, United States

Aaron Wilhelm   Interconnected and Integrated Bioelectronics Lab, Department of Electrical and Computer Engineering, University of California, Los Angeles, CA, United States

Ting Zhang   Suzhou Institute of Nano-tech and Nano-bionics, Chinese Academy of Sciences, Beijing, China

Yong Zhong   Division of Sensor and Actuator Systems, Department of Physics, Chemistry and Biology (IFM), Linköping University, Linköping, Sweden

Preface

We are delighted to introduce the very first book on *Wearable Bioelectronics*, to serve the global community with topical critical and tutorial reviews covering aspects of bioelectronic technology and engineering.

Wearable technologies are one of the most important and recent breakthroughs in the bioelectronics field and have attracted considerable attention because of their potential to change classical and established approaches in medicine and biotechnology. Wearable bioelectronics offer huge promise due to their ease of miniaturization, the possibility of rapid and in situ analysis, and the potential for low-cost fabrication. With more innovation and further attention to overcome technical hurdles, novel approaches and methodologies are expected to open up new and exciting avenues for the maintenance of well-being and the delivery of personalized health care. However, achieving these paradigm shifts requires significant progress and research into new materials, interfaces, circuit designs, power sources, and data processing, together with new business models. With this book, we aim to survey recent trends in wearable bioelectronics and their implications for health-care applications. In Chapter 1, *Ting Zhang et al.* provide an overview of the importance of materials and systems for wearable designs, introducing the reader to different materials and how they influence device performance. The following chapters (Chapter 2 by *Emaminejad et al.* and Chapter 3 by *Parlak et al.*) piece together different types of wearable sensors, including physical and (bio)chemical sensors, to highlight and discuss challenges, early breakthroughs, and key developments in point-of-care diagnostics. These chapters also draw attention to sample handling strategies for various wearable sensor systems. In Chapter 4, *Alina Sekretaryova* stresses the importance of powering strategies for wearable bioelectronic devices and outlines various different approaches. Moving toward applying these principles to develop innovative devices for the bioelectronic world, *Dahiya et al.* review the fascinating field of e-skin for health care in Chapter 5, and *Suh et al.* introduce the new concept of wearable devices for thermotherapies in Chapter 6. Finally, *Jager et al.* describe textile-based artificial muscles in Chapter 7, where electronic methods are employed to yield functional wearable devices. Each of these chapters concludes with a discussion of key examples in their respective areas and their implications in the field of wearable bioelectronics.

We hope you enjoy this book as much as we have enjoyed putting it together. It remains for us to thank all the contributing authors for their enthusiasm and patience and the editorial publishing team of Elsevier for all diligent work, and particularly Joshua Mearns and Kayla Dos Santos for enabling the publication of this book.

Onur Parlak, Anthony P.F. Turner, Alberto Salleo

CHAPTER 1

Materials, systems, and devices for wearable bioelectronics

Shuqi Wang[1], Yuanyuan Bai[1], Ting Zhang*
Suzhou Institute of Nano-tech and Nano-bionics, Chinese Academy of Sciences, Beijing, China

Chapter Outline

1.1 Introduction

Wearable bioelectronics, research on sophisticated state-of-the-art wearable devices which enable real-time monitoring of individuals' physiological parameters, has attracted much interest from researchers and clinicians in the recent years [1–5]. Researchers and clinicians believe that wearable devices could not only lead to significant improvements in personal health monitoring, to track one's metabolic status in real time for timely and effective diagnosis and treatment of diseases, but also bring tremendous benefits by building more advanced health-care systems. By using sophisticated wearables, a wide range of physical and (bio) chemical signals such as heart rate, blood pressure, respiration, body motion, body temperature, electrophysiological signs [e.g., electrocardiogram (ECG) and electroencephalogram (EEG)],

---

*Corresponding author.
[1] These authors contributed equally.

Wearable Bioelectronics. https://doi.org/10.1016/B978-0-08-102407-2.00002-3

and biofluids' (e.g., sweat, tears, saliva) components (e.g., electrolytes and metabolites) are available for real-time monitoring with clinical or health-care importance [6–9]. This makes it possible for portable and systematic home monitoring, which holds the promise to be used for remote medicine practices by connecting with the Internet of Things [10].

Wearable bioelectronic devices are basically represented by several components including the sensor module, processing module, communication module, and powering module, which are required to be mounted on soft skin, curved surfaces, or moving joints. Therefore, flexibility and stretchability are essential for their intimate and comfortable wearability. Thanks to the progress in this field, dedicated operating system, low-power wireless technologies, miniaturized and flexible sensor units that meet the requirements for wearable bioelectronics are available now. In the recent years, several groups have bridged the gap between those technologies and developed fully integrated wearable bioelectronic device prototypes for on-body physiological signal analysis [11–13]. However, the development of wearable sensors and systems is still in its infancy, researchers have been engaged in developing the technologies of sensing, computing, and processing to enable wearable bioelectronics to revolutionize the way medicine and health care are practiced.

This chapter focuses on the essential component of the flexible/stretchable sensor module in wearable bioelectronic device. Traditional sensors consisted of transducer (e.g., conductive electrode, semiconductor, piezoelectric, and piezoresistive materials) and active materials (e.g., sensitive inorganic materials, enzyme, ion-selective membrane) are rigid and planar (the hybrid materials of sensors have high Young's modulus about 100 GPa), which are mechanically incompatible with soft and curvilinear human body (human tissues have low Young's modulus from < 10 kPa of brain to hundreds kPa of skin), resulting in unreliable results due to the mismatch with skin [3]. Advances have been made in the recent years to develop flexible and stretchable sensors that can be attached intimately to the clothing or directly mounted on the skin for stable and accurate measurements. The following part of this chapter will address the latest strategies of using high-quality materials, novel processing approaches, and special configuration designs for fabrication of flexible/stretchable sensors. Moreover, lightweight wearable bioelectronic devices which can be conformably worn on human body for not only physical activities and vital signs monitoring (e.g., heart rate, respiration, body motion, body temperature), but also for biochemical signal analysis at molecular level (e.g., pH, electrolytes, metabolites) are demonstrated. Challenges and future prospects of flexible sensors are also discussed.

1.2 Materials and structural design for flexible/stretchable sensors

Conformal contact between flexible/stretchable sensor devices and human body can be achieved by matching the mechanical properties of the devices with those of the human tissues. The mounted sensor devices should maintain stable electrical properties under certain level of deformation (e.g., strain tolerance of more than 80% on knuckle, 50% on knee joint, and 30% on arm angle) [4, 14]. Generally, mechanical flexibility and stretchability can be achieved by using intrinsically flexible/stretchable materials, or by special structural design. Various intrinsically flexible/stretchable materials such as elastomeric polymers and nanocomposites have been used as substrates, active elements, and stretchable electrodes for wearable bioelectronics. Besides, advances in the development of nanomaterials have enabled a broad range of functional/active sensing materials to change from bulk rigid material to deformable nanomaterials. Other than these, the special structural design approach shows fascinating ability to engineer the traditional bulk rigid materials (metal and semiconductor) into "flexible/stretchable" electronic component by processing rigid materials as thin films or introducing special structures like serpentine, fractal, helical, and wavy ribbons [15–18]. The specially designed electronic devices can accommodate external deformations while maintaining electrical properties [16]. The following sections summarize commonly used materials and structural design for flexible/stretchable sensors.

1.2.1 Flexible/stretchable substrate

A flexible/stretchable substrate plays an important role in integrating various sensors and actuators for wearable bioelectronics. To provide significant weight and thickness decrease of traditional electronics, and afford compatible interfaces with human tissues to offer the potential for large-area, multimodal, and multipoint sensing on curvilinear surfaces [4], the mechanical properties of the substrate are particularly important. Other aspects including transparency, thermal stability, and chemical resistance should also be taken

Table 1.1: Characteristics of typical flexible substrate materials.

Materials	Stretchable/ bendable	Transparency/ dielectric constant	Thermal Stability/coefficient of thermal expansion	Chemical resistance
PI	Bendable	Low transparency (yellow color) 2.8–3.5	Resist temperature ($<450°C$) $\approx 5 \times 10^{-5}$/K	Weak acids and alkali Ethanol and acetone
PET	Bendable	High transparency ($>85\%$) 2.5–3.5	Resist temperature ($<100°C$) $\approx 7 \times 10^{-5}$/K	Dissolvable in acetone
PEN	Bendable	High transparency ($>85\%$) 2.9–3.2	Resist temperature ($<180°C$) $\approx 2 \times 10^{-5}$/K	Easily permeated by oxygen and water
Silicone (PDMS, Ecoflex)	Stretchable	High transparency ($>95\%$) 2.3–2.8	Resist temperature ($<100°C$) $\approx 30 \times 10^{-5}$/K	Ethanol and acetone (in short time)
Metal foil	Bendable	No Good conductivity	Resist temperature ($\approx 250°C$) Thermal stable	Ethanol and acetone Moisture and oxygen
Paper	Bendable	No 2.3–3.0	Resist temperature ($<100°C$)	No

into consideration for selecting appropriate substrate materials. The chemical and physical properties of typical flexible substrate materials are summarized in Table 1.1.

Among various polymer substrates, polyimide (PI) has been broadly used due to the characteristics like lightweight, flexible, and easy processing and most importantly, PI has a T_g of 275–450°C [19], endowing it with an excellent thermal stability to maintain its performance and slowdown the degradation. Besides, PI has good chemical resistance to weak acids/alkalis, and commonly used organic solvents like alcohols and acetone, making it compatible with the manufacturing processes of micro-electromechanical system (MEMS). However, despite that the stretchability of PI could reach over 120%, a relatively large force is usually needed to stretch it, which restricts its application fields. In addition, normally PI is yellow colored with low transmittance to visible light, making it not suitable for transparent devices. In contrast, polyethylene terephthalate (PET) and polyethylene naphthalate (PEN) are colorless materials with high transmittance (> 85%) to visible light. However, PET and PEN has much lower working temperature limit with a T_g of only 120°C and 150°C [19], respectively, and they present poor flexibility with a stretchability of only 1.8%–2.7%.

Commercially available silicone elastomers, such as polydimethylsiloxane (PDMS) and Ecoflex, are the most commonly used flexible and stretchable substrate materials, due to the merits including excellent biocompatibility, high stretchability, and good processability at low temperatures. Creating microstructures on PDMS films can endow the sensing devices with larger stretchability, higher sensitivity, and faster response time than unstructured PDMS films [20–23]. During a typical fabrication procedure, a micropatterned mold is first prepared using MEMS processing technology, and then degassed and premixed PDMS liquid of the base and cross-linker is spin coated onto the mold, thermally cured, and peeled off from the mold to obtain PDMS film with inversed micropattern. The MEMS technology can create various microstructures including hemispheres, pyramids, microrods, and microlines with high accuracy and reproducibility, but are somehow of high cost. In contrast, some natural materials with microstructures on the surfaces, like lotus leaf [22] and silk-based textiles [24] have been used as cost-effective molds. The versatile textile molds not only provide luxuriant microstructures, but also produce anisotropic microstructures on PDMS films, which will be beneficial for creating smart flexible sensors that can detect the direction of the excitation source.

Besides the synthetic materials, some natural flexible/stretchable materials have also been incorporated as substrates for wearable electronics. For example, textile-based clothing is an essential item of human daily life which plays the role of protection and aesthetics. In the recent years, smart textiles integrated with sensing, monitoring, and information-processing devices have been proposed as a new class of wearable electronic systems for innovative applications in the military, public safety, health care, space exploration, sports, and consumer fitness fields [25–27]. Silk is an intriguing and abundant biomaterial as substrates of flexible electronics, with the advantages of mechanical flexibility, biocompatibility, and biodegradability, which can provide new opportunities for implantable and surgical devices [28]. There are also many new strategies to fabricate paper-based sensors, conductive electronic art, interconnects and antennas, complementary metal-oxide-semiconductor (CMOS) inverters, etc. [29, 30]. Electronic components can be fabricated on paper directly by writing or printing. Paper is widely available and inexpensive, lightweight, flexible, and biodegradable, which offers many advantages for printable and disposable electronic devices.

1.2.2 Functional/active materials

Wearable sensors mounted on human body for physiological data monitoring should be performed with accuracy, repeatability, and stability during skin motion and deformation. Therefore, the functional and active sensor materials for flexible/stretchable sensor should be extensively studied and optimally selected. Active materials mainly refer to materials with specially required performance for functional elements in electronic devices, for example, materials with variable electrical properties to external stimuli (e.g., pressure, strain, humidity, temperature) for sensing. Graphene, carbon nanotubes (CNTs), metallic and semiconductive nanowires (NWs), conducting polymers, and polymer-based composites are some of the most commonly used active materials for wearable electronic devices including flexible sensors, batteries, and field-effect transistors (FETs).

1.2.2.1 Graphene

Graphene is a two-dimensional (2D) sheet of sp^2-hybridized carbon atoms packed in hexagonal structure, with extraordinary properties including high in-plane charge mobility ($\sim 2 \times 10^5 \, cm^2 V^{-1} s^{-1}$) [31], thermal conductivity ($\sim 5000 \, W \, m^{-1} K^{-1}$) [32], superior mechanical flexibility and stability (an in-plane tensile elastic strain of up to 25% and Young's modulus of $\sim 1 \, TPa$) [33], high restorability, and also good transparency to visible light (optical absorbance of 2.3% per layer) [34, 35]. Multiple techniques have been developed to produce graphene, such as mechanical/liquid-phase exfoliation, solution-based reduction of graphene oxide (GO), epitaxial growth, and chemical vapor deposition (CVD). The success in producing large-area, high-quality, and patterned graphene with unique properties has promoted the development of graphene-based flexible sensors, FETs, and many other flexible/stretchable electronic devices for wearable bioelectronics.

Mechanical exfoliation utilizes the friction and relative movement between an object and graphite to obtain thin layers of graphene. The method is simple, and can produce graphene samples with thickness down to a single layer. A carrier mobility in excess of $2 \times 10^5 \, cm^2 V^{-1} s^{-1}$ was achieved [31], which in principle would enable the fabrication of high-speed electronic devices even at today's integrated circuit (IC) channel lengths [34]. The very thin thickness of single-layered graphene combined with its unique ambipolarity also make it useful for single molecule detection (e.g., NO_2, NH_3, and H_2O) [36]. However, the mechanical exfoliation process is time consuming, low throughput, and not suitable for mass production. An improved method for high-yield production of graphene is the liquid-phase exfoliation of graphite [37, 38]. The graphene dispersions can be deposited on substrates, be formed into free-standing graphene films by vacuum filtering, or be incorporated into polymers to form composites [39–41], which have been demonstrated to be able to fabricate sensitive, high-strain, and high-rate bodily motion sensors [39].

Solution-based reduction of GO generally refers to creating stable aqueous GO dispersions and depositing GO films, which are then reduced either chemically or by means of thermal annealing to get reduced graphene oxide (r-GO) [34, 42]. Deposition of uniform and reproducible GO films is one key step to obtain high-quality graphene films, various techniques including drop casting, dip coating, spin coating, inject-printing [43], layer-by-layer assembly, and Langmuir-Blodgett (LB) assembly of GO sheets has been developed [42, 44–47]. Wafer-scale r-GO ultrathin films or graphene-based fibers could be obtained, which are useful for fabrication of wearable, highly sensitive strain sensors [48–51], and transparent wearable multifunctional electronic systems integrating stretchable sensors, actuators, light-emitting diodes, and other electronics [52]. Flexible noncontact sensing devices for human-machine interaction applications [53] flexible flash memory [45] and flexible electric circuits and hydrogen peroxide chemical sensors [43] have also been reported.

Epitaxial growth is to form multilayered graphene on single-crystal SiC substrate via sublimation of silicon atoms and reconfiguration of carbon atoms at high temperatures in ultrahigh vacuum or moderate vacuum conditions with controlled background gas [54, 55]. In contrast, the CVD technique uses organic molecules containing carbon as sources to form carbon-saturated surfaces on transition metal substrates at temperatures of hundreds to thousands of degree centigrade, which then decompose into thin layers of graphene upon cooling. Various transition metals have been reported for growing graphene, including crystalline substrates like Ni [56], Pt, Ru, Cu, Co, Ir, Pd, Pt, Fe, Au, Rh, and polycrystalline Ni and Cu substrates. The experiments and theories about epitaxial and CVD growth of graphene are thoroughly reviewed by Tetlow et al. recently [57]. Both the two substrate-based techniques can produce high-quality wafer-scale graphene, which can also be patterned using standard lithography methods for microelectronic and wearable electronic applications [56, 58–60]. The remaining challenge is to conduct systematic studies about the process parameters (e.g., growth temperature and process parameters) to better control the film structure (e.g., strain, defect density, and number of layers) and prevent secondary crystal formation.

1.2.2.2 CNT

CNTs can be considered as sheets of graphene bent into a cylindrical shape forming one-dimensional (1D) nanostructure, which are classified into single-walled carbon nanotubes (SWCNTs) and multiwalled carbon nanotubes (MWCNTs) according to the number of graphene layers. Because of the unique 1D structure of CNT with large aspect ratio, individual CNT possesses high thermal conductivity, large Young's modulus and tensile strength, as well as favorable flexibility and elasticity [61–63], making CNTs quite suitable as reinforcing materials in composites. CNTs may be either metallic or semiconducting depending on its spatial chirality and diameter. Besides, the electronic property varies with mechanical deformation of CNTs, which means CNTs also possess interesting electromechanical properties. These unique properties endow CNTs with a great many potential applications in electronic devices and strain sensors [64, 65]. For better integration with electronic devices, CNTs are usually assembled into macroscopic forms; the intrinsic properties of individual CNT would be lost to some degree, while new properties would be imparted as well. In the recent years, much effort has been devoted to fabricating flexible macroscopic CNT materials (e.g., films [66], fibers [67]) and related electronic devices for wearable electronics [65, 68–70].

Macroscopic CNT films are commonly produced using CVD technique. The growth is often carried out on rigid substrates since high growing temperatures are required, and either randomly distributed or aligned [66, 71–73]. CNT films can be obtained by controlling the growth parameters. The CNT films can also be produced at low temperatures ($< 100°C$) by directly depositing CNT dispersions onto a substrate by dip coating, spray coating [69], spin coating, "LB" deposition, vacuum filtration [74], self-assembly, or electrophoretic deposition. The deposition can be carried out directly on flexible substrates, or be transferred to other highly flexible substrates with the assistance of a stamp or an energy source like laser, heat, or microwave for flexible or wearable electronics [75]. For example, randomly distributed SWCNT films with modified microstructure were directly deposited on PDMS by spray coating, which can accommodate strains of up to 150% as electrodes for pressure/strain sensors [69]. Aligned SWCNT thin films grown by CVD technique were transferred to dog-bone-shaped PDMS substrates to form strain sensors that are capable of measuring strains up to 280% for human motion detection [76]. Other flexible devices including flexible circuits, flexible displays, flexible solar cells, skin-like pressure sensors, and conformable radio frequency identification (RFID) tags have also been demonstrated [77].

Macroscopic CNT fibers (or yarns, strands, threads, ropes) with aligned and even super-aligned CNTs can be produced by several approaches, mainly including wet spinning of SWCNT fibers from nanotube dispersions [35, 45, 78], dry-state spinning of SWCNT and MWCNT fibers from nanotube forests grown by CVD technique [79–83], and twisting/rolling of CNT films [50, 84]. Mechanical strength and flexibility are usually enhanced compared with individual CNTs [81, 85, 86], and by slight over-twisting of CNT yarns to make spring-like ropes, significant elongations, and sustain tensile strains of up to 285% was achieved [87]. Those macroscopic fibers have been used for various wearable devices [42], such as strain sensors, field electron emitters, electrochemical actuators, supercapacitors, and also been woven into self-supporting nanotube sheets [88] or smart textiles [35, 42] for wearable electronics.

1.2.2.3 Semiconductor NWs

Semiconductor NWs, such as Si, Ge, CdS, GaAs, In_2O_3, and CdSe, exhibit interesting mechanical flexibility, piezoresistivity, and optical transparency compared with their bulk counterparts through shape, size, and atomic-composition control, and have been broadly used as materials for FETs, sensors, photodetectors, high-speed circuitry in flexible, and printable electronics [49].

CVD is commonly used to grow semiconductor wires, which is a "bottom-up" approach to grow NWs with desired atomic composition but random orientation. To achieve highly aligned, parallel arrays, the NWs are then harvested and suspended in an organic solvent for the assembly on the desired substrate. Some generic approaches, such as flow-assisted alignment [89], LB assembly, bubble-blown techniques, and electric-field-directed assembly, have been developed for the assembly of NWs on various substrates. However, certain limitations mainly including the scalability, uniformity, and/or the complexity of the processes for use in certain applications still exist. To obtain large-scale and controllable assembly of highly aligned NW parallel arrays, the contact printing technology has been developed by Javey et al. to direct transfer the NWs from the growth to the desired substrate (receiver) [48]. Patterned printing can be achieved by using receiver substrates with lithographically pre-patterned photoresist [48, 90], electron-beam resist [48], or molecular monolayer resist [91]. NW superstructures for integrated electronic and photonic nanotechnologies can also be realized through a multistep printing process [92–94]. Another way to fabricate patterned arrays semiconductor NWs is the "top-down" approach mainly involving conventional lithographic techniques and anisotropic chemical etching with high-quality bulk semiconductor wafers. Elastomeric stamps can be used to transfer the wire arrays to plastic substrates [95, 96].

Various oriented semiconductor NW thin films could be produced at room temperature using the two techniques discussed above, which have been exploited as promising channel materials to build FETs/thin film transistors (TFTs) on plastic substrates for wearable, printable, and disposable electronics. For example, Goldman et al. reported the fabrication of high-performance TFTs on plastics using oriented Si NW thin films or CdS nanoribbons as semiconducting channels [43]. Rogers et al. reported mechanical flexible metal-semiconductor FETs built with GaAs wires [97] and demonstrated their ability to build various elemental units of functional circuits on plastic substrates including inverters and logic gates and diodes [98]. By sequential and repeated transfer printing of semiconductor wires, lateral distributed and vertically stacked layers of NW FETs can be fabricated on plastic substrates for heterogeneous three-dimensional (3D) multifunctional electronic applications [1, 99]. A series of transistor-based electronic devices and circuits, such as flexible pressure-sensor arrays integrated with Gi/Ge NW-array FETs as the active-matrix backplane for low-voltage macroscale artificial skin application [100]. Transistors based on In_2O_3 for detection of NO_2 down to ppb levels [101]. Image sensor circuitry integrated with optically active CdSe NW-based photodiodes and high-mobility Ge/Si NW-based transistors that is capable of detecting and amplifying an optical signal with high sensitivity and precision [94] has also been demonstrated. The FETs generally use the printing and transfer technique to assemble oriented NW thin films as the channel, and the conventional microfabrication processing to fabricate the contact materials and gate dielectrics. In the future, all-printed FETs and FET-based devices and circuitry might be developed to simplify the fabrication process and further reduce the cost.

1.2.2.4 Polymers

Polymers have been widely used as active materials in flexible sensors for wearable electronics for years due to their excellent mechanical flexibility/stretchability and diversity in species. Several kinds of polymers frequently used are described below, including piezoelectric polymers, pyroelectric polymers, conducting polymers, and dielectric elastomers (DEs).

Piezoelectric polymers are polymers that can generate electric charges on the surface under pressure/strain thus convert mechanical energy into electrical energy, while pyroelectric polymers are polymers that can generate electric charges changes on the surface under temperature changes thus convert thermal energy into electrical energy. In this way, piezoelectric and pyroelectric polymers are quite suitable materials for self-powered pressure/strain/temperature sensors. Polyvinylidene fluoride (PVDF) and its copolymer with trifluoroethylene P(VDF-TrFE) are not only piezoelectric but also pyroelectric, and with the merits of superior mechanical flexibility and ease of processing, they have been used in flexible sensors for detection of pressure [102–105], strain [106, 107], or temperature [108]. Sometimes, piezoelectric ceramic nanopowders such as $BaTiO_3$ and $PbTiO_3$ are introduced to form nanocomposites for performance improvement [59, 109]. The polymers are mainly fabricated in the form of thin films, with electrodes on the surfaces to form planar capacitors. Under applied pressure, strain, or temperature, voltage responses at the electrodes are generated to achieve sensing. Commonly, the electrodes can be connected to the gate of a transistor amplifier to read out the sensing signals [59, 105]. For example, Stadlober reported a smart active-matrix sensor array based on P(VDF-TrFE), which was connected to an electrochemical transistor or an organic thin film transistor (OTFT) as the read-out unit to form a touchless control interface [105]. The devices are printable and flexible, but have large areas and complicated structures. Correspondingly, Lee and coworkers [103, 107–109] developed flexible OTFTs integrated directly with P(VDF-TrFE) and P(VDF-TrFE)-BaTiO$_3$ as the gate dielectric layers. The sensing mechanism can be explained as follows: under applied pressure, strain, or temperature, the remnant polarization or equivalent voltage inside the piezoelectric/pyroelectric gate dielectric changes, which modulates the intensity of charges at the semiconductor channel/gate dielectric interface and changes the source-drain read-out current. The devices can not only detect pressure/strain or temperature separately [104, 107, 108], but also be able to respond to static/dynamic pressure/strain and temperature simultaneously and disproportionally [103, 109], which show great potential to be applied as multifunctional e-skins for biomonitoring of humans and robotics. These pressure/ strain or temperature sensors, however, still require input power to drive the OTFT devices. Contrastively, high-performance piezoelectric devices based on free-standing sheets of aligned electrospun nanofibers of P(VDF-TrFE) have been developed by Rogers et al., which are flexible, lightweight, and self-powered, providing prominent application opportunities in wearable electronics.

Conducting polymers, such as poly(3,4-ethylenedioxythiophene):polystyrene sulfonate acid (PEDOT:PSS), polypyrrole (PPy), and ionic hydrogels, play an important role in flexible conductors, electrodes, pressure/strain sensors, etc. PEDOT:PSS is commercially available as an aqueous dispersion of two ionomers: PEDOT and PSS. PEDOT:PSS thin films can be obtained by spin coating or printing for organic electronic applications as transparent conductors in electroluminescent devices or conductive layers in OTFTs [110]. Carlo et al. reported a low-cost flexible polymeric sensor fabricated with PEDOT:PSS thin film on PI substrate, which had a gauge factor (GF) of 17.8 ± 4 that well above the typical value for commercially available flexible metallic strain gauges on PI substrates [111]. The sensor also exhibited a linear response in resistance to bending angle from 0 degree to 60 degree, and a high reproducibility with low hysteresis. PEDOT:PSS can also be electrospun into nanofibers by mixing with a spinable polymer polyvinyl alcohol (PVA) [112]. Strain sensors fabricated with the electrospun PEDOT:PSS-PVA nanofibers on PI substrates have been reported by Zhao et al., which exhibited excellent stability, fast response, and a high GF of up to about 396. The capability to detect the bending of a finger was demonstrated for tiny and quick human motion monitoring. Other intrinsically conductive polymer, for example, PPy with hollow-sphere microstructure, is also used for resistive pressure sensor for detection of pressures of less than 1 Pa with a short response time, good reproducibility, excellent cycling stability, and temperature-stable sensing [113]. Ionic polymers, such as hydrogels and ionogels, have also been exploited as highly stretchable, fully transparent, and sometimes, biocompatible and self-healing materials for wearable electronics. Generally, hydrogels are cross-linked macromolecule networks filled with water. By tuning the way and degree of cross-linking of the polymer networks, the hydrogel can be stretched beyond 20 times its initial length along with high fracture energy of $\sim 9000 \, \mathrm{J \, m^{-2}}$, comparable to that of natural rubber [114]. Besides, water plays a crucial role in keeping the flexibility as well as conductivity of hydrogels. Humectants are usually introduced to enhance the water retention capacity of hydrogels, while coating helps prevent the loss and gain of water due to the daily fluctuation of ambient relative humidity (RH) [7, 115]. With water, ions can transport in hydrogels over long distances and at high speeds. Hydrogel-based ionic cables that can transmit electrical signals up to 100 MHz [116] and transparent hydrogel electrodes capable of driving artificial muscles [8, 26, 117] have been demonstrated both experimentally and theoretically. Suo et al. developed ionic transparent ionic skin based on hydrogels, which can monitor large deformation (strain of 1%–500%), dynamic bending of fingers, and pressure of touch as low as 1 kPa [118]. Recently, a bioinspired mineral hydrogel was exploited by Wu et al. as a self-healable and mechanical adaptable ionic skin, which can detect subtle pressure changes for monitoring human motions such as gentle finger bending, throat motion, and blood pressure [119].

DEs, which are insulating polymers with low mechanical modulus and high elasticity, such as PDMS and acrylic rubbers, are ideal materials for the dielectric layers of capacitive pressure and strain sensors with parallel-plate capacitor structures. DEs can be directly used in the form of planar thick films. A wide strain range of 1%–300% was realized by the sensors using PDMS as the dielectric layer and CNTs as the electrodes, which had a sensitivity smaller than 1 and a response time of ≤ 100 ms [24]. While Suo et al. have expanded the detection range of strain to 1%–500% and lowered the minimum detection pressure down to 1 kPa by using a kind of "very-high-bond" acrylic rubber as the dielectric layer and ionic hydrogel as the electrodes [118]. The developed sensory sheets can work as highly stretchable, transparent, and biocompatible ionic skins for wearable or implantable electronics. To further lower the detection limit and enlarge the sensitivity of capacitive pressure sensor, dielectric layers with specially designed structures are developed. For example, Bao et al. reported a pressure sensor with porous PDMS combined with air gap as the dielectric layer that was capable of detecting a pressure as low as 2.5 Pa, with an average sensitivity of 0.7 kPa^{-1} in the pressure region < 1 kPa [120]. The group also reported pressure sensors based on PDMS with microhairy structures, which had sensitivities between 0.55 and 0.58 kPa^{-1} [121]. Pressure sensors based on OTFTs with microstructured PDMS as the gate dielectrics were also developed by Bao and coworkers [122, 123]. A maximum sensitivity of 8.4 kPa^{-1} and a short response time of < 10 ms was achieved. However, the sensitivity of these OTFT sensors is still limited by the elasticity of the rubber-based gate dielectrics. Di and Zhu et al. demonstrated an OTFT-based pressure sensor with an air gap dielectric layer and suspended gate electrode, which shown an ultrahigh sensitivity of 192 kPa^{-1}, a low limit-of-detection pressure of < 0.5 Pa, and a short response time of < 10 ms [124]. These high-performance pressure sensors can be fabricated in large area and be used as promising intelligent elements in wearable electronics.

1.2.2.5 Elastomeric nanocomposites

Conductive nanoparticles (e.g., graphene [21, 125] and carbon black [126–128]), NWs (e.g., Ag NWs [5], CNTs [129–134], and carbon nanofibers [135]), or polymers (e.g., PPy [136] and PEDOT:PSS [31]) can be introduced as fillers into insulating plastic rubber matrix to form elastomeric nanocomposites with tunable electrical and mechanical properties for flexible electronics. As the load of conductive filler increases, resistance of the nanocomposite decreases. When the filler load reaches a critical value, named the percolation threshold, resistance of the nanocomposite decreases drastically due to the formation of percolating networks, causing electric conduction of the material. After that, resistivity of the nanocomposite does not increase much, or sometimes, even decreases with the increasing of filler load, which might result from the introduction of air gaps [137]. Nanocomposites with conductive filler load lower or just higher than the percolation threshold commonly exhibit variable resistance with strain (or piezoresistivity), which are potential as sensing materials for pressure/strain sensors, and the specific performances of which depend on a couple of parameters, such as the material type and morphology, concentration and dispersion of the conductive filler, as well as the filler/matrix interactions [138]. Based on the above principles, it is possible to obtain high piezoresistivity, superior mechanical flexibility or stretchability, as well as multifunctionality in elastomeric nanocomposites. For example, Ko et al. reported multifunctional stretchable electronic skins based on MWCNT/PDMS nanocomposites with interlocked microdome structures [130, 131], which are capable of detecting various mechanical stimuli including normal, shear, stretching, bending, and twisting forces. The electronic skin can detect lateral strain over the range of 0%–120% with a sensitivity as high as 9617, normal pressure of $0.2\,Pa$–$59\,kPa$ with a sensitivity of $15.1\,kPa^{-1}$, and shear force of 0–$3\,N$ with a sensitivity of $0.15\,N^{-1}$ (applied normal pressure: $58.8\,kPa$). Petras et al. reported flexible multifunctional sensors based on CNT/polyurethane (PU) nanocomposites which are not only able to detect mechanical strain over the range of 0%–400% with a sensitivity of nearly 69, but also to detect organic solvent vapors including ethanol and heptane [133, 134].

1.2.3 Stretchable electrodes

Conductors are materials with low resistivity (or high conductivity) that allow the flow of electric charges. Commonly, resistance (conductance) of a conductor increases (decreases) under strain due to the appearance of cracks in conductive paths. For wearable electronics, stretchable electrodes or conductors that could maintain high conductance over a large strain are essential for transmitting signals as electrical interconnects. Available stretchable electrodes or conductors include metal films, NWs, carbon-based nanomaterials, conducting polymers and nanocomposites, and ionic conductors.

Metal is the most conventional conductor with low resistivity of 10^{-8}–$10^{-6}\,\Omega\,m$. However, free-standing metal thin films usually have high Young's modulus of tens to hundreds of GPa and poor ductility with small net elongation typically less than a few percent [69, 70, 139–142]. By contrast, metal thin films fully bonded to polymer substrates can theoretically deform uniformly to large strains, despite that experimentally the failure strains are strongly influenced by several factors such as the adhesion strength between the film and substrate, the metal film quality, and thickness. Generally, stronger interface adhesion, thicker metal film lead to larger failure strain [143–146]. Most polymer-supported metal thin films sustain elongations of 10% [2, 72, 147], while a few can be stretched up to 20% [60, 145, 146], but only few with a thickness up to 1 μm can reach strain beyond 50% [148]. To acquire reversibly stretchable conductors with more stable conductance over large strains, serpentine electroplated metal wires have been developed. For example, Chen et al. reported tortuous Au wires encased by PDMS elastomer, which were able to accommodate much higher linear strains (~54%) compared with that of straight Au wires (~2.4%) [58]. Similarly, Schnakenberg et al. reported meander Au patterns covalently bonded to extra soft PDMS (Young's modulus of 50 kPa), which could sustain static strain up to 60%. Furthermore, Vanfleteren et al. compared the stretchability of elliptical, "U" shape, and horseshoe-shaped Au interconnects embedded in silicone elastomer, and the modeling results showed that a horseshoe-like shape was the optimal, while the experimental results showed that circuit of narrow metallizations could have a stretchability above 100% [56]. Highly stretchable geometrical metal thin films can be produced by using structured substrates. For example, Lacour et al. deposited Au thin film on soft microcellular PU foam, which exhibited conformability and large stretchability of 120%, much higher than those of Au thin films on plain PU (~25%) and less softer PU foam (~55%) [149]. Suo et al. developed wavy/buckled Au strips by using prestretched PDMS substrates, which could sustain strains ranging from 10% to 100% [150]. By metallization of silicone wires maintained under twisting and stretching constraints, and then releasing the system, helical Au tracks were produced, which were electrically stable within strain range of 0%–43% [19]. Other techniques to produce geometrical metal thin films have also been reported, for example, Suo and coworkers developed highly stretchable and transparent Au nanomesh electrodes on elastomers using grain boundary lithography, which showed a modest change in sheet resistance to a strain of up to 160% [63]. These highly stretchable geometrical metallizations have been demonstrated as interconnects for epidermal electronics [151].

Metal NWs (e.g., Ag and Cu NWs) with high electrical conductivity and aspect ratio can form elastic films of percolation networks on plastic substrates which are quite promising as transparent and flexible electrode materials [38, 75, 152–155]. The conductivity and transparency of NW network films are greatly influenced by the film thickness and the NW aspect ratio. Commonly, increasing thickness leads to increasing conductivity (till saturation) but decreasing film transparency [38], while high NW aspect ratio is critical for achieving both high conductivity and transparency [156]. For example, with the same sheet resistance (10 Ω/□), networks of long Ag NWs (20–50 μm) had a transparency of about 80%, improved by 5%–10% within the visible light range than that of short Ag NW (4–10 μm) networks [156]. Mechanical flexibility of NW network films is also related to the film thickness and the NW aspect ratio [152], but the dominating factors are the mechanical properties of the substrates and the interface interactions. Ag NW networks on PET substrates remain conductive upon bending up to 160 degree, while by casting liquid polymer monomer onto prefabricated Ag NW network on a flat substrate and then curing the polymer, Ag NWs can be partially buried in the polymer, resulting in strong interface interactions and a flexibility of the NW/polymer comparable to that of pure polymer [155, 157]. The main drawback of the Ag NW electrode is its scarcity and high price. Therefore, metal NWs using less expensive and more abundant materials are being developed. For example, films of Cu NWs with a sheet resistance of 15 $\Omega/\square$, a transmittance of 65%, superior flexibility with no change in sheet resistance after 1000 bending cycles have been reported, which are potential as flexible and transparent electrode materials [154]. However, the problem of aggregation of the NWs needs to be solved, and Cu NWs with higher aspect ratio are required.

1.2.4 Structural approaches for flexibility/stretchability

Inorganic electronic materials (e.g., metals and semiconductors) possess outstanding properties as electrodes, sensors, interconnects, contact pads, transistors, and diodes. However, their brittleness makes them tend to fracture under a very little tensile strain (1%), so it is hard to incorporate them directly onto flexible/stretchable substrates [158]. It is reported that once the thickness and size of rigid inorganic materials are reduced to nanometer level, they become deformable and flexible [159]. To achieve tolerance to certain levels of deformation on flexible/stretchable substrate, thin films and special structural configuration design of rigid materials have been developed. Basically, two forms of structural configurations have been widely used: one is out-of-plane buckling structures by compressive buckling strategy (a prestrained substrate during thin film deposition followed by strain release method), including wavy and island-bridge design [158, 160]; the other is in-plane self-similar serpentine or fractal interconnects design [161, 162], as shown in Fig. 1.1A.

Out-of-plane buckling structures are fabricated by compressive buckling strategy, which commonly uses the transfer-printing technique to fabricate a thin film or island-bridge designed mesh layer of inorganic materials on a prestretched elastomeric substrate, and then release of the prestrain leads to formation of wave-like or island-bridge structures on the substrate, as illustrated in Fig. 1.1A(a). The main difference in the fabrication process of wave-like structure and island-bridge is that the island-bridge mesh is transfer printed onto a prestrained elastomeric substrate with strong chemical bonds at the locations of island (commonly as active area) and weak bonds at the locations of bridge (commonly as interconnect), and when release the prestrain, the bridge buckles out of the plane to accommodate the deformation, while the island experiences very small deformations [163]. However, the thin film layer of wave-like structure is all strongly bonded on the prestrained substrate.

Wavy structure can accommodate external deformations along the prestretched direction (including 1D wavy ribbons layout along one direction and 2D wavy layout in all directions, as shown in Fig. 1.1B) via changing the wavelength (λ) and amplitude (A) in the waves. Both theoretical and experimental results demonstrate that the wavelength and amplitude of wavy structure are well determined by Eq. (1.1) in small deformation:

$$\lambda = 2\pi h_f \left(\frac{\overline{E_f}}{3\overline{E_s}}\right)^{1/3} , A = h_f \sqrt{\frac{\varepsilon_{pre}}{\varepsilon_c} - 1}$$

$$(1.1)$$

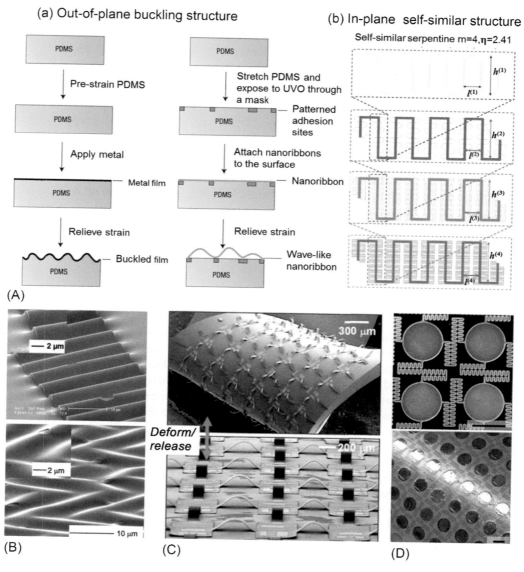

Fig. 1.1
See figure legend on next page.

In which h_f is the thickness of the rigid film, $\overline{E}_f$ is the Young's modulus of the film, $\overline{E}_s$ is the Young's modulus of the elastic substrate, ε_{pre} is the prestrain of the substrate, and ε_c is the critical strain to form wavy structure:

$$\varepsilon_c = \frac{1}{4}\left(\frac{3\overline{E}_s}{3\overline{E}_f}\right)^{2/3} \tag{1.2}$$

When $\varepsilon_{pre} < \varepsilon_c$, no wave forms. Once $\varepsilon_{pre} > \varepsilon_c$, wave-like structure will form and according to Eqs. (1.1), (1.2), the wavelengths of the wave-like structure are constant and strain independent. When the prestrain of the elastomeric substrate is relatively large, the wavelength will decrease with the increase of the prestrain [164]. Overall, by varying the material properties (e.g., moduli and thickness) of the rigid film and the compliant substrate, buckling wavy structure systems could be designed with controlled strain direction and level in stretchable electronics applications. Different films such as CNT [165], graphene [166], gold [167], platinum [168], and silver NW [169] are used to fabricate stretchable electronics. Wavy structures provide larger area coverage of active materials on the elastomeric substrate than the island-bridge, which is beneficial for sensors. However, most of them only offer large stretchability in one major direction or small stretchability in all direction on one plane [30]. In addition, the moduli mismatch between rigid film and the elastic substrate, the large strain concentration appearing on the peaks and valleys of the wavy structure could deteriorate the mechanical stability of the electronic device, which are still limitations for certain applications [170].

Fig. 1.1

(A) Structural configuration design strategies of rigid inorganic on stretchable substrate, including (a) out-of-plane buckling structure and (b) in-plane self-similar structure design. (B) Wave-like Si nanomembrane films on a compliant substrate, including 1D sinusoidal wave (*upper*) for 1D stretch/compression and herringbone wave (*below*) for 2D stretch/compression. (C) Out-of-plane mesh designs integrated with elastomeric substrate. (D) Al electrode pads and self-similar interconnects on Si wafer (*upper*) and the transfer printing on a sheet of silicone (*below*) for a stretchable Li-ion battery. *Part (A) reprinted with permission from X. Lu, Y. Xia, Electronic materials: buckling down for flexible electronics. Nat. Nanotechnol. 1 (2006) 163–164 and Y. Zhang, H. Fu, Y. Su, S. Xu, H. Cheng, J.A. Fan, K.-C. Hwang, J.A. Rogers, Y. Huang, Mechanics of ultra-stretchable self-similar serpentine interconnects. Acta Mater., 61 (2013) 7816–7827; (B) reprinted with permission from J. Song, H. Jiang, Y. Huang, J.A. Rogers, Mechanics of stretchable inorganic electronic materials. J. Vac. Sci. Technol. A, 27 (2009) 1107–1125; (C) reprinted with permission from D.-H. Kim, J. Song, W.M. Choi, H.-S. Kim, R.-H. Kim, Z. Liu, Y.Y. Huang, K.C. Hwang, Y.-W. Zhang, J.A. Rogers, Materials and noncoplanar mesh designs for integrated circuits with linear elastic responses to extreme mechanical deformations. Proc. Natl. Acad. Sci. 105 (2008) 18675–18680; (D) reprinted with permission from S. Xu, Y. Zhang, J. Cho, J. Lee, X. Huang, L. Jia, J.A. Fan, Y. Su, J. Su, H. Zhang, H. Cheng, B. Lu, C. Yu, C. Chuang, T.-I. Kim, T. Song, K. Shigeta, S. Kang, C. Dagdeviren, I. Petrov, P.V. Braun, Y. Huang, U. Paik, J.A. Rogers, Stretchable batteries with self-similar serpentine interconnects and integrated wireless recharging systems. Nat. Commun. 4 (2013) 1543.*

An island-bridge design has been developed to increase the stretchability of the inorganic electronics comparing to wavy structure, which requires the interconnects (bridge) to be stretchable and suspended out-of-plane, while the island to be rigid, as shown in Fig. 1.1C [160]. The maximum strain in the interconnect is

$$\varepsilon_{bridge}^{max} = 2\pi \frac{h_{bridge}}{L_{bridge}^0} \sqrt{\frac{\varepsilon_{pre}}{1+\varepsilon_{pre}}} \tag{1.3}$$

In which L_{bridge}^0 is the distance between islands before relaxation, h_{bridge} is the interconnect thickness, and ε_{pre} is the prestrain of the substrate. Eq. (1.3) shows that the maximum strain in the bridge is proportional to the ratio of the interconnect thickness to its length, h_{bridge}/L_{bridge}^0. To increase the stretchability of the interconnects, the maximum strain in the interconnects should be reduced, therefore, thin and long interconnects are preferred. For island, the maximum strain is

$$\varepsilon_{island}^{max} \approx 2\pi \frac{\left(1-v_{island}^2\right) E_{bridge} h_{bridge}^3}{E_{island} h_{island}^2 L_{bridge}^0} \sqrt{\frac{\varepsilon_{pre}}{1+\varepsilon_{pre}}} \tag{1.4}$$

In which h_{island} is the island thickness, v_{island} is the Poisson's ratio of the island, and E_{bridge} and E_{island} is the Young's modulus of the interconnect and the island, respectively. Eq. (1.4) shows that stiff and thick island could reduce its strain. As experimental and theoretical studies concluded that long interconnects, short islands, large prestrain could increase both the stretchability and compressibility of the island-bridge system.

To further increase the deformability of the island-bridge system, serpentine interconnects have been developed because they are much longer than straight interconnects. Moreover, serpentine interconnects could be stretched much further when the applied strain reaches the prestrain because structure twist exists to accommodate further deformation. Recently, more advanced 3D out-of-plane buckling design including free-standing helical structure [171], paper folding based spatial structures [64], porous sponge [172], and complex mesostructures [173] have been developed for deformable and stretchable electronics. Within this out-of-plane design, various electronic materials of high moduli can be applied to fabricate stretchable devices, including sensors, energy harvesting, and storage device [51, 174, 175].

Out-of-plane buckling structures can markedly broaden the stretchability and deformability of the flexible electronics. However, the methods involve expensive and complex fabrication processes. Besides, they may easily be broken by scratching from surface, which not suit with well-processed flat technology such as screen printing, lithography in traditional electronics. Therefore, in-plane design of 2D structure would be a good solution for constructing flexible and stretchable electronics. Serpentine structures as a typical in-plane layout have been widely designed and fully fabricated onto elastic substrate as interconnects/electrodes, which can accommodate an exceptional level of large applied strain without physical damage compared with traditional straight structures [56]. The mechanism to accommodate mechanical strain well is to rationally control the geometric parameters of the serpentine, including wire width, thickness, arc radius and angle, and so on [176]. The systematical simulations and experimental measurements of this structure have been deeply investigated by John Rogers' group [176, 177]. More advanced in-plane layouts are also developed. For example, a typical self-similar serpentine fractal structure (Fig. 1.1A(b)) shows multiple scale repeated "U"-shaped units [162]. This type of self-similar design expands the lithium-ion battery to a biaxial stretchability of up to ~300%, which possesses improved level of stretchability compared with traditional networks of periodic serpentine structures with a given spacing between adjacent islands. Moreover, the system can reach even higher stretchability by increasing the fractal order (self-similar orders) of the system, and also can be engineered to accommodate strain along a selected dimension, biaxial, radial, and other deformation modes [46]. These strategies enable thin films of hard electronic materials on flexible and stretchable substrates to be designed for various (bio)electronic devices such as mechanical sensors, radio frequency antennas, heating devices, and so on [178–181]. Future applications lie in broadening the material versatility to other functional materials such as high-quality semiconductors, piezoelectric materials, and 2D layered materials [182].

1.3 Flexible/stretchable sensor devices for wearable bioelectronics

Wearable bioelectronics enables the noninvasive and real-time detection of human physiological information, which mainly includes two categories, one is the physical stimuli signals such as body temperature, heart rate, wrist pulse, respiration, electrophysiological signal (ECG and EEG), and body motions of human activity (subtle movement of face, swallowing and large bending movement of hands, arms, legs, etc.) and the other is biological/chemical stimuli signals, mainly referring to body fluids (sweat, tears, and saliva). For physical signals, plenty of flexible and stretchable physical sensors including pressure/strain sensors, temperature sensors have been widely developed in the recent years and have shown great application prospects in fitness monitoring, human-machine interfaces, electronic skin (e-skin), and medical diagnostics [4, 29, 65, 183, 184]. Relatively, the developments of (bio)chemical sensors that directly contact with skin for continuous monitoring of biochemical signals are limited, which is due to their complexities in fabrication and performance (molecular level of sensitivity, selectivity, stability of wearable sensors, sample complexity, etc.) [11]. Great efforts have been made to develop wearable flexible and stretchable (bio)chemical sensors in the recent years to obtain more comprehensive, molecular-level information of human body, such as wearable ion-selective electrode sensors, enzyme-based biosensors, wearable microfluidic sensors, and so on. The following part of this chapter will present advanced flexible and stretchable physical and (bio)chemical sensor devices based on the above strategies for wearable bioelectronics.

1.3.1 Pressure/strain sensors

Flexible and stretchable pressure or strain sensors are widely used to monitor human motions, heart rate, blood pressure, respiration rate, and other mechanical changes of skin. Generally speaking, pressure sensors are used to detect the pressure produced by human body ranging from low regime ($< 10\,kPa$, e.g., intracranial pressure and intraocular pressure), medium regime ($< 100\,kPa$, e.g., heartbeat, wrist pulse, blood pressure wave, respiration rate, phonation vibration, etc.), and high regime ($> 100\,kPa$, foot pressure) [183]. While, strain sensors are widely employed in human activity monitoring to measure the mechanical deformation of human body ranging from small-scale motions (e.g., breath, swallowing, speaking and subtle movements of face, etc.) to large-scale motions (e.g., bending of joints and muscle movements, etc.). Theoretically, both pressure sensor and strain sensor are mechanical sensors that convert the structural deformations of the sensor materials into electric signal changes, which are commonly based on piezoresistive, capacitive, or piezoelectric mechanism. Their unique performance of sensitivity, workable range, response/recovery speed, etc., mainly depends on the micro/nanostructural design and the material properties (nanomaterials and mechanism).

Piezoresistive-based flexible and stretchable pressure/strain sensors are typically made of soft or stretchable substrates combined with conductive sensing materials, which can produce signal changes in electrical resistance when applied pressure or strain. The simplicity and low cost in both the fabrication process and the transduction mechanism make them the most widely reported pressure/strain sensors for wearable bioelectronics. Piezoresistive effect is caused by the change in the resistance of the sensor material under a structural deformation. The resistance R of the conductive materials is given by $R = (\rho L)/A$, where ρ, L, and A represent the resistivity, length, and the cross-sectional area, respectively. In the case of the strain sensor, the relative resistance change is written as $\Delta R/R = (1 + 2\nu)\varepsilon + \Delta\rho/\rho$, where ν is Poisson's ratio and ε is the applied strain. The sensitivity of a strain or pressure sensor is named as GF, defined as $(\Delta R/R)/P$ for the pressure sensor (P is the intensity of pressure) and $(\Delta R/R)/\varepsilon$ for the strain sensor. When the resistivity of materials such as some metal and metal alloys remains constant, the resistance change mainly depends on the geometry change ($\Delta R/R = (1 + 2\nu)\varepsilon$) under the applied strain, which can only increase by a few times, resulting in a typical GF of ~ 2 [185]. While for some materials such as semiconductor, CNT, graphene, and some other nanomaterials, the resistance change depends on both the geometry and the resistivity, thus the resistance can change by several orders of magnitudes with a high sensitive GF [6, 76, 186]. Therefore, a piezoresistive pressure or strain sensor is designed according to several factors, including the geometry or structure of the sensor, the resistivity of the materials and the contact resistance R_c (caused by contact interface/area change) between different sensing elements.

Traditional piezoresistive materials for pressure/strain sensors are conductive rubbers, which are fabricated by incorporating conductive filler materials (such as carbon nanomaterials, metal nanoparticles and NWs or conductive polymers, etc.) into elastomer composites [PDMS, thermoplastic elastomers (TPE), PU, etc.], as the above descriptions in Section 1.2.2. However, the early sensors with planar structure do not exhibit satisfactory response speed and sensitivity in the low-pressure range (<10 kPa) [187]. In the recent years, many advanced micro/nanostructural designs for the contact interface of the pressure sensors have been proposed to achieve high sensitivity, fast response speed, large working range as well as low-temperature sensitivity, based mainly on the contact resistance of R_c changes with the pressure force (expressed as $R_c \propto F^{-1/2}$) following a power law dependence [188]. For instance, a 3D micro-pyramid array PDMS polymeric surface coated with a layer of conductive PEDOT:PSS/PU composite polymer was proposed as the piezoresistive electrode, in which the pressure-induced geometrical change incurred by the conductive electrode could be maximized [31]. As shown in Fig. 1.2A, the pyramid structure could greatly enhance the pressure sensitivity of the sensor comparing to that of an unstructured film, attributing to the change in the resistance of the contact interface (R_{CI}) and the piezoresistive electrode (R_{PE}) under the pressure. The sensor also exhibits nearly nine times more sensitive than its capacitive counterpart. As a result, the sensitivity is enhanced enough to detect the pressure of a 93-mg object (23 Pa) at 40% with a sensitivity of 10.3 kPa^{-1}. Based on the above microstructural sensor model, various special structural designs of the polymeric surface have been demonstrated to fabricate the flexible piezoresistive sensors, including some nature-inspired microstructures. An interesting interlocked structure-based platform that is commonly formed by facing two layers of hair-like array [189], dome-like array [130, 131], or pyramid array [61] to each other have been widely used to enhance the sensitivity of the sensors. This interlocking design can not only increase the sensitivity, but also enable the sensor to detect different mechanical loadings (pressure, shear, and torsion) according to the distinguishable GFs [189]. Their high sensitivities are mainly attributed to the percolating changes in the tunneling currents between the two interlocked structures. The high sensitivity of the pressure sensor can also be achieved by using nature structural molds, the microstructures existing on some plant surface (lotus, mimosa, rose, etc.) or textile (silk) can be directly used as the templates for fabricating structured electrode with low-cost, simplicity, and large area [190–193].

Piezoresistive strain sensors are applied to monitor body strain ranging from low-strain skin motions (induced by breath, swallowing, speaking, and subtle movements of face) to large strain body movement (e.g., bending and straightening of body joints), where high sensitivity as well as high stretchability are required. (Graphene, CNTs, or carbon blacks)-polymer composite have been widely employed as stretchable strain sensors, which exhibit an excellent performance in stretchability, sensitivity, and multifunctionality [21, 194]. The experimental and simulating results indicate that the tunneling resistance change effect is

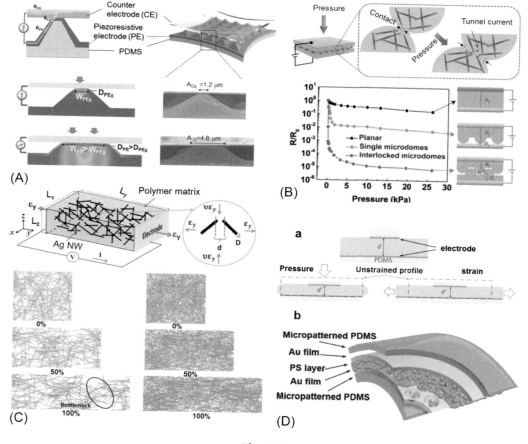

Fig. 1.2

(A) Circuit model (*top*) and finite element analysis (*below*) used to derive the sensing principle of the resistive pressure sensor, which relies on the change of the pyramid's geometry in response to pressure. (B) Interlocked microdome arrays-based CNT/PDMS pressure sensor and the comparison of pressure sensitivities of different sensor structures. (C) AgNWs-PDMS-based stretchable strain sensor with a 3D network resistor model under different strains. (D) (a) Schematic representation showing a stretchable capacitor after being placed under pressure (*left*) and being stretched (*right*). (b) Capacitive sensors with micropatterned PDMS/Au electrodes and PS microspheres dielectric layer. *Part (A) reprinted with permission from C.L. Choong, M.B. Shim, B.S. Lee, S. Jeon, D.S. Ko, T.H. Kang, J. Bae, S.H. Lee, K.E. Byun, J. Im, Y.J. Jeong, C.E. Park, J.J. Park, U.I. Chung, Highly stretchable resistive pressure sensors using a conductive elastomeric composite on a micropyramid array. Adv. Mater. 26 (2014) 3451–3458; (B) reprinted with permission from J. Park, Y. Lee, J. Hong, M. Ha, Y.D. Jung, H. Lim, S.Y. Kim, H. Ko, Giant tunneling piezoresistance of composite elastomers with interlocked microdome arrays for ultrasensitive and multimodal electronic skins. ACS Nano 8 (2014) 4689–4697.; (C) reprinted with permission from M. Amjadi, A. Pichitpajongkit, S. Lee, S. Ryu, I. Park, Highly stretchable and sensitive strain sensor based on silver nanowire-elastomer nanocomposite. ACS Nano 8 (2014) 5154–5163; (D-a) reprinted with permission from D.J. Lipomi, M. Vosgueritchian, B.C.K. Tee, S.L. Hellstrom, J.A. Lee, C.H. Fox, Z.N. Bao, Skin-like pressure and strain sensors based on transparent elastic films of carbon nanotubes. Nat. Nanotechnol. 6 (2011) 788–792 and (D-b) reprinted with permission from T. Li, H. Luo, L. Qin, X. Wang, Z. Xiong, H. Ding, Y. Gu, Z. Liu, T. Zhang, Flexible capacitive tactile sensor based on micropatterned dielectric layer. Small 12 (2016) 5042–5048.*

the main mechanism of the piezoresistivity in CNTs-polymer nanocomposite strain sensors, where tunneling refers to the crossing of charged carries through a nonconductive barrier. For example, CNT to CNT junctions are separated from direct electrical connection by the polymer matrix, within a cutoff distance, electrons can tunnel through and form quantum tunneling junctions [4, 195, 196]. The composite's resistance increases exponentially when the distance between neighboring nanomaterials is extended under an applied strain, explained by the tunneling resistance equation of Simmons' theory [5, 196]. In addition, microstructure-based strain sensor could significantly increase and affect the tunneling resistance at the contact spots, as shown in Fig. 1.2B [130]. Moreover, CNTs and graphene could be regarded as elastic nanomaterials that are folded or entangled in the polymer-based composite, when a strain is applied, they tend to unfold other than slide in the axial direction, which is different from the disconnection mechanism of rigid nanomaterials inside the polymer [6, 196]. While for the disconnection mechanism-based strain sensors, a typical AgNWs-PDMS composites formed percolation network platform is shown in Fig. 1.2C [5]. The junctions between two NWs could be classified into three categories depending on their distances including (i) complete contact with no contact resistance, (ii) tunneling junction within a certain cutoff distance, and (iii) complete disconnection between NWs. Calculation results and experimental data show that the disconnection flowing of the NWs increases gradually with the applied strain, which greatly increases the resistance of the film, while the number of tunneling junctions is very low. It could be concluded that the strain sensor with high number density of NWs exhibits better connectivity between NWs, which results in a highly linear behavior with low resistance upon stretching, due to that the electrical resistance is dependent on the number of the disconnected NWs. On the contrary, the strain sensor with high resistance showing nonlinear behavior is not dominated by the number of disconnection of the NWs, but is due to that the topology of percolating NWs changes from homogeneous network to inhomogeneous network which limits the electrical current, as shown in Fig. 1.2C.

Capacitive-based stretchable pressure or strain sensors typically consist of a dielectric layer of elastomer sandwiched by two parallel layers of conductive electrodes. Based on the equation of the plate capacitor ($C = \varepsilon A/d$, where ε is the permittivity of the dielectric layer, A is the effective area of the electrode, and d is the distance between the top and bottom layer), any stimulus which can cause a change in ε, A, or d will be measured through the capacitance change. Therefore, the capacitive-based pressure sensor commonly detects an applied pressure according to the changes in d as well as in the capacitance, while the strain sensor may detect the stretching and shear forces via variation of both A and d. Several factors are critical for constructing a sensitive and stretchable capacitive-based pressure or strain sensor, including the compressibility of the dielectric materials, interface properties between the electrode layer and dielectric layer, and also the stretchable and conductive electrode. Compressibility is directly related with the sensitivity of the sensors, thus, low mechanical modulus materials such as PDMS, Ecoflex, and PU have widely been used as the highly compressible dielectric. To enhance the compressibility of the low-modulus elastomer-based dielectric layer and improve the sensitivity of the sensors, microstructuralizing the elastomers as the dielectric materials are widely investigated [121, 190, 197]. For example, the sensitivity of a pyramid-structured PDMS dielectric layer-based pressure sensor shows 30 times greater than that of the unstructured device [122]. The electrode layer also could be microstructured, and when being combined with the PS microspheres dielectric layer, as shown in Fig. 1.2D, the sensitivity of this microstructured PDMS/Au pressure sensor is 20 times greater than that of the unstructured sensor [190]. Constructing a stable interface, stretchable and conductive electrode is important for achieving high performance of stretchable pressure/strain sensor. Traditional Au film-based flexible sensors are prone to cracks. A good strategy is to embed the conductive materials such as CNTs, graphene, and metal NWs networks into the elastomers as the electrode layers, which has shown greatly enhanced stretchability and stability for capacitive-type sensors [122, 157, 198–200].

Piezoelectric-based pressure/strain sensors are dependent on the piezoelectricity of materials which can generate electrical charges that are proportional to the applied pressure/strain. Piezoelectric pressure/strain sensors possess ultrafast (transient) response speed and high sensitivity, additionally, they show low-power consumption, and even self-power ability, therefore, they have shown great advantages in constructing advanced ultrathin, lightweight, and self-powered wearable electronics [201]. Inorganic materials such as ZnO, lead contained materials [lead zirconate titanate (PZT), PbTiO$_3$], barium titanate (BaTiO$_3$) with large piezoelectric coefficients have been widely used for pressure sensors. However, the brittleness and stiffness nature of the inorganic materials is not well comparable with the flexible and stretchable polymers. Polymer-based piezoelectric materials such as PVDF, P(VDF-TrFE) have been intensively investigated for their good flexibility, but their piezoelectric coefficients are commonly lower than those of the inorganic materials (more properties of piezoelectric polymer are introduced in Section 1.2.2), and the low voltage and force generation capabilities have greatly limited their applications. To improve both the flexibility and piezoelectric effect of the device, strategies such as the combination of the inorganic piezoelectric nanomaterials with flexible polymer in the form of nanocomposites [186, 202, 203], and the modification of polymer-based piezoelectric materials with inorganic additives are developed [18, 204, 205]. For example, integrating ZnO NWs with PU fiber could achieve high stretchability (tolerable strain up to 150%) and multifunctional sensing of strain, temperature, and UV [202]. A mixture of P(VDF-TrFE) and BaTiO$_3$ nanoparticles is directly used as the gate dielectric and P(VDF-TrFE) as the channel to the physically responsive FET platform [109]. The nanocomposites could enhance the electro-physical coupling effects and improve the stability of their stimuli-responsive properties. As a result, the device is able to analyze two stimuli as pressure (or strain) and temperature simultaneously and disproportionally, additionally, the device can response to dynamic and static force conditions (piezoelectric sensors usually only detect dynamic force), which make them useful for practical applications [103].

In addition to the above demonstrated pressure/strain sensors, some nature-inspired sensing mechanism-based devices have also been developed. For example, inspired by the geometry and function of the sensory organ of the spider, which has crack-shaped slits embedded in the exoskeleton located near the leg joint that can ultrasensitively detect small external force variations, a flexible sensor based on nanoscale crack junctions is developed and can achieve ultrahigh sensitivity to strain (GF > 2000 in the 0%–2% strain range), as shown in Fig. 1.3A [206]. The sensor is fabricated by depositing a Pt layer on top of a viscoelastic polyurethane acrylate (PUA) followed by a mechanically bending with various radii of curvature to form controlled cracks in the Pt film. The ultrahigh mechanosensitivity is attributed to the disconnection-reconnection process undergone by the zip-like nanoscale crack junctions under strain/vibration, as shown in Fig. 1.3A(g). Inspired by nature gradient structure in tree roots growing and architecture designing with gradient suspension cable for force balance, a thickness-gradient film strategy is proposed to construct a strain sensor which could achieve both high sensitivity and large strain sensors range [207]. The thickness-gradient CNT film is fabricated by a dip-casting process with a designed mask via the self-spinning effect, as shown in Fig. 1.3B. The thick ring region of the gradient CNT film is brittle so that it could be broken first when applied a small strain, which enables the sensor to exhibit high sensitivity. The thin film inside the gradient shows conductive network, therefore, it could accommodate large strain. This strain sensor possesses a GF as high as 161 ($\varepsilon < 2\%$), 9.8 (avg., $2\% < \varepsilon < 15\%$), and 0.58 ($\varepsilon > 15\%$) for different strain phases. Additionally, the strain sensors can withstand uniaxial strain of more than 150% and isotropic strain of more than 75%, which show great potential in weak sound detection applications.

1.3.2 Temperature sensors

Body temperature monitoring is important for clinical diagnosis and health management. Wearable platform enables the continuous and invasive measuring body temperature changes to prevent injuries caused by abnormal health conditions such as fever, infections, and other thermal-related syndromes. Additionally, a wearable temperature sensor is a necessary element used to calibrate other temperature-sensitive devices such as piezoelectric/pyroelectric-based pressure/strain sensors and enzyme-based biochemical sensors [54, 107]. To fabricate a wearable temperature sensor that can meet the requirements of skin-comfortability and long-term spatiotemporal monitoring, several important characteristics should be achieved, including high accuracy ($\pm 0.1°C$ from 37°C to 39°C, and $\pm 0.2°C$ both below 37°C and above 39°C), fast response, wide working range (commonly 25–40°C for on-body monitoring), long-term stability, soft, biocompatibility, and lightweight [208]. Commonly, wearable temperature sensor devices are based on resistive temperature detectors (RTDs) that integrated on flexible/stretchable substrates, thermally sensitive resistors (thermistors)-based composites, and other mechanism-based detectors.

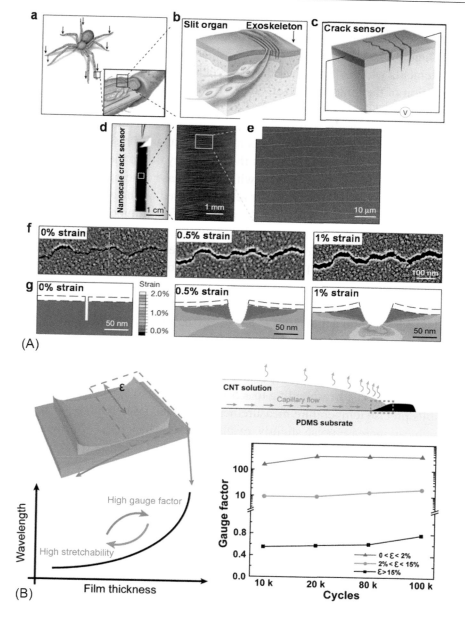

Fig. 1.3
See figure legend on next page.

RTDs integrated on flexible substrates are the most commonly used temperature sensor platform because of their simplicity and low cost [183]. Pure metal materials such as platinum (Pt), gold (Au), nickel (Ni), copper (Cu), and aluminum (Al) are used as the sensing transducer elements which operate based on the changes in electrical resistance of a metal with the variation of the temperature [36, 209–212]. The equation is given as $R(T) = R(T_0) (1 + \alpha \Delta T)$, where $R(T)$ and $R(T_0)$ are the resistances of the metal at temperature T and T_0 (reference temperature), respectively; ΔT is $T - T_0$; α is the temperature coefficient of resistance (TCR), which represents the percentage change of resistance per degree Kelvin ($\%K^{-1}$) and can be used to quantify the sensitivity of the thermistor [52, 213]. The resistance of a RTD usually increases with the increase of temperature (i.e., positive temperature coefficient) in an almost linear relation. Based on the above theory, metals in the form of thin film or wire combined with special configuration designs (such as buckling structure, serpentine layout which presented in above section) have been embedded in the flexible or stretchable substrate for wearable temperature sensors. As shown in Fig. 1.4A, an ultrathin, compliant skin-like RTD device is fabricated for precise and continuous thermal characterization of human skin [214]. The sensor relying on the TCR property of the Cr/Au metal thin film (5 nm/50 nm) with a thin (50 nm) and narrow (20 μm) serpentine feature design is first supported by a thin (PVA) elastomeric substrate, and is subsequently directly integrated onto the human skin (Fig. 1.4A(b)). The filamentary mesh, serpentine design, and the ultrathin device dimensions could act together to minimize local strains in the sensors and interconnects during deformation (a uniaxial strain of 10%, the average strains developed at the sensors are < 0.02%, corresponding to < 50 mK shift in the apparent temperature). The sensor exhibits precise temperature measurement even when used on human skin in hospital settings which can increase noise slightly, resulting in a precision of ∼ 23 mK sampled at 2 Hz ($n = 300$) or ∼ 14 mK sampled at 0.5 Hz ($n = 75$). A 4×4 RTD sensors array could be directly

Fig. 1.3
(A) Schematic illustrations and images of an ultra-mechanosensitive nanoscale crack junction-based sensor inspired by the spider sensory system. (a) The images of the sensory slit organs in the vicinity of the leg joint of a spider for the detection of external forces and vibrations. (b) The slits are connected to the nervous system to monitor vibrations. (c) Illustration of the crack-based sensor and its measurement scheme. (d) Image of the spider-inspired sensor with a cracked, 20 nm-thick Pt layer formed by bending with a 1 mm radius of curvature. (e) SEM image of the boxed region of the right-hand image in (d). (f) The zip-like crack junctions SEM image for different applied strains. (g) Finite-element modelling results of crack interfacial deformation. (B) Schematic illustrations of the thickness-gradient-based strain sensor with the self-pinning effect fabrication process and the GF of the sensor at various strains and circles. *Part (A) reprinted with permission from D. Kang, P.V. Pikhitsa, Y.W. Choi, C. Lee, S.S. Shin, L. Piao, B. Park, K.-Y. Suh, T.-I. Kim, M. Choi, Ultrasensitive mechanical crack-based sensor inspired by the spider sensory system. Nature 516 (2014) 222 and (B) reprinted with permission from Z. Liu, D. Qi, P. Guo, Y. Liu, B. Zhu, H. Yang, Y. Liu, B. Li, C. Zhang, J. Yu, B. Liedberg, X. Chen, Thickness-gradient films for high gauge factor stretchable strain sensors. Adv. Mater. 27 (2015) 6230–6237.*

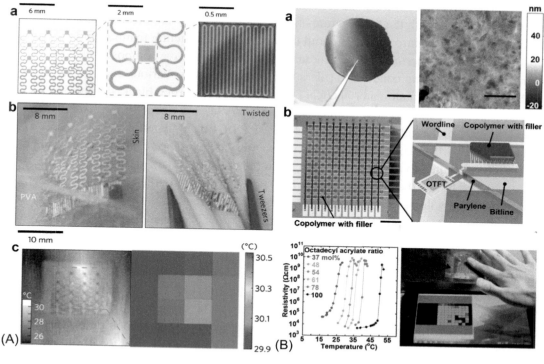

Fig. 1.4

(A) A 4×4 RTD sensor array with serpentine features of thin gold on (a) thin elastic sheets or (b) directly integrates on skin. (c) Infrared image of a device mounted on the skin of the human wrist (*left*) and map of temperature (*right*), where each pixel represents the reading of one sensor in the array. (B) Copolymer with graphite filler-based thermistor temperature sensor. (a) Photograph and AFM image of the surface of the film. (b) Illustration of a flexible large-area active-matrix sensor with 12×12 temperature pixels. (c) Temperature dependence of the resistivity of the copolymer with filler with various comonomer compositions (*left*) and the temperature mapping after touching the sensor sheet with a finger. *Part (A) reprinted with permission from R.C. Webb, A.P. Bonifas, A. Behnaz, Y. Zhang, K.J. Yu, H. Cheng, M. Shi, Z. Bian, Z., Liu, Y.-S. Kim, W.-H. Yeo, J.S. Park, J. Song, Y. Li, Y. Huang, A.M. Gorbach, J.A. Rogers, Ultrathin conformal devices for precise and continuous thermal characterization of human skin. Nat. Mater. 12 (2013) 938 and (B) reprinted with permission from T. Yokota, Y. Inoue, Y. Terakawa, J. Reeder, M. Kaltenbrunner, T. Ware, K. Yang, K. Mabuchi, T. Murakawa, M. Sekino, W. Voit, T. Sekitani, T. Someya, Ultraflexible, large-area, physiological temperature sensors for multipoint measurements. Proc. Natl. Acad. Sci. U. S. A. 112 (2015) 14533–14538.*

mounted onto the skin and used to map the temperature distribution, the results shown in Fig. 1.4A(c) reveal a spatial map of temperature (right) that matches well with the image obtained by the infrared camera (left). This wearable temperature sensor device provides real-time, clinical quality data for continuous health/wellness assessment.

Thermistor-based flexible temperature sensors are also dependent on the resistance change of the sensor element with the temperature change. However, they are much different from the flexible RTD temperature sensors in both the material and structure features and the working principles. Flexible thermistors are generally based on conductive composite materials fabricated by dispersing conductive fillers into polymer matrix. Various conductive fillers such as carbon-based nanomaterials (CNT, rGO, graphene, carbon black, graphite, etc.) [74, 215–217], metal particles (Ni micro- or nanoparticles and fibers, PtNPs, AuNPs, etc.) [36, 218, 219], and conductive polymers (PEDOT:PSS, PPy, polyaniline, etc.) [220, 221] are dispersed in PDMS, PU, PI, copolymers, and so on. The resistance changes of the composites are mainly attributed to the structure changes in the conductive percolation network of the fillers induced by the thermal expansion of the polymer matrix upon temperature change. Due to the large volume expansion ability of the polymer matrix, the conductive composite-based thermistor temperature sensors exhibit much larger TCR than that of RTDs sensors fabricated on a flexible substrate, which can eliminate the need for amplification circuitry of the external equipment to directly record the signal. For example, graphite particles (2–3 μm) are added as conductive fillers to a semicrystalline acrylate copolymer (octadecyl acrylate and butyl acrylate) to reach over a percolation conduction, Fig. 1.4B(a) shows the photograph and atomic force micrographs of the composites [217]. The semicrystalline polymers can display six orders of magnitude in the change of resistivity near their melting points over just a few degrees because that they can transfer from crystalline phase to amorphous phase and, therefore, lead to the large volume expansion and increase the interval distance of conductive fillers. As Fig. 1.4B(c) shows, by vary the mixing ratio of two polymers, the melting point varies systematically, which indicates that this temperature sensor system can easily tune the melt temperature for different human applications (as the physiological temperatures range from 32°C at the fingertips to over 42°C in the core during hyperpyrexia) [57]. The sensors offer an ideal solution to measure temperature over a large area with high spatial resolution, high sensitivity of 0.1°C or less (20 mK), and fast response time of 100 ms. Ultraflexible sensor pads for real-time temperature mapping are demonstrated in Fig. 1.4B(b), where green and black pixels represent large and small current, respectively.

Wearable temperature sensors could also be fabricated by other approaches. For instance, pyroelectric materials of P(VDF-TrFE) could be used as a gate-insulator layer in a flexible organic field-effect transistor (OFET) for temperature-sensing application [108, 109]. The temperature response of the device is mainly attributed to the pyroelectric property (refers to the electric polarization of certain materials to generate a transient voltage in response to the temperature changes) of the highly crystalline P(VDF-TrFE) layer, rather than to temperature-dependent changes in the other parameters, such as field-effect mobility, gate capacitance, and contact resistance. Thermal diodes containing p-n junctions could detect temperature at numerous locations because that their signals placed in an array can be obtained via scanning across the array, which are mainly attributed to the attractive feature of a diode that the current flows only from the anode to the cathode and thus isolates one diode sensor from the others electrically during the scanning [66, 214, 222]. The attractive property of the diode-based sensors could enable them to detect the temperature distributions on a small surface with high resolution, which are highly required for microthermal systems.

1.3.3 (Bio)chemical sensors

Monitoring (bio)chemical molecular in body biofluids (blood, urine, saliva, sweat, tears, and skin interstitial fluid) is well known as a gold standard to achieve more comprehensive information about a human's well-being. However, the current laboratory-based analytical methods mostly rely on blood sampled by invasive and painful means, which are not only inconvenient for elderly, neonatal or patients when frequent blood sampling is requested, but also making them bear risks of infection during the blood sampling process. As much effort has been made in shifting health care from centralized hospital-based patient care to home-based personal management, noninvasive, real-time, and continuous analyte monitoring is of particular importance in personalized diagnostic applications [12, 15]. Therefore, wearable (bio)chemical sensor platforms for noninvasive body fluids measurement appear to be an essential approach to collect the vital molecular-level health information in a real-time and continuous way, which is of great importance as a technological leap comparing to physical sensors demonstrated in the above section [68].

(Bio)chemical sensors are the devices that can transform biological (amino acid, protein, DNA, RNA, cells, bacteria, etc.) and chemical molecular (metal ion, glucose, gas molecular, salt, etc.) information into analytically useful signals (electrical, optical, calorimetric, piezoelectric, etc.). The devices usually consist of two main functional units: an analyte-sensitive receptor and a transducer, while a biosensor refers to the receptor that is made of biological recognition elements such as enzyme, aptamer, antibody, DNA, and so on. Over decades, (bio)chemical sensors have been widely developed and used as ideal alternatives to the bulky, expensive analytical instruments (such as ion and gas chromatography, atomic absorption spectroscopy, and so on) in analytical applications for medical diagnosis, food quality control, industry, environmental monitoring owing to their high performance, portability, simplicity, and low cost [223]. However, there are still multiple challenges faced by (bio)chemical sensors during their normal use, especially for wearable (bio)electronic applications. For instances, the traditional (bio)chemical sensors commonly built with rigid materials and substrates are apparently incompatible with flexible and soft platform, not to speak of their performances at moving state on soft skin. Wearable (bio)chemical sensors should be well and comfortably mounted on soft, curvilinear skin while maintaining their mechanical robustness and performance stability at the same time, so that to achieve accurate, health-related information. Therefore, flexible and stretchable (bio)chemical sensors are much needed. Additionally, (bio)chemical sensors are even more complicated than the physical sensors in many aspects. (Bio)chemical sensors are usually sort into several categories, including reaction-based catalytic sensors (enzymes and other active catalysts), selective binding-based bio-affinity sensors (DNA, aptamer, and antibody-based sensors), and other selective mechanism-based sensors (ion-selective sensors, gas sensors, etc.). Due to their continuous exposure to the body fluids and interact or binding with analyte, most of the sensors need frequent calibration to correct the signal drift, which is incompatible with wearable platform for continuous monitoring [11]. Especially in the case of bio-affinity sensors, which need long incubation time and necessary washing steps, so that the wearable bio-affinity sensors have not yet been reported. Furthermore, the stability of biosensors for long-term storage and use (i.e., the stability of enzymes, antibodies, DNA, etc. in ambient environment), the sensitivity for low analyte concentration in very small sampling volumes (e.g., glucose concentration in tear commonly two orders of magnitude lower than that in blood), the response time for real-time dynamic concentration change (long response time could result unfaithful or wrong data), biocompatibility of the flexible and soft sensors, and so on, all these factors are key challenges that have to be addressed for wearable (bio) chemical sensor. Recently, much effort has been made in developing wearable (bio)chemical sensor platforms to measure a broad range of health-related molecular including electrolytes (Na^+, K^+, Cl^-, etc.) [14, 25, 55, 224–226], metabolites (glucose, lactate, uric acid, alcohol, etc.) [227–231], heavy metals [34, 232], pH [10, 62], and so on in various body fluids such as sweat, tears, and saliva. However, wearable (bio)chemical sensors are still in their infancy and those developments cannot match with the rapid progress and commercial success achieved by wearable physical sensors [11].

Noninvasive detection of glucose in sweat, tears, saliva, and interstitial fluids is the most studied wearable biosensor platform because of the frequent need for diabetics to monitor their glucose level in daily life. The most successful glucose biosensor is the glucose oxidase (GOx)-based electrochemical amperometric sensor, which has been widely employed in most commercial handheld glucose analyzer [233]. To construct a GOx-based amperometric glucose sensor, the key element is to fabricate the effective electron transfer strategy between GOx and electrode surface. Mediator-based "second-generation" glucose biosensor is the most used platform, which mainly rely on a nonphysiological electron acceptor that can shuttle electrons from the redox center of GOx to the surface of the electrode. This platform could be conveniently produced by simple methods like screen-printing technology, which relies on the inks containing GOx, mediator, binding agents, membranes, and other necessary reagents. For example, tattoo-based GOx sensor is fabricated by employing printable Prussian Blue as the mediator transducer and chitosan as the polymeric matrix for immobilizing the GOx on the transducer surface, as shown in Fig. 1.5A [13]. Due to the simplicity of the device and the efficient electrochemical performance, the glucose sensor device could be fabricated on the highly soft skin-like substrate, together with a reverse iontophoresis electrode for glucose detection in extracted interstitial fluids. This tattoo-based system exhibits attractive wearable noninvasive glucose monitoring ability; however, the key challenges toward

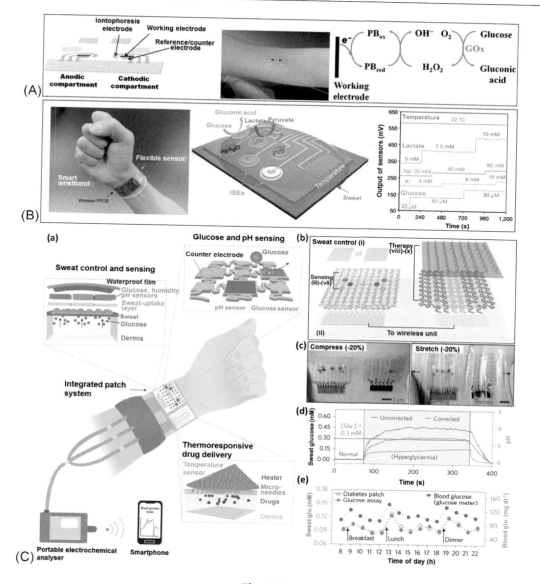

Fig. 1.5

(A) Tattoo-based platform for noninvasive glucose sensing with an iontophoretic-sensing system and a Prussian Blue electrodes applied to a human subject. (B) Images and schematic illustrations of the fully integrated wearable sensors array for multiplexed perspiration analysis. (C) Schematic illustrations (a) and corresponding images (b), (c) of the Graphene-hybrid-based electrochemical devices and thermoresponsive drug delivery microneedles system form diabetes patch. Glucose monitoring with pH calibration in artificial sweat (d) and one-day monitoring in sweat and blood of a human subject (e). *Part (A) reprinted with permission from Bandodkar et al. [13]; (B) reprinted with permission from Gao et al. [54]; (C) reprinted with permission from Lee et al. [229].*

long-term continuous operation still remain. Enzyme-based glucose sensors can also be integrated on flexible transparent polymer substrate in the form of a contact lens, which would be the ideal vehicle for continuous glucose monitoring in tears [231, 234]. Due to the direct contact with eyes, the GOx-based glucose sensor is fabricated with the "first-generation" principle by detecting hydrogen peroxide produced from the oxidation of glucose by immobilized GOx in a titania sol-gel layer and a nafion permselective film for minimal irritation.

Wearable enzyme-based biosensors mounted on skin may be effected by temperature variation due to their influences on enzyme activities. Multiple sensors array including temperature sensor, GOx-based glucose sensor, lactate oxidase-based lactate sensor, ion-selective electrode-based Na^+ and K^+ sensor, together with flexible printed circuit board containing electric signal conditioning, processing and wireless transmission units are integrated on a single flexible PET substrate for sweat analysis, as shown in Fig. 1.5B [54]. The sensor array can in situ monitoring several sweat metabolites and electrolytes simultaneously, as well as the skin temperature to calibrate the response of the enzyme-based sensors. The fully integrated wearable system needs no external analysis procedures, which enables a real-time assessment of the physiological state of human engaged in prolonged indoor and outdoor physical activities. To go further, it is desirable to achieve clinically accurate and continuous glucose monitoring in connection to closed-loop system for optimal insulin delivery, which has been achieved with implantable sensors and represents the first example of personalized medicine. A more sophisticated wearable patch for sweat-based diabetes monitoring and feedback therapy has been developed, as shown in Fig. 1.5C [229]. The patch consists of multiple modules including: sweat-control components (a sweat-uptake layer and waterproof film) for efficient sweat sampling; sensing components (humidity, glucose, pH, and tremor sensors) for more sensitive and accurate measurement; therapeutic components (microneedles, a heater and a temperature sensor) for thermally activated drug delivery, as shown in Fig. 1.5C(a)–(c). First, a bilayer of Au serpentine mesh and gold-doped CVD graphene is constructed on PDMS as the electrode materials which can ensure high conductivity, mechanical reliability (Fig. 1.5C(d)) and optical transparency for more stable electrical signal transfer, improved electrochemical activity and a semitransparent skin-like appearance with deformable configuration. The gold-doped graphene hybrid exhibits better electrochemical performance for both the Prussian Blue-based GOx glucose sensor and the PEDOT-based humidity sensor due to its large electrochemical active surface area and low interfacial impedance. The humidity sensor monitors the RH changes based on the impedance changes in the interdigitated PEDOT electrodes to determine the starting point for glucose and pH sensing. While the pH sensor is used to correct the pH-dependent deviation of the enzyme-based glucose sensor (Fig. 1.5C(e)). Daily glucose monitoring in situ with the patch (red circles) compared with a commercial glucose assay kit (red dots) are well match presented in Fig. 1.5C(f). Additionally, the sweat glucose concentration changes (red, left y-axis) were reportedly well correlated with those of the blood glucose concentration (blue, right y-axis) with a correlation factor of ~0.017 (the ratio of the sweat glucose concentration to the blood glucose concentration). The therapeutic components could be triggered by the real-time glucose monitoring data when the glucose concentration reaches to the hyperglycemia state (0.3 mM sweat glucose level corresponding to a 300-mg dL^{-1} blood glucose level). The microneedles are composed of a bioresorbable polymer [polyvinyl pyrrolidone (PVP)] in combination with a pharmacological agent coated with a layer of thermally active bioresorbable PCM (tridecanoic acid). Thermal actuation triggered by the embedded heater above the transition temperature will melt the PCM and release drug into the bloodstream. This sweat patch system combined with sweat monitoring and transcutaneous drug delivery could achieve a closed-loop, point-of-care treatment for diabetes, which shows great opportunities for health-care applications.

1.4 Conclusions and perspectives

In the above sections, we mainly highlight the materials and configuration strategies as well as working principles of flexible and stretchable sensors for wearable bioelectronics in the recent years. Tremendous efforts have been made to develop effective sensor devices with an excellent mechanical deformability that can conformably coverage nonplanar and soft surface of human skin and exhibit sensitive, accurate response to physiological stimuli. As a conclusion, mainly two kinds of approaches are used to achieve these characteristics, one is to engineer traditional rigid high-performance sensor materials in the form of ultrathin, microstructure, or with special configuration design to enable electronic devices to accommodate external deformations; the other one is to develop intrinsically flexible and stretchable functional materials with good electronic properties. Throughout the above section, it gives us the idea of that the newly developed intrinsically flexible and stretchable functional materials (including conducting polymers, piezoelectric polymers, pyroelectric polymers, etc.) could not yet replace the traditional materials due to their insufficient performance in electronics [170]. On the contrary, the combination of those flexible, stretchable, lightweight, and transparent polymer with rigid electronic materials via rational structure design have shown great potential for flexible and stretchable sensor devices. Indeed, many flexible and stretchable sensors have already exceeded the properties of natural sensing mechanisms in many respects. The stretchability of electronic skin (e-skin) exceeds that of human skin for many times [21, 65], and some superior ability such as spatial resolution, superwide detection range, ultrahigh sensitivity, and high accuracy are available [29, 214]. However, the main gap still exists regarding to the multifunction, biocompatibility, self-healing, highly integrated capabilities, and other merits comparing to nature sensors on human body. Additional properties such as self-power and biodegradability are also desirable for smart applications in wearable bioelectronics. As wearable biochemical sensors could provide more directly molecular-level information about human health condition than physical sensors, much attention should be focused on developing wearable biochemical sensors for noninvasive, continuous, and low-cost personalized health monitoring. Wearable biochemical sensors face more challenges such as calibration-free, user-independent, long-term stability, and so on. Future efforts are aiming at addressing these challenges as well as integrating the corresponding electronic system for powering the sensor, signal processing, and wireless communication on a flexible wearable platform and performing a large-scale health-related data-mining study.

References

[1] S. Bauer, Flexible electronics: sophisticated skin, Nat. Mater. 12 (2013) 871–872.

[2] P. Bonato, Wearable sensors and systems, IEEE Eng. Med. Biol. Mag. 29 (2010) 25–36.

[3] D.H. Kim, N.S. Lu, R. Ma, Y.S. Kim, R.H. Kim, S.D. Wang, J. Wu, S.M. Won, H. Tao, A. Islam, K.J. Yu, T.I. Kim, R. Chowdhury, M. Ying, L.Z. Xu, M. Li, H.J. Chung, H. Keum, M. McCormick, P. Liu, Y.W. Zhang, F.G. Omenetto, Y.G. Huang, T. Coleman, J.A. Rogers, Epidermal electronics, Science 333 (2011) 838–843.

[4] T. Someya, Z.N. Bao, G.G. Malliaras, The rise of plastic bioelectronics, Nature 540 (2016) 379–385.

[5] X.W. Wang, Z. Liu, T. Zhang, Flexible sensing electronics for wearable/attachable health monitoring, Small 13 (2017) 1602790.

[6] M. Amjadi, K.U. Kyung, I. Park, M. Sitti, Stretchable, skin-mountable, and wearable strain sensors and their potential applications: a review, Adv. Funct. Mater. 26 (2016) 1678–1698.

[7] A.J. Bandodkar, I. Jeerapan, J. Wang, Wearable chemical sensors: present challenges and future prospects, ACS Sens. 1 (2016) 464–482.

[8] S. Choi, H. Lee, R. Ghaffari, T. Hyeon, D.-H. Kim, Recent advances in flexible and stretchable bio-electronic devices integrated with nanomaterials, Adv. Mater. 28 (2016) 4203–4218.

[9] T.Q. Trung, N.E. Lee, Flexible and stretchable physical sensor integrated platforms for wearable human-activity monitoring and personal healthcare, Adv. Mater. 28 (2016) 4338–4372.

[10] J. Wei, How wearables intersect with the cloud and the internet of things considerations for the developers of wearables, IEEE Consum. Electron. Mag. 3 (2014) 53–56.

[11] W. Gao, S. Emaminejad, H.Y.Y. Nyein, S. Challa, K. Chen, A. Peck, H.M. Fahad, H. Ota, H. Shiraki, D. Kiriya, D.-H. Lien, G.A. Brooks, R.W. Davis, A. Javey, Fully integrated wearable sensor arrays for multiplexed in situ perspiration analysis, Nature 529 (2016) 509–514.

[12] D.-H. Kim, R. Ghaffari, N. Lu, J.A. Rogers, Flexible and stretchable electronics for biointegrated devices, Annu. Rev. Biomed. Eng. 14 (2012) 113–128.

[13] S. Xu, Y. Zhang, L. Jia, K.E. Mathewson, K.I. Jang, J. Kim, H. Fu, X. Huang, P. Chava, R. Wang, S. Bhole, L. Wang, Y.J. Na, Y. Guan, M. Flavin, Z. Han, Y. Huang, J.A. Rogers, Soft microfluidic assemblies of sensors, circuits, and radios for the skin, Science 344 (2014) 70–74.

[14] R. Maiti, L.-C. Gerhardt, Z.S. Lee, R.A. Byers, D. Woods, J.A. Sanz-Herrera, S.E. Franklin, R. Lewis, S.J. Matcher, Carré, M. J., In vivo measurement of skin surface strain and sub-surface layer deformation induced by natural tissue stretching, J. Mech. Behav. Biomed. Mater. 62 (2016) 556–569.

[15] D.-Y. Khang, H. Jiang, Y. Huang, J.A. Rogers, A stretchable form of single-crystal silicon for high-performance electronics on rubber substrates, Science 311 (2006) 208–212.

[16] D.-H. Kim, J. Song, W.M. Choi, H.-S. Kim, R.-H. Kim, Z. Liu, Y.Y. Huang, K.-C. Hwang, Y.-W. Zhang, J.A. Rogers, Materials and noncoplanar mesh designs for integrated circuits with linear elastic responses to extreme mechanical deformations, Proc. Natl. Acad. Sci. 105 (2008) 18675–18680.

[17] Y. Won, A. Kim, W. Yang, S. Jeong, J. Moon, A highly stretchable, helical copper nanowire conductor exhibiting a stretchability of 700%, NPG Asia Mater. 6 (2014) e132.

[18] W.-H. Yeo, Y.-S. Kim, J. Lee, A. Ameen, L. Shi, M. Li, S. Wang, R. Ma, S.H. Jin, Z. Kang, Y. Huang, J.A. Rogers, Multifunctional epidermal electronics printed directly onto the skin, Adv. Mater. 25 (2013) 2773–2778.

[19] Y.S. Rim, S.H. Bae, H.J. Chen, N. De Marco, Y. Yang, Recent progress in materials and devices toward printable and flexible sensors, Adv. Mater. 28 (2016) 4415–4440.

[20] C.L. Choong, M.B. Shim, B.S. Lee, S. Jeon, D.S. Ko, T.H. Kang, J. Bae, S.H. Lee, K.E. Byun, J. Im, Y.J. Jeong, C.E. Park, J.J. Park, U.I. Chung, Highly stretchable resistive pressure sensors using a conductive elastomeric composite on a micropyramid array, Adv. Mater. 26 (2014) 3451–3458.

[21] Y. Gu, X.W. Wang, W. Gu, Y.J. Wu, T. Li, T. Zhang, Flexible electronic eardrum, Nano Res. 10 (2017) 2683–2691.

[22] T. Li, H. Luo, L. Qin, X. Wang, Z. Xiong, H. Ding, Y. Gu, Z. Liu, T. Zhang, Flexible capacitive tactile sensor based on micropatterned dielectric layer, Small 12 (2016) 5042–5048.

[23] S.C.B. Mannsfeld, B.C.K. Tee, R.M. Stoltenberg, C.V.H.H. Chen, S. Barman, B.V.O. Muir, A.N. Sokolov, C. Reese, Z.N. Bao, Highly sensitive flexible pressure sensors with microstructured rubber dielectric layers, Nat. Mater. 9 (2010) 859–864.

[24] X.W. Wang, Y. Gu, Z.P. Xiong, Z. Cui, T. Zhang, Silk-molded flexible, ultrasensitive, and highly stable electronic skin for monitoring human physiological signals, Adv. Mater. 26 (2014) 1336–1342.

[25] J.T. Di, X.H. Zhang, Z.Z. Yong, Y.Y. Zhang, D. Li, R. Li, Q.W. Li, Carbon-nanotube fibers for wearable devices and smart textiles, Adv. Mater. 28 (2016) 10529–10538.

[26] M.G. Honarvar, M. Latifi, Overview of wearable electronics and smart textiles, J. Text. Inst. 108 (2017) 631–652.

[27] W. Weng, P.N. Chen, S.S. He, X.M. Sun, H.S. Peng, Smart electronic textiles, Angew. Chem. Int. Ed. 55 (2016) 6140–6169.

[28] B.W. Zhu, H. Wang, W.R. Leow, Y.R. Cai, X.J. Loh, M.Y. Han, X.D. Chen, Silk fibroin for flexible electronic devices, Adv. Mater. 28 (2016) 4250–4265.

[29] X.Q. Liao, Z. Zhang, Q.L. Liao, Q.J. Liang, Y. Ou, M.X. Xu, M.H. Li, G.J. Zhang, Y. Zhang, Flexible and printable paper-based strain sensors for wearable and large-area green electronics, Nanoscale 8 (2016) 13025–13032.

[30] H. Liu, H.B. Qing, Z.D. Li, Y.L. Han, M. Lin, H. Yang, A. Li, T.J. Lu, F. Li, F. Xu, Paper: a promising material for human-friendly functional wearable electronics, Mater. Sci. Eng. R Rep. 112 (2017) 1–22.

[31] K.I. Bolotin, K.J. Sikes, Z. Jiang, M. Klima, G. Fudenberg, J. Hone, P. Kim, H.L. Stormer, Ultrahigh electron mobility in suspended graphene, Solid State Commun. 146 (2008) 351–355.

[32] A.A. Balandin, S. Ghosh, W.Z. Bao, I. Calizo, D. Teweldebrhan, F. Miao, C.N. Lau, Superior thermal conductivity of single-layer graphene, Nano Lett. 8 (2008) 902–907.

[33] C. Lee, X.D. Wei, J.W. Kysar, J. Hone, Measurement of the elastic properties and intrinsic strength of monolayer graphene, Science 321 (2008) 385–388.

[34] M.J. Allen, V.C. Tung, R.B. Kaner, Honeycomb carbon: a review of graphene, Chem. Rev. 110 (2010) 132–145.

[35] R.R. Nair, P. Blake, A.N. Grigorenko, K.S. Novoselov, T.J. Booth, T. Stauber, N.M.R. Peres, A.K. Geim, Fine structure constant defines visual transparency of graphene, Science 320 (2008) 1308.

[36] F. Schedin, A.K. Geim, S.V. Morozov, E.W. Hill, P. Blake, M.I. Katsnelson, K.S. Novoselov, Detection of individual gas molecules adsorbed on graphene, Nat. Mater. 6 (2007) 652–655.

[37] Y. Hernandez, V. Nicolosi, M. Lotya, F.M. Blighe, Z.Y. Sun, S. De, I.T. McGovern, B. Holland, M. Byrne, Y.K. Gun'ko, J.J. Boland, P. Niraj, G. Duesberg, S. Krishnamurthy, R. Goodhue, J. Hutchison, V. Scardaci, A.C. Ferrari, J.N. Coleman, High-yield production of graphene by liquid-phase exfoliation of graphite, Nat. Nanotechnol. 3 (2008) 563–568.

[38] U. Khan, A. O'neill, M. Lotya, S. De, J.N. Coleman, High-concentration solvent exfoliation of graphene, Small 6 (2010) 864–871.

[39] C.S. Boland, U. Khan, C. Backes, A. O'neill, J. McCauley, S. Duane, R. Shanker, Y. Liu, I. Jurewicz, A.B. Dalton, J.N. Coleman, Sensitive, high-strain, high-rate bodily motion sensors based on graphene-rubber composites, ACS Nano 8 (2014) 8819–8830.

[40] U. Khan, P. May, A. O'neill, J.N. Coleman, Development of stiff, strong, yet tough composites by the addition of solvent exfoliated graphene to polyurethane, Carbon 48 (2010) 4035–4041.

[41] K.R. Paton, E. Varrla, C. Backes, R.J. Smith, U. Khan, A. O'neill, C. Boland, M. Lotya, O.M. Istrate, P. King, T. Higgins, S. Barwich, P. May, P. Puczkarski, I. Ahmed, M. Moebius, H. Pettersson, E. Long, J. Coelho, S.E. O'brien, E.K. McGuire, B.M. Sanchez, G.S. Duesberg, N. Mcevoy, T.J. Pennycook, C. Downing, A. Crossley, V. Nicolosi, J.N. Coleman, Scalable production of large quantities of defect-free few-layer graphene by shear exfoliation in liquids, Nat. Mater. 13 (2014) 624–630.

[42] V.C. Tung, M.J. Allen, Y. Yang, R.B. Kaner, High-throughput solution processing of large-scale graphene, Nat. Nanotechnol. 4 (2009) 25–29.

[43] L. Huang, Y. Huang, J.J. Liang, X.J. Wan, Y.S. Chen, Graphene-based conducting inks for direct inkjet printing of flexible conductive patterns and their applications in electric circuits and chemical sensors, Nano Res. 4 (2011) 675–684.

[44] L.J. Cote, F. Kim, J.X. Huang, Langmuir-Blodgett assembly of graphite oxide single layers, J. Am. Chem. Soc. 131 (2009) 1043–1049.

[45] S.T. Han, Y. Zhou, C.D. Wang, L.F. He, W.J. Zhang, V.A.L. Roy, Layer-by-layer-assembled reduced graphene oxide/gold nanoparticle hybrid double-floating-gate structure for low-voltage flexible flash memory, Adv. Mater. 25 (2013) 872–877.

[46] X.L. Li, G.Y. Zhang, X.D. Bai, X.M. Sun, X.R. Wang, E. Wang, H.J. Dai, Highly conducting graphene sheets and Langmuir-Blodgett films, Nat. Nanotechnol. 3 (2008) 538–542.

[47] J.H. Wu, Q.W. Tang, H. Sun, J.M. Lin, H.Y. Ao, M.L. Huang, Y.F. Huang, Conducting film from graphite oxide nanoplatelets and poly(acrylic acid) by layer-by-layer self-assembly, Langmuir 24 (2008) 4800–4805.

[48] Y. Cheng, R.R. Wang, J. Sun, L. Gao, A stretchable and highly sensitive graphene-based fiber for sensing tensile strain, bending, and torsion, Adv. Mater. 27 (2015) 7365–7371.

[49] X.M. Li, T.T. Yang, Y. Yang, J. Zhu, L. Li, F.E. Alam, X. Li, K.L. Wang, H.Y. Cheng, C.T. Lin, Y. Fang, H.W. Zhu, Large-area ultrathin graphene films by single-step marangoni self-assembly for highly sensitive strain sensing application, Adv. Funct. Mater. 26 (2016) 1322–1329.

[50] Q. Liu, M. Zhang, L. Huang, Y.R. Li, J. Chen, C. Li, G.Q. Shi, High-quality graphene ribbons prepared from graphene oxide hydrogels and their application for strain sensors, ACS Nano 9 (2015) 12320–12326.

[51] C.Y. Yan, J.X. Wang, W.B. Kang, M.Q. Cui, X. Wang, C.Y. Foo, K.J. Chee, P.S. Lee, Highly stretchable piezoresistive graphene-nanocellulose nanopaper for strain sensors, Adv. Mater. 26 (2014) 2022–2027.

[52] M.K. Choi, I. Park, D.C. Kim, E. Joh, O.K. Park, J. Kim, M. Kim, C. Choi, J. Yang, K.W. Cho, J.H. Hwang, J.M. Nam, T. Hyeon, J.H. Kim, D.H. Kim, Thermally controlled, patterned graphene transfer printing for transparent and wearable electronic/optoelectronic system, Adv. Funct. Mater. 25 (2015) 7109–7118.

[53] X.W. Wang, Z.P. Xiong, Z. Liu, T. Zhang, Exfoliation at the liquid/air interface to assemble reduced graphene oxide ultrathin films for a flexible noncontact sensing device, Adv. Mater. 27 (2015) 1370–1375.

[54] W.A. De Heer, C. Berger, X.S. Wu, P.N. First, E.H. Conrad, X.B. Li, T.B. Li, M. Sprinkle, J. Hass, M.L. Sadowski, M. Potemski, G. Martinez, Epitaxial graphene, Solid State Commun. 143 (2007) 92–100.

[55] K.V. Emtsev, A. Bostwick, K. Horn, J. Jobst, G.L. Kellogg, L. Ley, J.L. Mcchesney, T. Ohta, S.A. Reshanov, J. Rohrl, E. Rotenberg, A.K. Schmid, D. Waldmann, H.B. Weber, T. Seyller, Towards wafer-size graphene layers by atmospheric pressure graphitization of silicon carbide, Nat. Mater. 8 (2009) 203–207.

[56] K.S. Kim, Y. Zhao, H. Jang, S.Y. Lee, J.M. Kim, K.S. Kim, J.H. Ahn, P. Kim, J.Y. Choi, B.H. Hong, Large-scale pattern growth of graphene films for stretchable transparent electrodes, Nature 457 (2009) 706–710.

[57] H. Tetlow, J.P. De Boer, I.J. Ford, D.D. Vvedensky, J. Coraux, L. Kantorovich, Growth of epitaxial graphene: theory and experiment, Phys. Rep. 542 (2014) 195–295.

[58] C. Berger, Z.M. Song, X.B. Li, X.S. Wu, N. Brown, C. Naud, D. Mayou, T.B. Li, J. Hass, A.N. Marchenkov, E.H. Conrad, P.N. First, W.A. De Heer, Electronic confinement and coherence in patterned epitaxial graphene, Science 312 (2006) 1191–1196.

[59] Y.H. Kim, S.J. Kim, Y.J. Kim, Y.S. Shim, S.Y. Kim, B.H. Hong, H.W. Jang, Self-activated transparent all-graphene gas sensor with endurance to humidity and mechanical bending, ACS Nano 9 (2015) 10453–10460.

[60] Y. Wang, L. Wang, T.T. Yang, X. Li, X.B. Zang, M. Zhu, K.L. Wang, D.H. Wu, H.W. Zhu, Wearable and highly sensitive graphene strain sensors for human motion monitoring, Adv. Funct. Mater. 24 (2014) 4666–4670.

[61] B.G. Demczyk, Y.M. Wang, J. Cumings, M. Hetman, W. Han, A. Zettl, R.O. Ritchie, Direct mechanical measurement of the tensile strength and elastic modulus of multiwalled carbon nanotubes, Mater. Sci. Eng. 334 (2002) 173–178.

[62] E.W. Wong, P.E. Sheehan, C.M. Lieber, Nanobeam mechanics: elasticity, strength, and toughness of nanorods and nanotubes, Science 277 (1997) 1971–1975.

[63] B.I. Yakobson, C.J. Brabec, J. Bernholc, Nanomechanics of carbon tubes: instabilities beyond linear response, Phys. Rev. Lett. 76 (1996) 2511–2514.

[64] R.H. Baughman, A.A. Zakhidov, W.A. De Heer, Carbon nanotubes—the route toward applications, Science 297 (2002) 787–792.

[65] W. Obitayo, T. Liu, A review: carbon nanotube-based piezoresistive strain sensors, J. Sens. 15 (2012) 652438.

[66] D.N. Futaba, K. Hata, T. Yamada, T. Hiraoka, Y. Hayamizu, Y. Kakudate, O. Tanaike, H. Hatori, M. Yumura, S. Iijima, Shape-engineerable and highly densely packed single-walled carbon nanotubes and their application as super-capacitor electrodes, Nat. Mater. 5 (2006) 987–994.

[67] B. Vigolo, A. Penicaud, C. Coulon, C. Sauder, R. Pailler, C. Journet, P. Bernier, P. Poulin, Macroscopic fibers and ribbons of oriented carbon nanotubes, Science 290 (2000) 1331–1334.

[68] D.J. Cohen, D. Mitra, K. Peterson, M.M. Maharbiz, A highly elastic, capacitive strain gauge based on percolating nanotube networks, Nano Lett. 12 (2012) 1821–1825.

[69] D.J. Lipomi, M. Vosgueritchian, B.C.K. Tee, S.L. Hellstrom, J.A. Lee, C.H. Fox, Z.N. Bao, Skin-like pressure and strain sensors based on transparent elastic films of carbon nanotubes, Nat. Nanotechnol. 6 (2011) 788–792.

[70] T. Yamada, Y. Hayamizu, Y. Yamamoto, Y. Yomogida, A. Izadi-Najafabadi, D.N. Futaba, K. Hata, A stretchable carbon nanotube strain sensor for human-motion detection, Nat. Nanotechnol. 6 (2011) 296–301.

[71] W.A. Deheer, W.S. Bacsa, A. Chatelain, T. Gerfin, R. Humphreybaker, L. Forro, D. Ugarte, Aligned carbon nanotube films—production and optical and electronic-properties, Science 268 (1995) 845–847.

[72] W.A. Deheer, A. Chatelain, D. Ugarte, A carbon nanotube field-emission electron source, Science 270 (1995) 1179–1180.

[73] S.S. Fan, M.G. Chapline, N.R. Franklin, T.W. Tombler, A.M. Cassell, H.J. Dai, Self-oriented regular arrays of carbon nanotubes and their field emission properties, Science 283 (1999) 512–514.

[74] X.W. Wang, G.H. Li, R. Liu, H.Y. Ding, T. Zhang, Reproducible layer-by-layer exfoliation for free-standing ultrathin films of single-walled carbon nanotubes, J. Mater. Chem. 22 (2012) 21824–21827.

[75] T. Yamada, Y. Yamamoto, Y. Hayamizu, A. Sekiguchi, H. Tanaka, K. Kobashi, D.N. Futaba, K. Hata, Torsion-sensing material from aligned carbon nanotubes wound onto a rod demonstrating wide dynamic range, ACS Nano 7 (2013) 3177–3182.

[76] A.J. Bandodkar, W. Jia, J. Wang, Tattoo-based wearable electrochemical devices: a review, Electroanalysis 27 (2015) 562–572.

[77] A.R. Madaria, A. Kumar, F.N. Ishikawa, C.W. Zhou, Uniform, highly conductive, and patterned transparent films of a percolating silver nanowire network on rigid and flexible substrates using a dry transfer technique, Nano Res. 3 (2010) 564–573.

[78] J. Wang, J.T. Jiu, M. Nogi, T. Sugahara, S. Nagao, H. Koga, P. He, K. Suganuma, A highly sensitive and flexible pressure sensor with electrodes and elastomeric interlayer containing silver nanowires, Nanoscale 7 (2015) 2926–2932.

[79] Y.Y. Shang, X.D. He, Y.B. Li, L.H. Zhang, Z. Li, C.Y. Ji, E.Z. Shi, P.X. Li, K. Zhu, Q.Y. Peng, C. Wang, X.J. Zhang, R.G. Wang, J.Q. Wei, K.L. Wang, H.W. Zhu, D.H. Wu, A.Y. Cao, Super-stretchable spring-like carbon nanotube ropes, Adv. Mater. 24 (2012) 2896–2900.

[80] N.S. Lu, C. Lu, S.X. Yang, J. Rogers, Highly sensitive skin-mountable strain gauges based entirely on elastomers, Adv. Funct. Mater. 22 (2012) 4044–4050.

[81] R.M. Niu, G. Liu, C. Wang, G. Zhang, X.D. Ding, J. Sun, Thickness dependent critical strain in submicron Cu films adherent to polymer substrate, Appl. Phys. Lett. 90 (2007) 161907.

[82] A. Crew, D.C. Cowell, J.P. Hart, Development of an anodic stripping voltammetric assay, using a disposable mercury-free screen-printed carbon electrode, for the determination of zinc in human sweat, Talanta 75 (2008) 1221–1226.

[83] T. Guinovart, G. ValdéS-Ramírez, J.R. Windmiller, F.J. Andrade, J. Wang, Bandage-based wearable potentiometric sensor for monitoring wound pH, Electroanalysis 26 (2014) 1345–1353.

[84] H.B. Huang, F. Spaepen, Tensile testing of free-standing Cu, Ag and Al thin films and Ag/Cu multilayers, Acta Mater. 48 (2000) 3261–3269.

[85] Q. Sun, W. Seung, B.J. Kim, S. Seo, S.W. Kim, J.H. Cho, Active matrix electronic skin strain sensor based on piezopotential-powered graphene transistors, Adv. Mater. 27 (2015) 3411–3417.

[86] N. Hu, Y. Karube, M. Arai, T. Watanabe, C. Yan, Y. Li, Y.L. Liu, H. Fukunaga, Investigation on sensitivity of a polymer/carbon nanotube composite strain sensor, Carbon 48 (2010) 680–687.

[87] H. Jiang, D.-Y. Khang, J. Song, Y. Sun, Y. Huang, J.A. Rogers, Finite deformation mechanics in buckled thin films on compliant supports, Proc. Natl. Acad. Sci. 104 (2007) 15607–15612.

[88] J. Kim, W.R. De Araujo, I.A. Samek, A.J. Bandodkar, W. Jia, B. Brunetti, T.R.L.C. PaixãO, J. Wang, Wearable temporary tattoo sensor for real-time trace metal monitoring in human sweat, Electrochem. Commun. 51 (2015) 41–45.

[89] M. Zhang, K.R. Atkinson, R.H. Baughman, Multifunctional carbon nanotube yarns by downsizing an ancient technology, Science 306 (2004) 1358–1361.

[90] S. Wang, Y. Wu, Y. Gu, T. Li, H. Luo, L.-H. Li, Y. Bai, L. Li, L. Liu, Y. Cao, H. Ding, T. Zhang, Wearable sweatband sensor platform based on gold nanodendrite array as efficient solid contact of ion-selective electrode, Anal. Chem. 89 (2017) 10224–10231.

[91] M. Kubo, X.F. Li, C. Kim, M. Hashimoto, B.J. Wiley, D. Ham, G.M. Whitesides, Stretchable microfluidic radiofrequency antennas, Adv. Mater. 22 (2010) 2749.

[92] M.H. Miao, Yarn spun from carbon nanotube forests: production, structure, properties and applications, Particuology 11 (2013) 378–393.

[93] Y. Huang, X.F. Duan, Q.Q. Wei, C.M. Lieber, Directed assembly of one-dimensional nanostructures into functional networks, Science 291 (2001) 630–633.

[94] J. Fontes, Chapter 20—Temperature sensors A2, in: J.S. Wilson (Ed.), Sensor Technology Handbook, Newnes, Burlington, 2005.

[95] Y. Zhang, S. Wang, X. Li, J.A. Fan, S. Xu, Y.M. Song, K.-J. Choi, W.-H. Yeo, W. Lee, S.N. Nazaar, B. Lu, L. Yin, K.-C. Hwang, J.A. Rogers, Y. Huang, Experimental and theoretical studies of serpentine microstructures bonded to prestrained elastomers for stretchable electronics, Adv. Funct. Mater. 24 (2014) 2028–2037.

[96] Y. Huang, W. Dong, T. Huang, Y. Wang, L. Xiao, Y. Su, Z. Yin, Self-similar design for stretchable wireless LC strain sensors, Sensors Actuators A Phys. 224 (2015) 36–42.

[97] J.A. Fan, W.-H. Yeo, Y. Su, Y. Hattori, W. Lee, S.-Y. Jung, Y. Zhang, Z. Liu, H. Cheng, L. Falgout, M. Bajema, T. Coleman, D. Gregoire, R.J. Larsen, Y. Huang, J.A. Rogers, Fractal design concepts for stretchable electronics, Nat. Commun. 5 (2014) 3266.

[98] J.A. Rogers, T. Someya, Y. Huang, Materials and mechanics for stretchable electronics, Science 327 (2010) 1603–1607.

[99] J.M. Feng, R. Wang, Y.L. Li, X.H. Zhong, L. Cui, Q.J. Guo, F. Hou, One-step fabrication of high quality double-walled carbon nanotube thin films by a chemical vapor deposition process, Carbon 48 (2010) 3817–3824.

[100] M.L. Hammock, A. Chortos, B.C.K. Tee, J.B.H. Tok, Z.A. Bao, 25th Anniversary article: the evolution of electronic skin (E-Skin): a brief history, design considerations, and recent progress, Adv. Mater. 25 (2013) 5997–6037.

[101] H. Yao, A.J. Shum, M. Cowan, I. Lähdesmäki, B.A. Parviz, A contact lens with embedded sensor for monitoring tear glucose level, Biosens. Bioelectron. 26 (2011) 3290–3296.

[102] Z.Y. Fan, J.C. Ho, T. Takahashi, R. Yerushalmi, K. Takei, A.C. Ford, Y.L. Chueh, A. Javey, Toward the development of printable nanowire electronics and sensors, Adv. Mater. 21 (2009) 3730–3743.

[103] A. Javey, S. Nam, R.S. Friedman, H. Yan, C.M. Lieber, Layer-by-layer assembly of nanowires for three-dimensional, multifunctional electronics, Nano Lett. 7 (2007) 773–777.

[104] X. Xiao, L. Yuan, J. Zhong, T. Ding, Y. Liu, Z. Cai, Y. Rong, H. Han, J. Zhou, Z.L. Wang, High-strain sensors based on ZnO nanowire/polystyrene hybridized flexible films, Adv. Mater. 23 (2011) 5440–5444.

[105] X. Lu, Y. Xia, Electronic materials: buckling down for flexible electronics, Nat. Nanotechnol. 1 (2006) 163–164.

[106] J.W. Lee, R. Xu, S. Lee, K.-I. Jang, Y. Yang, A. Banks, K.J. Yu, J. Kim, S. Xu, S. Ma, S.W. Jang, P. Won, Y. Li, B.H. Kim, J.Y. Choe, S. Huh, Y.H. Kwon, Y. Huang, U. Paik, J.A. Rogers, Soft, thin skin-mounted power management systems and their use in wireless thermography, Proc. Natl. Acad. Sci. 113 (2016) 6131–6136.

[107] L.B. Hu, W. Yuan, P. Brochu, G. Gruner, Q.B. Pei, Highly stretchable, conductive, and transparent nanotube thin films, Appl. Phys. Lett. 94 (2009) 161108.

[108] R.S. Timsit, Electrical contact resistance: properties of stationary interfaces, IEEE Trans. Compon. Packag. Technol. 22 (1999) 85–98.

[109] M. Shimojo, A. Namiki, M. Ishikawa, R. Makino, K. Mabuchi, A tactile sensor sheet using pressure conductive rubber with electrical-wires stitched method, IEEE Sensors J. 4 (2004) 589–596.

[110] M. Zirkl, A. Sawatdee, U. Helbig, M. Krause, G. Scheipl, E. Kraker, P.A. Ersman, D. Nilsson, D. Platt, P. Bodo, S. Bauer, G. Domann, B. Stadlober, An all-printed ferroelectric active matrix sensor network based on only five functional materials forming a touchless control interface, Adv. Mater. 23 (2011) 2069–2074.

[111] I. Graz, M. Krause, S. Bauer-Gogonea, S. Bauer, S.P. Lacour, B. Ploss, M. Zirkl, B. Stadlober, S. Wagner, Flexible active-matrix cells with selectively poled bifunctional polymer-ceramic nanocomposite for pressure and temperature sensing skin, J. Appl. Phys. 106 (2009) 034503.

[112] J. Park, Y. Lee, J. Hong, Y. Lee, M. Ha, Y. Jung, H. Lim, S.Y. Kim, H. Ko, Tactile-direction-sensitive and stretchable electronic skins based on human-skin-inspired interlocked microstructures, ACS Nano 8 (2014) 12020–12029.

[113] S. Wagner, S.P. Lacour, J. Jones, P.H.I. Hsu, J.C. Sturm, T. Li, Z.G. Suo, Electronic skin: architecture and components, Physica E 25 (2004) 326–334.

[114] X. Feng, B.D. Yang, Y.M. Liu, Y. Wang, C. Dagdeviren, Z.J. Liu, A. Carlson, J.Y. Li, Y.G. Huang, J.A. Rogers, Stretchable ferroelectric nanoribbons with wavy configurations on elastomeric substrates, ACS Nano 5 (2011) 3326–3332.

[115] N.T. Tien, S. Jeon, D.I. Kim, T.Q. Trung, M. Jang, B.U. Hwang, K.E. Byun, J. Bae, E. Lee, J.B.H. Tok, Z.N. Bao, N.E. Lee, J.J. Park, A flexible bimodal sensor array for simultaneous sensing of pressure and temperature, Adv. Mater. 26 (2014) 796–804.

[116] A. Cazale, W. Sant, F. Ginot, J.C. Launay, G. Savourey, F. Revol-Cavalier, J.M. Lagarde, D. Heinry, J. Launay, P. Temple-Boyer, Physiological stress monitoring using sodium ion potentiometric microsensors for sweat analysis, Sens. Actuators B Chem. 225 (2016) 1–9.

[117] Y. Huang, X.F. Duan, C.M. Lieber, Nanowires for integrated multicolor nanophotonics, Small 1 (2005) 142–147.

[118] K. Nan, H. Luan, Z. Yan, X. Ning, Y. Wang, A. Wang, J. Wang, M. Han, M. Chang, K. Li, Y. Zhang, W. Huang, Y. Xue, Y. Huang, Y. Zhang, J.A. Rogers, Engineered elastomer substrates for guided assembly of complex 3D mesostructures by spatially nonuniform compressive buckling, Adv. Funct. Mater. 27 (2017).

[119] Y.Y. Bai, Y.H. Jiang, B.H. Chen, C.C. Foo, Y.C. Zhou, F. Xiang, J.X. Zhou, H. Wang, Z.G. Suo, Cyclic performance of viscoelastic dielectric elastomers with solid hydrogel electrodes, Appl. Phys. Lett. 104 (2014) 062902.

[120] P. Lee, J. Lee, H. Lee, J. Yeo, S. Hong, K.H. Nam, D. Lee, S.S. Lee, Ko, S. H., Highly stretchable and highly conductive metal electrode by very long metal nanowire percolation network, Adv. Mater. 24 (2012) 3326–3332.

[121] S. Befahy, S. Yunus, T. Pardoen, P. Bertrand, M. Troosters, Stretchable helical gold conductor on silicone rubber microwire, Appl. Phys. Lett. 91 (2007) 141911.

[122] T. Li, Z.Y. Huang, Z.C. Xi, S.P. Lacour, S. Wagner, Z. Suo, Delocalizing strain in a thin metal film on a polymer substrate, Mech. Mater. 37 (2005) 261–273.

[123] Y. Zhang, H. Fu, Y. Su, S. Xu, H. Cheng, J.A. Fan, K.-C. Hwang, J.A. Rogers, Y. Huang, Mechanics of ultra-stretchable self-similar serpentine interconnects, Acta Mater. 61 (2013) 7816–7827.

[124] A.M.V. Mohan, J.R. Windmiller, R.K. Mishra, J. Wang, Continuous minimally-invasive alcohol monitoring using microneedle sensor arrays, Biosens. Bioelectron. 91 (2017) 574–579.

[125] S. Wang, L.-P. Xu, X. Zhang, Ultrasensitive electrochemical biosensor based on noble metal nanomaterials, Sci. Adv. Mater. 7 (2015) 2084–2102.

[126] M.F.F. Li, H.Y. Li, W.B. Zhong, Q.H. Zhao, D. Wang, Stretchable conductive polypyrrole/polyurethane (PPY/PU) strain sensor with netlike microcracks for human breath detection, ACS Appl. Mater. Interfaces 6 (2014) 1313–1319.

[127] T. Li, Z. Suo, Deformability of thin metal films on elastomer substrates, Int. J. Solids Struct. 43 (2006) 2351–2363.

[128] M. Hommel, O. Kraft, Deformation behavior of thin copper films on deformable substrates, Acta Mater. 49 (2001) 3935–3947.

[129] Y.P. Zang, F.J. Zhang, D.Z. Huang, X.K. Gao, C.A. Di, D.B. Zhu, Flexible suspended gate organic thin-film transistors for ultra-sensitive pressure detection, Nat. Commun. 6 (2015) 6269.

[130] S. De, T.M. Higgins, P.E. Lyons, E.M. Doherty, P.N. Nirmalraj, W.J. Blau, J.J. Boland, J.N. Coleman, Silver nanowire networks as flexible, transparent, conducting films: extremely high DC to optical conductivity ratios, ACS Nano 3 (2009) 1767–1774.

[131] L.B. Hu, H.S. Kim, J.Y. Lee, P. Peumans, Y. Cui, Scalable coating and properties of transparent, flexible, silver nanowire electrodes, ACS Nano 4 (2010) 2955–2963.

[132] R.-H. Kim, M.-H. Bae, D.G. Kim, H. Cheng, B.H. Kim, D.-H. Kim, M. Li, J. Wu, F. Du, H.-S. Kim, S. Kim, D. Estrada, S.W. Hong, Y. Huang, E. Pop, J.A. Rogers, Stretchable, transparent graphene interconnects for arrays of microscale inorganic light emitting diodes on rubber substrates, Nano Lett. 11 (2011) 3881–3886.

[133] S.P. Lacour, S. Wagner, Z. Huang, Z. Suo, Stretchable gold conductors on elastomeric substrates, Appl. Phys. Lett. 82 (2003) 2404–2406.

[134] A.L. Volynskii, S. Bazhenov, O.V. Lebedeva, N.F. Bakeev, Mechanical buckling instability of thin coatings deposited on soft polymer substrates, J. Mater. Sci. 35 (2000) 547–554.

[135] B. Su, S. Gong, Z. Ma, L.W. Yap, W. Cheng, Mimosa-inspired design of a flexible pressure sensor with touch sensitivity, Small 11 (2015) 1886–1891.

[136] C. Keplinger, J.-Y. Sun, C.C. Foo, P. Rothemund, G.M. Whitesides, Z. Suo, Stretchable, transparent, ionic conductors, Science (New York, N.Y.) 341 (2013) 984–987.

[137] C.A.O. Henning, F.W. Boswell, J.M. Corbett, Mechanical-properties of vacuum-deposited metal-films. 2. Nickel films, Acta Metall. 23 (1975) 187–192.

[138] A.B. Dalton, S. Collins, E. Munoz, J.M. Razal, V.H. Ebron, J.P. Ferraris, J.N. Coleman, B.G. Kim, R.H. Baughman, Super-tough carbon-nanotube fibres—these extraordinary composite fibres can be woven into electronic textiles, Nature 423 (2003) 703.

[139] L.M. Ericson, H. Fan, H.Q. Peng, V.A. Davis, W. Zhou, J. Sulpizio, Y.H. Wang, R. Booker, J. Vavro, C. Guthy, A.N.G. Parra-Vasquez, M.J. Kim, S. Ramesh, R.K. Saini, C. Kittrell, G. Lavin, H. Schmidt, W.W. Adams, W.E. Billups, M. Pasquali, W.F. Hwang, R.H. Hauge, J.E. Fischer, R.E. Smalley, Macroscopic, neat, single-walled carbon nanotube fibers, Science 305 (2004) 1447–1450.

[140] T. Takahashi, K. Takei, J.C. Ho, Y.L. Chueh, Z.Y. Fan, A. Javey, Monolayer resist for patterned contact printing of aligned nanowire arrays, J. Am. Chem. Soc. 131 (2009) 2102.

[141] Y.Y. Bai, B.H. Chen, F. Xiang, J.X. Zhou, H. Wang, Z.G. Suo, Transparent hydrogel with enhanced water retention capacity by introducing highly hydratable salt, Appl. Phys. Lett. 105 (2014) 151903.

[142] D.S. Gray, J. Tien, C.S. Chen, High conductivity elastomeric electronics, Adv. Mater. 16 (2004) 393.

[143] Z.Y. Lei, Q.K. Wang, S.T. Sun, W.C. Zhu, Wu, P. Y., A bioinspired mineral hydrogel as a self-healable, mechanically adaptable ionic skin for highly sensitive pressure sensing, Adv. Mater. 29 (2017).

[144] S. Park, H. Kim, M. Vosgueritchian, S. Cheon, H. Kim, J.H. Koo, T.R. Kim, S. Lee, G. Schwartz, H. Chang, Z.A. Bao, Stretchable energy-harvesting tactile electronic skin capable of differentiating multiple mechanical stimuli modes, Adv. Mater. 26 (2014) 7324–7332.

[145] N.S. Lu, X. Wang, Z.G. Suo, J. Vlassak, Metal films on polymer substrates stretched beyond 50%, Appl. Phys. Lett. 91 (2007) 221909.

[146] M. Gonzalez, F. Axisa, M.V. Buicke, D. Brosteaux, B. Vandevelde, J. Vanfleteren, Design of metal interconnects for stretchable electronic circuits, Microelectron. Reliab. 48 (2008) 825–832.

[147] T. Yokota, Y. Inoue, Y. Terakawa, J. Reeder, M. Kaltenbrunner, T. Ware, K. Yang, K. Mabuchi, T. Murakawa, M. Sekino, W. Voit, T. Sekitani, T. Someya, Ultraflexible, large-area, physiological temperature sensors for multipoint measurements, Proc. Natl. Acad. Sci. U. S. A. 112 (2015) 14533–14538.

[148] F. Lux, Models proposed to explain the electrical-conductivity of mixtures made of conductive and insulating materials, J. Mater. Sci. 28 (1993) 285–301.

[149] Y. Joo, J. Byun, N. Seong, J. Ha, H. Kim, S. Kim, T. Kim, H. Im, D. Kim, Y. Hong, Silver nanowire-embedded PDMS with a multiscale structure for a highly sensitive and robust flexible pressure sensor, Nanoscale 7 (2015) 6208–6215.

[150] W. Wu, X. Wen, Z.L. Wang, Taxel-addressable matrix of vertical-nanowire piezotronic transistors for active and adaptive tactile imaging, Science 340 (2013) 952–957.

[151] J.H. Ahn, H.S. Kim, K.J. Lee, S. Jeon, S.J. Kang, Y.G. Sun, R.G. Nuzzo, J.A. Rogers, Heterogeneous three-dimensional electronics by use of printed semiconductor nanomaterials, Science 314 (2006) 1754–1757.

[152] C.H. Yang, B. Chen, J.J. Lu, J.H. Yang, J. Zhou, Y.M. Chen, Z. Suo, Ionic cable, Extreme Mech. Lett. 3 (2015) 59–65.

[153] R.R. Keller, J.M. Phelps, D.T. Read, Tensile and fracture behavior of free-standing copper films, Mater. Sci. Eng. 214 (1996) 42–52.

[154] F. Xu, Y. Zhu, Highly conductive and stretchable silver nanowire conductors, Adv. Mater. 24 (2012) 5117–5122.

[155] H. Lee, T.K. Choi, Y.B. Lee, H.R. Cho, R. Ghaffari, L. Wang, H.J. Choi, T.D. Chung, N. Lu, T. Hyeon, S.H. Choi, D.H. Kim, A graphene-based electrochemical device with thermoresponsive microneedles for diabetes monitoring and therapy, Nat. Nanotechnol. 11 (2016) 566–572.

[156] P. Kassal, J. Kim, R. Kumar, W.R. De Araujo, I.M. Steinberg, M.D. Steinberg, J. Wang, Smart bandage with wireless connectivity for uric acid biosensing as an indicator of wound status, Electrochem. Commun. 56 (2015) 6–10.

[157] K. Takei, W. Honda, S. Harada, T. Arie, S. Akita, Toward flexible and wearable human-interactive health-monitoring devices, Adv. Healthc. Mater. 4 (2015) 487–500.

[158] Y.G. Sun, D.Y. Khang, F. Hua, K. Hurley, R.G. Nuzzo, J.A. Rogers, Photolithographic route to the fabrication of micro/nanowires of III-V semiconductors, Adv. Funct. Mater. 15 (2005) 30–40.

[159] Y.Z. Xie, Y. Liu, Y.D. Zhao, Y.H. Tsang, S.P. Lau, H.T. Huang, Y. Chai, Stretchable all-solid-state supercapacitor with wavy shaped polyaniline/graphene electrode, J. Mater. Chem. A 2 (2014) 9142–9149.

[160] H. Guo, M.-H. Yeh, Y.-C. Lai, Y. Zi, C. Wu, Z. Wen, C. Hu, Z.L. Wang, All-in-one shape-adaptive self-charging power package for wearable electronics, ACS Nano 10 (2016) 10580–10588.

[161] M. Gradisar, L. Lack, Relationships between the circadian rhythms of finger temperature, core temperature, sleep latency, and subjective sleepiness, J. Biol. Rhythm. 19 (2004) 157–163.

[162] J. Wang, Electrochemical glucose biosensors, Chem. Rev. 108 (2008) 814–825.

[163] Y. Liu, K. He, G. Chen, W.R. Leow, X. Chen, Nature-inspired structural materials for flexible electronic devices, Chem. Rev. 117 (2017) 12893–12941.

[164] W.B. Lu, M. Zu, J.H. Byun, B.S. Kim, T.W. Chou, State of the art of carbon nanotube fibers: opportunities and challenges, Adv. Mater. 24 (2012) 1805–1833.

[165] S.K. Mahadeva, S. Yun, J. Kim, Flexible humidity and temperature sensor based on cellulose–polypyrrole nanocomposite, Sensors Actuators A Phys. 165 (2011) 194–199.

[166] D.I. Kim, T.Q. Trung, B.U. Hwang, J.S. Kim, S. Jeon, J. Bae, J.J. Park, N.E. Lee, A sensor array using multifunctional field-effect transistors with ultrahigh sensitivity and precision for bio-monitoring, Sci. Rep. 5 (2015).

[167] N.T. Tien, Y.G. Seol, L.H.A. Dao, H.Y. Noh, N.E. Lee, Utilizing highly crystalline pyroelectric material as functional gate dielectric in organic thin-film transistors, Adv. Mater. 21 (2009) 910.

[168] S.S. Yao, Y. Zhu, Wearable multifunctional sensors using printed stretchable conductors made of silver nanowires, Nanoscale 6 (2014) 2345–2352.

[169] D.H. Zhang, Z.Q. Liu, C. Li, T. Tang, X.L. Liu, S. Han, B. Lei, C.W. Zhou, Detection of NO2 down to ppb levels using individual and multiple In2O3 nanowire devices, Nano Lett. 4 (2004) 1919–1924.

[170] P. Slobodian, P. Riha, P. Saha, A highly-deformable composite composed of an entangled network of electrically-conductive carbon-nanotubes embedded in elastic polyurethane, Carbon 50 (2012) 3446–3453.

[171] R.C. Webb, A.P. Bonifas, A. Behnaz, Y. Zhang, K.J. Yu, H. Cheng, M. Shi, Z. Bian, Z. Liu, Y.-S. Kim, W.-H. Yeo, J.S. Park, J. Song, Y. Li, Y. Huang, A.M. Gorbach, J.A. Rogers, Ultrathin conformal devices for precise and continuous thermal characterization of human skin, Nat. Mater. 12 (2013) 938.

[172] P. Slobodian, P. Riha, R. Benlikaya, P. Svoboda, D. Petras, A flexible multifunctional sensor based on carbon nanotube/polyurethane composite, IEEE Sensors J. 13 (2013) 4045–4048.

[173] I.M. Graz, D.P.J. Cotton, S.P. Lacour, Extended cyclic uniaxial loading of stretchable gold thin-films on elastomeric substrates, Appl. Phys. Lett. 94 (2009) 071902.

[174] P. Le Floch, X. Yao, Q. Liu, Z. Wang, G. Nian, Y. Sun, L. Jia, Z. Suo, Wearable and washable conductors for active textiles, ACS Appl. Mater. Interfaces 9 (2017) 25542–25552.

[175] J. Jeon, H.-B.-R. Lee, Z. Bao, Flexible wireless temperature sensors based on Ni microparticle-filled binary polymer composites, Adv. Mater. 25 (2013) 850–855.

[176] A.J. Bandodkar, W. Jia, C. Yardımcı, X. Wang, J. Ramirez, J. Wang, Tattoo-based noninvasive glucose monitoring: a proof-of-concept study, Anal. Chem. 87 (2015) 394–398.

[177] J. Song, H. Jiang, Y. Huang, J.A. Rogers, Mechanics of stretchable inorganic electronic materials, J. Vac. Sci. Technol. A 27 (2009) 1107–1125.

[178] Y.L. Li, I.A. Kinloch, A.H. Windle, Direct spinning of carbon nanotube fibers from chemical vapor deposition synthesis, Science 304 (2004) 276–278.

[179] T.Q. Trung, N.T. Tien, Y.G. Seol, N.-E. Lee, Transparent and flexible organic field-effect transistor for multi-modal sensing, Org. Electron. 13 (2012) 533–540.

[180] I.Y. Han, S.J. Kim, Diode temperature sensor array for measuring micro-scale surface temperatures with high resolution, Sensors Actuators A Phys. 141 (2008) 52–58.

[181] D. Solovei, J. Zak, P. Majzlikova, J. Sedlacek, J. Hubalek, Chemical sensor platform for non-invasive monitoring of activity and dehydration, Sensors 15 (2015) 1479–1495.

[182] A.J. Bandodkar, D. Molinnus, O. Mirza, T. Guinovart, J.R. Windmiller, G. ValdéS-Ramírez, F.J. Andrade, M.J. Schöning, J. Wang, Epidermal tattoo potentiometric sodium sensors with wireless signal transduction for continuous non-invasive sweat monitoring, Biosens. Bioelectron. 54 (2014) 603–609.

[183] Y. Wei, S. Chen, Y. Lin, Z. Yang, L. Liu, Cu-Ag core-shell nanowires for electronic skin with a petal molded microstructure, J. Mater. Chem. C 3 (2015) 9594–9602.

[184] Z. Liu, D. Qi, P. Guo, Y. Liu, B. Zhu, H. Yang, Y. Liu, B. Li, C. Zhang, J. Yu, B. Liedberg, X. Chen, Thickness-gradient films for high gauge factor stretchable strain sensors, Adv. Mater. 27 (2015) 6230–6237.

[185] C.-Y. Lee, F.-B. Weng, C.-H. Cheng, H.-R. Shiu, S.-P. Jung, W.-C. Chang, P.-C. Chan, W.-T. Chen, C.-J. Lee, Use of flexible micro-temperature sensor to determine temperature in situ and to simulate a proton exchange membrane fuel cell, J. Power Sources 196 (2011) 228–234.

[186] T.-P. Huynh, H. Haick, Self-healing, fully functional, and multiparametric flexible sensing platform, Adv. Mater. 28 (2016) 138–143.

[187] F. Xu, X. Wang, Y.T. Zhu, Y. Zhu, Wavy ribbons of carbon nanotubes for stretchable conductors, Adv. Funct. Mater. 22 (2012) 1279–1283.

[188] C. Pang, G.-Y. Lee, T.-I. Kim, S.M. Kim, H.N. Kim, S.-H. Ahn, K.-Y. Suh, A flexible and highly sensitive strain-gauge sensor using reversible interlocking of nanofibres, Nat. Mater. 11 (2012) 795–801.

[189] C.F. Guo, T.Y. Sun, Q.H. Liu, Z.G. Suo, Z.F. Ren, Highly stretchable and transparent nanomesh electrodes made by grain boundary lithography, Nat. Commun. 5 (2014).

[190] L. Cai, L. Song, P.S. Luan, Q. Zhang, N. Zhang, Q.Q. Gao, D. Zhao, X. Zhang, M. Tu, F. Yang, W.B. Zhou, Q.X. Fan, J. Luo, W.Y. Zhou, P.M. Ajayan, S.S. Xie, Super-stretchable, transparent carbon nanotube-based capacitive strain sensors for human motion detection, Sci. Rep. 3 (2013) 3048.

[191] W. Liu, Z. Chen, G. Zhou, Y. Sun, H.R. Lee, C. Liu, H. Yao, Z. Bao, Y. Cui, 3D porous sponge-inspired electrode for stretchable lithium-ion batteries, Adv. Mater. 28 (2016) 3578.

[192] B. Ploss, B. Ploss, F.G. Shin, H.L.W. Chan, C.L. Choy, Pyroelectric activity of ferroelectric PT/PVDF-TRFE, IEEE Trans. Dielectr. Electr. Insul. 7 (2000) 517–522.

[193] C.-Y. Lee, G.-W. Wu, W.-J. Hsieh, Fabrication of micro sensors on a flexible substrate, Sensors Actuators A Phys. 147 (2008) 173–176.

[194] B.H. Chen, Y.Y. Bai, F. Xiang, J.Y. Sun, Y.M. Chen, H. Wang, J.X. Zhou, Z.G. Suo, Stretchable and transparent hydrogels as soft conductors for dielectric elastomer actuators, J. Polym. Sci. Part B Polym. Phys. 52 (2014) 1055–1060.

[195] S. Park, M. Vosguerichian, Z.A. Bao, A review of fabrication and applications of carbon nanotube film-based flexible electronics, Nanoscale 5 (2013) 1727–1752.

[196] H. Vandeparre, Q.H. Liu, I.R. Minev, Z.G. Suo, S.P. Lacour, Localization of folds and cracks in thin metal films coated on flexible elastomer foams, Adv. Mater. 25 (2013) 3117–3121.

[197] G.R. Witt, The electromechanical properties of thin films and the thin film strain gauge, Thin Solid Films 22 (1974) 133–156.

[198] M. Zhang, S.L. Fang, A.A. Zakhidov, S.B. Lee, A.E. Aliev, C.D. Williams, K.R. Atkinson, R.H. Baughman, Strong, transparent, multifunctional, carbon nanotube sheets, Science 309 (2005) 1215–1219.

[199] W. Zhang, R. Zhu, V. Nguyen, R. Yang, Highly sensitive and flexible strain sensors based on vertical zinc oxide nanowire arrays, Sensors Actuators A Phys. 205 (2014) 164–169.

[200] G. Matzeu, C. O'quigley, E. McNamara, C. Zuliani, C. Fay, T. Glennon, D. Diamond, An integrated sensing and wireless communications platform for sensing sodium in sweat, Anal. Methods 8 (2016) 64–71.

[201] C. Yan, J. Wang, P.S. Lee, Stretchable graphene thermistor with tunable thermal index, ACS Nano 9 (2015) 2130–2137.

[202] C. Mattmann, F. Clemens, G. Troster, Sensor for measuring strain in textile, Sensors 8 (2008) 3719–3732.

[203] A.J. Bandodkar, V.W.S. Hung, W. Jia, G. Valdes-Ramirez, J.R. Windmiller, A.G. Martinez, J. Ramirez, G. Chan, K. Kerman, J. Wang, Tattoo-based potentiometric ion-selective sensors for epidermal pH monitoring, Analyst 138 (2013) 123–128.

[204] Z.B. Yu, Q.W. Zhang, L. Li, Q. Chen, X.F. Niu, J. Liu, Q.B. Pei, Highly flexible silver nanowire electrodes for shape-memory polymer light-emitting diodes, Adv. Mater. 23 (2011) 664–668.

[205] Z.B. Yu, L. Li, Q.W. Zhang, W.L. Hu, Q.B. Pei, Silver nanowire-polymer composite electrodes for efficient polymer solar cells, Adv. Mater. 23 (2011) 4453.

[206] Z.Y. Fan, J.C. Ho, Z.A. Jacobson, R. Yerushalmi, R.L. Alley, H. Razavi, A. Javey, Wafer-scale assembly of highly ordered semiconductor nanowire arrays by contact printing, Nano Lett. 8 (2008) 20–25.

[207] H.A.K. Toprakci, S.K. Kalanadhabhatla, R.J. Spontak, T.K. Ghosh, Polymer nanocomposites containing carbon nanofibers as soft printable sensors exhibiting strain-reversible piezoresistivity, Adv. Funct. Mater. 23 (2013) 5536–5542.

[208] J.Y. Sun, C. Keplinger, G.M. Whitesides, Z.G. Suo, Ionic skin, Adv. Mater. 26 (2014) 7608–7614.

[209] X.F. Duan, C.M. Niu, V. Sahi, J. Chen, J.W. Parce, S. Empedocles, J.L. Goldman, High-performance thin-film transistors using semiconductor nanowires and nanoribbons, Nature 425 (2003) 274–278.

[210] S. Kirchmeyer, K. Reuter, Scientific importance, properties and growing applications of poly(3,4-ethylenedioxythiophene), J. Mater. Chem. 15 (2005) 2077–2088.

[211] N.S. Liu, G.J. Fang, J.W. Wan, H. Zhou, H. Long, X.Z. Zhao, Electrospun PEDOT:PSS-PVA nanofiber based ultrahigh-strain sensors with controllable electrical conductivity, J. Mater. Chem. 21 (2011) 18962–18966.

[212] M. Amjadi, A. Pichitpajongkit, S. Lee, S. Ryu, I. Park, Highly stretchable and sensitive strain sensor based on silver nanowire-elastomer nanocomposite, ACS Nano 8 (2014) 5154–5163.

[213] G. Latessa, F. Brunetti, A. Reale, G. Saggio, A. Di Carlo, Piezoresistive behaviour of flexible PEDOT:PSS based sensors, Sens. Actuators B Chem. 139 (2009) 304–309.

[214] D.-H. Kim, N. Lu, R. Ghaffari, Y.-S. Kim, S.P. Lee, L. Xu, J. Wu, R.-H. Kim, J. Song, Z. Liu, J. Viventi, B. De Graff, B. Elolampi, M. Mansour, M.J. Slepian, S. Hwang, J.D. Moss, S.-M. Won, Y. Huang, B. Litt, J.A. Rogers, Materials for multifunctional balloon catheters with capabilities in cardiac electrophysiological mapping and ablation therapy, Nat. Mater. 10 (2011) 316.

[215] L. Li, Y. Bai, L. Li, S. Wang, T. Zhang, A superhydrophobic smart coating for flexible and wearable sensing electronics, Adv. Mater. 29 (2017).

[216] J. Heikenfeld, Bioanalytical devices: technological leap for sweat sensing, Nature 529 (2016) 475–476.

[217] W. Jia, A.J. Bandodkar, G. ValdéS-Ramírez, J.R. Windmiller, Z. Yang, J. Ramírez, G. Chan, J. Wang, Electrochemical tattoo biosensors for real-time noninvasive lactate monitoring in human perspiration, Anal. Chem. 85 (2013) 6553–6560.

[218] X.B. Zhang, K.L. Jiang, C. Teng, P. Liu, L. Zhang, J. Kong, T.H. Zhang, Q.Q. Li, S.S. Fan, Spinning and processing continuous yarns from 4-inch wafer scale super-aligned carbon nanotube arrays, Adv. Mater. 18 (2006) 1505.

[219] W.J. Ma, L.Q. Liu, R. Yang, T.H. Zhang, Z. Zhang, L. Song, Y. Ren, J. Shen, Z.Q. Niu, W.Y. Zhou, S.S. Xie, Monitoring a micromechanical process in macroscale carbon nanotube films and fibers, Adv. Mater. 21 (2009) 603.

[220] H.J. Lee, P. Zhang, J.C. Bravman, Tensile failure by grain thinning in micromachined aluminum thin films, J. Appl. Phys. 93 (2003) 1443–1451.

[221] Z. Yan, M. Han, Y. Yang, K. Nan, H. Luan, Y. Luo, Y. Zhang, Y. Huang, J.A. Rogers, Deterministic assembly of 3D mesostructures in advanced materials via compressive buckling: a short review of recent progress, Extreme Mech. Lett. 11 (2017) 96–104.

[222] Y.G. Sun, H.S. Kim, E. Menard, S. Kim, I. Adesida, J.A. Rogers, Printed arrays of aligned GaAs wires for flexible transistors, diodes, and circuits on plastic substrates, Small 2 (2006) 1330–1334.

[223] A. Peláiz-Barranco, P. Marin-Franch, Piezo-, pyro-, ferro-, and dielectric properties of ceramic/polymer composites obtained from two modifications of lead titanate, J. Appl. Phys. 97 (2005) 034104.

[224] L. Nanshu, S. Zhigang, J.J. Vlassak, The effect of film thickness on the failure strain of polymer-supported metal films, Acta Mater. 58 (2010) 1679–1687.

[225] K.K. Kim, S. Hong, H.M. Cho, J. Lee, Y.D. Suh, J. Ham, S.H. Ko, Highly sensitive and stretchable multidimensional strain sensor with prestrained anisotropic metal nanowire percolation networks, Nano Lett. 15 (2015) 5240–5247.

[226] C. Baur, J.R. Dimaio, E. McAllister, R. Hossini, E. Wagener, J. Ballato, S. Priya, A. Ballato, Jr., D. W. S., Enhanced piezoelectric performance from carbon fluoropolymer nanocomposites, J. Appl. Phys. 112 (2012) 124104.

[227] K. Koziol, J. Vilatela, A. Moisala, M. Motta, P. Cunniff, M. Sennett, A. Windle, High-performance carbon nanotube fiber, Science 318 (2007) 1892–1895.

[228] R. Yerushalmi, Z.A. Jacobson, J.C. Ho, Z. Fan, A. Javey, Large scale, highly ordered assembly of nanowire parallel arrays by differential roll printing, Appl. Phys. Lett. 91 (2007) 203104.

[229] J.Y. Sun, X.H. Zhao, W.R.K. Illeperuma, O. Chaudhuri, K.H. Oh, D.J. Mooney, J.J. Vlassak, Z.G. Suo, Highly stretchable and tough hydrogels, Nature 489 (2012) 133–136.

[230] B.E. Alaca, M.T.A. Saif, H. Sehitoglu, On the interface debond at the edge of a thin film on a thick substrate, Acta Mater. 50 (2002) 1197–1209.

[231] T. Glennon, C. O'quigley, M. Mccaul, G. Matzeu, S. Beirne, G.G. Wallace, F. Stroiescu, N. O'mahoney, P. White, D. Diamond, 'Sweatch': a wearable platform for harvesting and analysing sweat sodium content, Electroanalysis 28 (2016) 1283–1289.

[232] K. Takei, T. Takahashi, J.C. Ho, H. Ko, A.G. Gillies, P.W. Leu, R.S. Fearing, A. Javey, Nanowire active-matrix circuitry for low-voltage macroscale artificial skin, Nat. Mater. 9 (2010) 821–826.

[233] X. Liao, Q. Liao, Z. Zhang, X. Yan, Q. Liang, Q. Wang, M. Li, Y. Zhang, A highly stretchable ZnO@fiber-based multifunctional nanosensor for strain/temperature/UV detection, Adv. Funct. Mater. 26 (2016) 3074–3081.

[234] J. Song, Mechanics of stretchable electronics, Curr. Opin. Solid State Mater. Sci. 19 (2015) 160–170.

Further reading

[235] K.L. Jiang, Q.Q. Li, S.S. Fan, Nanotechnology: spinning continuous carbon nanotube yarns—carbon nanotubes weave their way into a range of imaginative macroscopic applications, Nature 419 (2002) 801.

[236] G.Y. Jung, E. Johnston-Halperin, W. Wu, Z.N. Yu, S.Y. Wang, W.M. Tong, Z.Y. Li, J.E. Green, B.A. Sheriff, A. Boukai, Y. Bunimovich, J.R. Heath, R.S. Williams, Circuit fabrication at 17 nm half-pitch by nanoimprint lithography, Nano Lett. 6 (2006) 351–354.

[237] D. Whang, S. Jin, Y. Wu, C.M. Lieber, Large-scale hierarchical organization of nanowire arrays for integrated nanosystems, Nano Lett. 3 (2003) 1255–1259.

[238] Y.G. Sun, J.A. Rogers, Fabricating semiconductor nano/microwires and transfer printing ordered arrays of them onto plastic substrates, Nano Lett. 4 (2004) 1953–1959.

[239] Y.G. Sun, S. Kim, I. Adesida, J.A. Rogers, Bendable GaAs metal-semiconductor field-effect transistors formed with printed GaAs wire arrays on plastic substrates, Appl. Phys. Lett. 87 (2005) 083501.

[240] A.B. Joshi, A.E. Kalange, D. Bodas, S.A. Gangal, Simulations of piezoelectric pressure sensor for radial artery pulse measurement, Mater. Sci. Eng. 168 (2010) 250–253.

[241] N.T. Tien, T.Q. Hung, Y.G. Seoul, D.I. Kim, N.E. Lee, Physically responsive field-effect transistors with giant electromechanical coupling induced by nanocomposite gate dielectrics, ACS Nano 5 (2011) 7069–7076.

[242] L.J. Pan, A. Chortos, G.H. Yu, Y.Q. Wang, S. Isaacson, R. Allen, Y. Shi, R. Dauskardt, Z.N. Bao, An ultra-sensitive resistive pressure sensor based on hollow-sphere microstructure induced elasticity in conducting polymer film, Nat. Commun. 5 (2014).

[243] C. Pang, J.H. Koo, A. Nguyen, J.M. Caves, M.G. Kim, A. Chortos, K. Kim, P.J. Wang, J.B.H. Tok, Z.A. Bao, Highly skin-conformal microhairy sensor for pulse signal amplification, Adv. Mater. 27 (2015) 634–640.

[244] G. Schwartz, B.C.K. Tee, J.G. Mei, A.L. Appleton, D.H. Kim, H.L. Wang, Z.N. Bao, Flexible polymer transistors with high pressure sensitivity for application in electronic skin and health monitoring, Nat. Commun. 4 (2013).

[245] J.T. Muth, D.M. Vogt, R.L. Truby, Y. Menguc, D.B. Kolesky, R.J. Wood, J.A. Lewis, Embedded 3D printing of strain sensors within highly stretchable elastomers, Adv. Mater. 26 (2014) 6307–6312.

[246] Y. Li, S.D. Luo, M.C. Yang, R. Liang, C.C. Zeng, Poisson ratio and piezoresistive sensing: a new route to high-performance 3D flexible and stretchable sensors of multimodal sensing capability, Adv. Funct. Mater. 26 (2016) 2900–2908.

[247] J. Park, Y. Lee, J. Hong, M. Ha, Y.D. Jung, H. Lim, S.Y. Kim, H. Ko, Giant tunneling piezoresistance of composite elastomers with interlocked microdome arrays for ultrasensitive and multimodal electronic skins, ACS Nano 8 (2014) 4689–4697.

[248] M.K. Shin, J. Oh, M. Lima, M.E. Kozlov, S.J. Kim, R.H. Baughman, Elastomeric conductive composites based on carbon nanotube forests, Adv. Mater. 22 (2010) 2663.

[249] C.A.O. Henning, F.W. Boswell, J.M. Corbett, Mechanical-properties of vacuum-deposited metal-films. 1. Copper-films, Acta Metall. 23 (1975) 177–185.

[250] C.A. Neugebauer, Tensile properties of thin, evaporated gold films, J. Appl. Phys. 31 (1960) 1096–1101.

[251] Y. Xiang, T. Li, Z.G. Suo, J.J. Vlassak, High ductility of a metal film adherent on a polymer substrate, Appl. Phys. Lett. (2005) 87.

[252] A.R. Rathmell, S.M. Bergin, Y.L. Hua, Z.Y. Li, B.J. Wiley, The growth mechanism of copper nanowires and their properties in flexible, transparent conducting films, Adv. Mater. 22 (2010) 3558.

[253] Y. Sun, J.A. Rogers, Inorganic semiconductors for flexible electronics, Adv. Mater. 19 (2007) 1897–1916.

[254] S. Xu, Y. Zhang, J. Cho, J. Lee, X. Huang, L. Jia, J.A. Fan, Y. Su, J. Su, H. Zhang, H. Cheng, B. Lu, C. Yu, C. Chuang, T.-I. Kim, T. Song, K. Shigeta, S. Kang, C. Dagdeviren, I. Petrov, P.V. Braun, Y. Huang, U. Paik, J.A. Rogers, Stretchable batteries with self-similar serpentine interconnects and integrated wireless recharging systems, Nat. Commun. 4 (2013) 1543.

[255] W.M. Choi, J. Song, D.-Y. Khang, H. Jiang, Y.Y. Huang, J.A. Rogers, Biaxially stretchable "wavy" silicon nanomembranes, Nano Lett. 7 (2007) 1655–1663.

[256] S.-H. Bae, Y. Lee, B.K. Sharma, H.-J. Lee, J.-H. Kim, J.-H. Ahn, Graphene-based transparent strain sensor, Carbon 51 (2013) 236–242.

[257] B.C.K. Tee, A. Chortos, R.R. Dunn, G. Schwartz, E. Eason, Z.A. Bao, Tunable flexible pressure sensors using microstructured elastomer geometries for intuitive electronics, Adv. Funct. Mater. 24 (2014) 5427–5434.

[258] D. Kang, P.V. Pikhitsa, Y.W. Choi, C. Lee, S.S. Shin, L. Piao, B. Park, K.-Y. Suh, T.-I. Kim, M. Choi, Ultrasensitive mechanical crack-based sensor inspired by the spider sensory system, Nature 516 (2014) 222.

[259] Q. Li, L.N. Zhang, X.M. Tao, X. Ding, Review of flexible temperature sensing networks for wearable physiological monitoring, Adv. Healthc. Mater. 6 (2017).

[260] M.D. Dankoco, G.Y. Tesfay, E. Benevent, M. Bendahan, Temperature sensor realized by inkjet printing process on flexible substrate, Mater. Sci. Eng. B 205 (2016) 1–5.

[261] C.-Y. Lee, A. Su, Y.-C. Liu, W.-Y. Fan, W.-J. Hsieh, In situ measurement of the junction temperature of light emitting diodes using a flexible micro temperature sensor, Sensors 9 (2009) 5068–5075.

[262] D.J. Lichtenwalner, A.E. Hydrick, A.I. Kingon, Flexible thin film temperature and strain sensor array utilizing a novel sensing concept, Sensors Actuators A Phys. 135 (2007) 593–597.

[263] S.Y. Hong, Y.H. Lee, H. Park, S.W. Jin, Y.R. Jeong, J. Yun, I. You, G. Zi, J.S. Ha, Stretchable active matrix temperature sensor array of polyaniline nanofibers for electronic skin, Adv. Mater. 28 (2016) 930–935.

[264] T.Q. Trung, S. Ramasundaram, S.W. Hong, N.-E. Lee, Flexible and transparent nanocomposite of reduced graphene oxide and P(VDF-TrFE) copolymer for high thermal responsivity in a field-effect transistor, Adv. Funct. Mater. 24 (2014) 3438–3445.

[265] D.-H. Kim, S. Wang, H. Keum, R. Ghaffari, Y.-S. Kim, H. Tao, B. Panilaitis, M. Li, Z. Kang, F. Omenetto, Y. Huang, J.A. Rogers, Thin, flexible sensors and actuators as 'instrumented' surgical sutures for targeted wound monitoring and therapy, Small 8 (2012) 3263–3268.

[266] A.J. Bandodkar, J. Wang, Non-invasive wearable electrochemical sensors: a review, Trends Biotechnol. 32 (2014) 363–371.

[267] M. Senior, Novartis signs up for Google smart lens, Nat. Biotechnol. 32 (2014) 856.

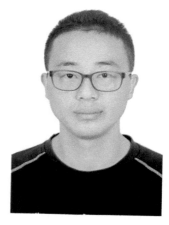

Shuqi Wang is currently a postdoctoral researcher in Suzhou Institute of Nano-Tech and Nano-Bionics at Chinese Academy of Sciences, People's Republic of China. He received his BSc in biotechnology (2010) and PhD in chemistry (2016) from the University of Science and Technology Beijing, China. His research interests focus on the synthesis of nanomaterials for electrochemical biosensors, and their application in wearable health monitoring.

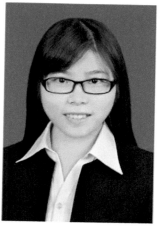

Yuanyuan Bai is currently a postdoctoral researcher in Suzhou Institute of Nano-Tech and Nano-Bionics at Chinese Academy of Sciences, People's Republic of China. She received her BSc and PhD in electronic science and technology from Xi'an Jiaotong University, China in 2010 and 2016, respectively. Her research interests focus on multifunctional smart sensing materials and devices, and their applications in wearable electronics.

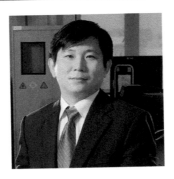

Ting Zhang is a professor in Suzhou Institute of Nano-Tech and Nano-Bionics at Chinese Academy of Sciences, People's Republic of China. He received his PhD from the University of California, Riverside in 2007. His research expertise is in the area of micro/nanosensors, nanomaterials, flexible electronics, and micro-manufacturing technology, especially in developing advanced nanomaterials for flexible electronics, and cost-effective, high-throughput, and manufacturable techniques for electronic nanosensors.

CHAPTER 2

Wearable chemical sensors

Bo Wang, Andrew Wilhelm, Aaron Wilhelm, Sanaz Pilehvar, Sina Moshfeghi, Phoenix Stout, Kamyar Salahi, Sam Emaminejad
Interconnected and Integrated Bioelectronics Lab, Department of Electrical and Computer Engineering, University of California, Los Angeles, CA, United States

Chapter Outline

Addressing our grand societal health-care challenges, in regard to both human suffering and the ever-growing cost of health care, necessitates a paradigm shift from generic and reactive medicine to personalized, proactive, and preventive medicine. Accordingly, wearable biomonitoring technologies play a critical role in promoting awareness and adoption of healthy lifestyles for disease prevention and enabling actionable feedback. Currently, commercialized wearable sensors and Internet of things (IoT) devices are only capable of tracking physical activities and vital signs, and fail to noninvasively access molecular-level biomarker information to provide insight into the body's dynamic chemistry.

In the present state, blood-based sensing techniques that provide direct measurements of circulating biomarkers cannot be scaled across the general population for individual-level daily monitoring (due to their invasive nature and risk of infection). Alternatively, other

Wearable Bioelectronics. https://doi.org/10.1016/B978-0-08-102407-2.00003-5

biofluids, which share biomarker partitioning pathways with blood (e.g., sweat and skin interstitial fluid, ISF), can be probed and accessed noninvasively [1–9]. Inherently, these noninvasive measurements are noisy due to the presence of confounders. Fortunately, with a combination of clever chemical sensor and device design as well as data analytics methods (leveraging the relatively high sampling rate), the interfering effect of the confounders can be mitigated to provide physiologically meaningful estimates of blood biomarker levels. Specifically, at the sensor level the following criteria must be considered to render undistorted biomarker readings [10–14]:

(1) Detection limit and sensitivity which are particularly challenging when targeting low concentration (~nanomolar range), yet clinically informative molecules such as hormones and neuroimmune protein markers. To address such challenges, signal amplification and background noise suppression strategies are needed at sensor design and signal processing stages.

(2) High selectivity toward the biomarker of interest in the presence of highly interfering species and in complex biofluid matrices. This fundamental requirement can be addressed by incorporating selective recognition elements to minimize false-positive readouts.

(3) Operational stability to facilitate reliable (semi)continuous/long-term monitoring. The recognition elements (e.g., enzymes) or other sensing components (e.g., mediators) are prone to biofouling as well as denaturation and degradation over time in ambient conditions, resulting in unintended signal shifts.

(4) Wearability requires biocompatible sensor interfaces to be miniaturized or alternatively to be patterned on a flexible substrate to allow for efficient and robust sampling and analysis of low volumes of biofluids (ISF and sweat).

To this end, chemical sensing interfaces are excellent candidates for performing wearable biomarker analysis due to their potential capabilities of addressing the aforementioned criteria and providing direct sample-to-answer readouts of target analytes. For this reason, electrochemical sensors present great potential for integration with existing commercialized wearable electronics (e.g., smart watches), as they inherently transduce concentrations into electrical signals that can be acquired and processed using conventional analog and digital integrated circuits. As a result, the envisioned (semi)continuous biofluid analysis can be performed seamlessly and without any user intervention [15, 16].

2.1 Target biomarker categories

Various biomarkers with impactful clinical relevance can be measured with chemical sensing interfaces. As shown in Table 2.1, examples of such biomarkers include electrolytes, metabolites, small molecules, and proteins and peptides [10, 11, 17].

Table 2.1: Example biomarker categories and their concentration ranges (e.g., in sweat).

Biomarker	Examples	Concentration range
Electrolytes	Na^+, K^+, Mg^{2+}, Cl^-, Ca^{2+}	1–100 mM
Metabolites	Glucose, Lactate, Urea, Alcohol	0.05–30 mM
Small molecules	Cortisol, Testosterone, Progesterone	0.1–700 nM
Proteins and peptide	Albumin, Cytokines, Neuropeptide Y	0.1–100 pM

2.1.1 Electrolytes

The informative electrolytes found in sweat and ISF include sodium, potassium, magnesium, calcium, and chloride [5–7]. Among them, chloride information in sweat has an established clinical utility with an FDA-approved collection procedure. Particularly, chloride levels in sweat are used as the basis for the diagnosis of cystic fibrosis (CF). CF is a genetic condition that disrupts the normal regulation of salt and fluids transportation in the body, resulting in elevated sweat chloride levels in CF patients [18–23]. Beyond this clinical application, and in the context of athletic performance monitoring, sweat electrolyte analysis (e.g., sodium and potassium) allows for tracking the electrolyte loss, which provides insight into the water homeostasis state of individuals (hydration and hyponatremia vs. hypernatremia) [24–27]. Additionally, the measurement of electrolytes, particularly calcium, can potentially be useful for monitoring the body's mineral homeostasis. Abnormal changes in calcium levels can negatively impact the normal function of the human body's organs and systems, resulting in disorders such as myeloma, acid-base balance disorder, cirrhosis, and renal failure [28–30].

2.1.2 Metabolites

Metabolites, such as glucose and lactate, have been heavily investigated in various physiological studies and monitoring their concentrations facilitates the detection of abnormalities and the promotion of self-awareness/behavioral modification [31, 32]. Specifically, the monitoring of glucose is important as currently more than 415 million adults are diabetic (with an economic burden of US $1.3 trillion annually) [33]. Currently, self-testing using standard finger-stick and invasive continuous glucose monitoring systems (with a glucose sensor inserted under the skin to analyze the tissue fluid) are the most prevalent methods of screening blood glucose level [8, 32]. However, both methods are invasive and inconvenient. Accordingly, providing noninvasive monitoring solutions allows for frequent and continuous monitoring of glucose levels, thus providing actionable feedback toward preventing the development of diabetes in prediabetic individuals. Glucose concentrations in sweat and ISF have been shown to correlate with blood glucose levels when properly retrieved [9]. Similarly, the correlation between lactate in ISF and blood has been explored, but the conclusion remains unclear most likely due to complex lactate generation sources and mechanisms. [34–38] Sweat lactate information could be uniquely useful for a variety of physiological applications, because it is a product of sweat gland energy metabolism. In the context of sweat-based analysis, the lactate molecules are primarily originated from the sweat gland metabolism (unlike the case for glucose, where the molecules are mostly originated from blood) [9, 35]. In this regard, sweat lactate levels can be used as a proxy measure of sweat gland activity and the body's thermoregulation state.

2.1.3 Hormones

Hormones play a critical role in mediating important mechanisms within the endocrine system and the body as a whole. The endocrine system regulates critical physiological processes, including metabolism, growth and development, tissue function, sexual function, reproduction, sleep, and mood. An example of a clinically informative hormone is cortisol, which plays a crucial role in maintaining the homeostasis of the hypothalamic-pituitary-adrenal (HPA) axis. This makes cortisol a promising biomarker for evaluating the HPA axis noninvasively as it is considered a stress marker [39–45]. Salivary cortisol has been extensively studied by the Trier Social Stress Test (TSST), which is the standardized protocol for studies of stress hormone reactivity. This important biomarker of the HPA axis is also present in ISF and sweat, with comparable concentration levels in saliva and plasma.

2.1.4 Proteins and peptides

Neuroimmune biomarkers, such as cytokines and neuropeptides, are an important class of protein and peptide biomarker molecules with impactful clinical applications. Previous studies have shown the presence of proinflammatory cytokines (IL-1α, IL1-β, IL-6, TNF-α, and IL-8) and neuropeptides [e.g., neuropeptide Y (NPY), substance P, and calcitonin-gene-related peptide] in sweat [46–50]. In addition, it has been demonstrated that these biomarkers have a high degree of correlation with respect to the corresponding levels in plasma [51]. Neuropeptides (e.g., NPY) also play an important role in the nervous system and regulate satiety, emotional state, vascular tone, and gastrointestinal secretion. NPY is a polypeptide macromolecule with antistress and antidepressive properties found in dermal nerve fibers, sweat glands, and hair follicles [50, 52]. In a sweat patch-based study, proinflammatory cytokines and NPY are shown to be significantly elevated in major depressive disorder (MDD) patients as compared to the control group, in which case the depressive symptomatology strongly correlated with biomarker levels [51, 52].

2.2 Suitable chemical sensing interfaces

Electrochemical sensing methods can be generally organized into three main categories on the basis of the nature of their transduced electrical signals (e.g., current, potential, and impedance) [53].

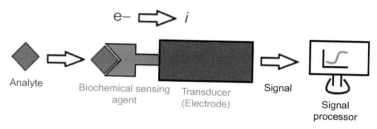

Fig. 2.1
Electrochemical transducer interface and operation for biosensing.

To construct a wearable electrochemical sensing interface with high sensitivity and specificity toward the target biomarkers, selective membranes, or biological recognition elements are utilized. As shown in Fig. 2.1, these elements recognize the biomarker of interest with high degree of specificity, and are often immobilized on a solid-state transducer interface, which converts biochemical reactions/interactions (originating from the presence of target biomarkers) into a measurable signal.

The design of the electrochemical sensing interface for the most part depends on the availability of suitable sensing layers and transduction methods that can reliably measure the biomarker of interest within its physiologically relevant concentration range in the target biofluid. For example, to quantify clinically relevant electrolytes (e.g., Na^+ and K^+, present in millimolar range), ion-selective electrodes (ISEs) are used as a sensing interface, where the transduced output voltage is measured using potentiometric methods. Additionally, to quantify metabolites such as glucose and lactate (present in micro- to millimolar range), enzymatic interfaces are used to measure the output of electrical current through amperometric approaches [53]. Furthermore, affinity-based sensing interfaces, which use antibody or aptamer molecules as their probe molecules, are suitable for chemical analysis of hormones and proteins that are typically in sub micromolar range. The following section expands on the wearable sensing approaches that use ion-selective, enzymatic, affinity-based, and emerging synthetic sensing layers.

2.2.1 Ion-selective electrodes

The use of ISEs, in a wearable format, has been demonstrated for the measurement of electrolytes, such as sodium (Na^+) and potassium (K^+) [5, 9]. In order to achieve selectivity, the electrode surface is modified with a membrane that allows only one type of ionic species (i.e., charged target) to pass through and accumulate near the surface of the working electrode. For example, Na ionophore X, valinomycin, and calcium ionophore (all coupled with a polyvinyl chloride membrane) are used as part of the sensing layer to allow for the passage and accumulation of Na^+, K^+, or Ca^{2+}, respectively [5, 9]. The accumulation of the ionic species results in an electrical potential difference across the membrane, which can be effectively probed by measuring the potential difference

Table 2.2: Wearable ion-selective chemical sensor.

Analyte	Recognition element	Analytical technique	Substrate	Refs.
H^+ (pH)	Polyaniline (PANI)	Potentiometry	PET	[27]
Ammonium	Nonactin ionophore-based ISE	Potentiometry	Tattoo paper	[54]
Sodium	Sodium ionophore-based ISE	Potentiometry	PET/Tattoo paper	[25, 55]
Potassium	Potassium ISE	Potentiometry	PET	[25]
Calcium	Calcium ISE	Potentiometry	PET	[27]
Chloride	Ag/AgCl electrode	Potentiometry	PET/PDMS	[17, 56]

between the working and reference electrodes. In this interface, the ISE's output voltage is logarithmically correlated to the concentration of the target ions in the solution; this follows from the Nernst equation, which describes the charge distribution near the electrode's surface.

Table 2.2 provides examples of ISEs that have been demonstrated in a wearable format [5, 9, 10]. The clinical and physiological utility of the ISE-based sensors have been validated through testing human subjects. For example, Emaminejad et al. [17] introduced, for the first time, a wearable sweat-based disease monitoring wristband which utilized ISE-based Na^+ and Cl^- sensors (patterned on polyethylene terephthalate, PET). In particular, they demonstrated with their platform that CF patients exhibited elevated levels of Na^+ and Cl^- ions compared to healthy individuals. Additionally, in a separate work [25], they used their ISE-based sensors to measure the electrolyte profiles of subjects engaged in prolonged outdoor physical exercise. Based on the measured profiles, the subjects who were not continuously hydrating presented a Na^+ profile distinct from that of those who were hydrating, demonstrating the potential use case of sweat electrolyte monitoring for athletic applications.

2.2.2 Enzymatic sensors

Efforts in developing enzymatic sensors have been primarily focused on glucose monitoring for personal diabetes management, which in turn has led to the successful commercialization of fingerstick-based and continuous glucose monitoring products.

The enzymatic interface incorporates enzymes (e.g., oxidase) as catalyst agents to selectively lower the energy barrier of the conversion of the specific target (or substrate) to an intermediary product, thus accelerating the chain of reactions needed to produce a measurable signal (Fig. 2.2). In this way, enzymes effectively act as a biorecognition element. Typically, enzymatic sensors exploit hydrogen peroxide (H_2O_2) as an intermediary product, the

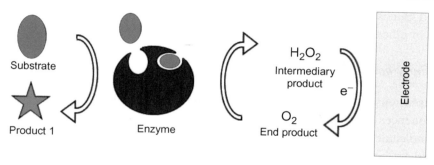

Fig. 2.2
Schematic diagram of the operation of an enzymatic biosensor.

electro-oxidization/reduction of which (as the last reaction step) generates/consumes electrons. The resultant change in the number of electrons is proportional to the concentration of the target in the solution and can be measured using amperometric techniques. Amperometry is based on maintaining a constant voltage across a working and reference electrode pair and monitoring the change in current.

It is noteworthy that the development of intermediary product (e.g., H_2O_2) conversion/sensing interfaces is critical to achieve a robust enzymatic sensor. The optimal working potential for H_2O_2 detection is usually around 0.7 V. However, this relatively high potential also results in the electro-oxidization of a large number of electroactive species (e.g., ascorbic acid and uric acid) which would mask the desired signal. To solve this problem, mediator agents such as Prussian Blue (PB) are incorporated in the sensing layer to reduce the working potential for H_2O_2 detection [25].

Table 2.3 provides examples of enzymatic sensors that have been demonstrated in a wearable format.

The clinical and physiological utility of enzymatic sensors has been validated through testing on human subjects. For example, Emaminejad et al. [17] utilized an enzymatic glucose sensor to demonstrate the elevation of sweat glucose upon the consumption of 30 g of glucose in subjects who had been fasting for 12 h prior to the glucose intake. Similarly, a wearable

Table 2.3: Enzyme-based wearable chemical sensors.

Analyte	Recognition element	Analytical technique	Substrate	Refs.
Glucose	Glucose Oxidase	Amperometry	PET	[25, 57, 58]
Lactate	Lactate Oxidase	Amperometry	PET	[25, 59, 60]
Uric acid	Uricase	Amperometry	PET	[61]
Alcohol	Alcohol Oxidase	Amperometry	Tattoo paper	[62]

sweat-based glucose monitoring device was developed by Kim et al. [63] to study the correlation of glucose in sweat and blood in the context of physical exercise.

2.2.3 Affinity-based chemical sensors

Affinity-based sensors that incorporate conventional antibody molecules and emerging aptamer sequences as biorecognition elements are suitable for targeting a variety of proteins and small molecules (e.g., hormones). Currently, immunoassays that utilize surface-immobilized antibody probe molecules are commonly used to measure a wide range of target molecules in various biofluids. The underlying sensing mechanisms of the established immunoassays can be adapted to perform wearable chemical analysis (e.g., by rendering label-free sensing). In this regard, Prasad et al. developed a ZnO-thin-film-functionalized sensing interface to target IL-6 [64]. In this work, room temperature ionic liquids were incorporated in the sensing layer to facilitate prolonged stable sensing. In a separate work, they also demonstrated an electrochemical immunosensor to target cortisol in sweat. For this purpose, cortisol antibodies were coupled to MoS_2 nanosheets patterned on a flexible substrate to produce a non-faradaic interface [65].

Recently, the potential use of aptamer sequences as probe molecules for wearable chemical analysis has been shown by Lin et al. [66]. In particular, they functionalized the graphene-based channel of a field-effect transistor with aptamers that are specific toward tumor necrosis factor-α (TNF-α, an inflammatory cytokine molecule). In this implementation, the aptamer experiences conformation change upon binding to TNF-α. As a result of this structural change, the negatively charged TNF-α and oligonucleotide complex are brought to the close proximity of the graphene surface, resulting in the modulation of the drain-source current. This sensing interface was patterned on a flexible SiO_2-coated polyethylene naphthalate polymer substrate.

2.2.4 Synthetic receptor-based chemical sensors

The reliance on probe molecules in enzymatic and affinity-based sensors limits the diversity of the measurable targets in sweat due to the unviability of biological probe molecules. Therefore, synthetic receptor-based probes can be considered as an alternative. In this regard, the properties of the synthetic receptors can be tuned to resolve the practical challenges of wearable chemical analysis in terms of the reproducibility and stability of the sensors during the operation.

Molecularly imprinted polymers (MIPs) have emerged as suitable synthetic receptor candidates. Fabrication of MIP-based sensing interfaces commonly includes polymerization of monomers in the presence of a template (target analyte), followed by template elution, resulting in cavity-like features in the polymer layer. The formed cavities serve as artificial receptors for the target analyte (Fig. 2.3). Compared to biomolecule probe candidates, MIPs are speculated to present a high level of stability in varying pH and temperature conditions

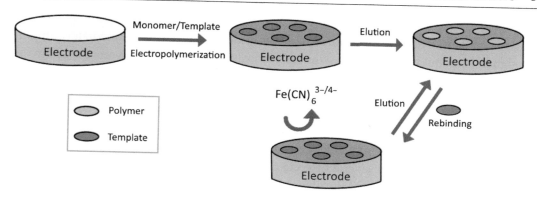

Fig. 2.3
Schematic diagram of molecularly imprinted polymers.

[67–69]. Recently, Parlak et al. reported an MIP-based sensing interface on a flexible elastomer substrate [70]. In their approach, functional monomer and cross-linkers were copolymerized in the presence of template cortisol molecules. The intended cortisol binding sites were exposed after a mechanical-grinding step and elution of the template from the MIPs matrix with a wash solution. The intended sensing operation of the MIP-based sensor was demonstrated by conducting cortisol measurements in sweat samples.

2.3 Electrochemical sensor integration

For reliable wearable chemical sensing, microfluidic interfaces and electronic integration strategies are required for biofluid delivery and seamless signal processing/transmission, respectively [4].

2.3.1 Microfluidic interfaces

Several research groups have developed a variety of interfaces for the in situ collection and delivery of sweat to the sensor surface. The reported interfaces are based on absorbent pads, textile patches, and polydimethylsiloxane (PDMS)-based microfluidic housings [71–73]. The substrates used in these devices are flexible to maintain close contact with the skin for robust sensing and to ensure the users' comfort in wearing such devices for an extended period of time. For example, a wearable, microfluidic-based device has been developed by Rogers et al. that collects and transports sweat within the device for analysis [73]. The device was successfully tested during extended physical activity (bicycle racing).

2.3.2 Electronic integration

Wearable sensing is prone to external interference, originating from various sources such as artifacts from user motion and electromagnetic interference, which would distort the biomarker readings. To address this issue, analog and digital signal conditioning and processing circuits need to be coupled with a transducer interface to immediately amplify the signal, filter out the noise, and wirelessly transmit the digitally converted readings. In theory, the readout circuitry can be miniaturized to mm-scale and integrated into a single IC chip; however, IC manufacturing is time and cost intensive, making IC design unsuitable for rapid and inexpensive prototyping to test design specifications. In contrast, commercially available chips can be interconnected in a modular fashion to meet high-level specifications. A drawback to the use of commercial chips is that a device requiring diverse electronic functionalities may require several discrete chips and peripherals to be incorporated into the design, enlarging the size of the electronic system (beyond cm-scale). Thus, for a wearable device to be practical, it may be necessary to develop electronic systems on flexible substrates. To this end, a wearable microfluidic system utilizing a thin elastomeric enclosure consisting of electronic components connected via free-floating connectors was developed by Xu et al. [74]. The electronic components selectively attach to the elastomeric substrate and the microfluidic channels are implemented in a way to minimize mechanical strain. These techniques allow the overall device to have similar characteristics (e.g., elasticity, moduli, and thickness) as human skin, allowing for a better fit and a higher level of integration.

Similarly, Emaminejad et al. [17, 25, 75] used a flexible printed circuit board (FPCB) to develop a mechanically flexible electronic system. Consisting of more than 10 IC chips that allow for sensing across 5 different measurement channels, the device was able to conduct a multiplexed measurement of sweat biomarkers. This scalable integration strategy allowed for the incorporation of additional complex operations such as iontophoresis (in the follow-up work), rendering a fully integrated wearable system capable of performing autonomous sweat extraction and sensing [17].

2.4 Practical design considerations for wearable biomarker analysis

One of the major challenges of wearable biomarker analysis is the variations in ambient and environmental parameters, which affect the sensor response. Such parameters include skin temperature and biofluid ionic strength/pH. For example, in the case of enzyme-based sensing, the increased skin temperature leads to enhanced enzyme activity, resulting in a larger electrical current output for a given concentration of target analyte. Therefore, by not compensating for the increased temperature, the sweat glucose content may be exaggerated. To mitigate such interfering effects, in situ calibration strategies may be helpful. To this end, Emaminejad et al. demonstrated an in situ calibration strategy where the measured skin temperature was used to correct the glucose and lactate enzymatic sensor readouts [25, 75]. In their approach, the skin temperature information was obtained with the aid of a resistive-based temperature sensor, which was patterned onto the same substrate as the enzymatic sensors.

Furthermore, an important consideration for devising sensor development strategy is the simultaneous measurement of a panel of biomarkers in order to provide a comprehensive view of an individual's health and to unravel interdependent and complex physiological functions. Specifically, in the context of sweat-based analysis, multiplexed sensing allows for decoupling the effect of multivariate mechanisms that contribute to the sweat secretion process. This in turn necessitates the creation of multiplexed sensing interfaces, which can be packed in compact array formats to meet the spatial constraints imposed by the envisioned wearable applications. To this end, Emaminejad et al. reported a fully integrated sensor array for in situ multiplexed sweat analysis of a group of metabolites and electrolytes [17, 25, 75]. In their approach, the independent and selective operation of individual sensors is preserved during multiplexed measurements by electrically decoupling the operating points of each sensor's interface. Such multiplexed sensors are extremely helpful in performing large-scale studies efficiently, because they allow the clinicians to simultaneously investigate the clinical utility of a group of biomarkers.

Additionally, providing adequate biofluid sample volume is a prerequisite to reliable chemical analysis. For example, in the context of sweat-based analysis, currently, the majority of the demonstrated wearable sensing platforms rely on exercise-based sweat generation to access biomarkers. However, this intense and continuous physical activity is not suitable for general population health monitoring. To this end, Emaminejad et al. demonstrated a chemically enhanced and miniaturized iontophoresis interface for autonomous in situ sweat extraction and analysis [17]. Iontophoresis involves the use of minimal levels of electrical current to deliver stimulating agonists (packed in a hydrogel, placed in between the iontophoresis electrode and skin) to sweat glands. This method was also applied in the context of sweat alcohol sensing by Kim et al. [62].

References

[1] A.J. Bandodkar, I. Jeerapan, J. Wang, Wearable chemical sensors: present challenges and future prospects, ACS Sens. 1 (2016) 464–482, https://doi.org/10.1021/acssensors.6b00250.
[2] A. Tricoli, G. Neri, Miniaturized bio-and chemical-sensors for point-of-care monitoring of chronic kidney diseases, Sensors 18 (2018) 942, https://doi.org/10.3390/s18040942.
[3] S. Ajami, F. Teimouri, Features and application of wearable biosensors in medical care, J. Res. Med. Sci. 20 (2015) 1208, https://doi.org/10.4103/1735-1995.172991.
[4] W. Gao, G.A. Brooks, D.C. Klonoff, Wearable physiological systems and technologies for metabolic monitoring. J. Appl. Physiol. 124 (2018) 548–556, https://doi.org/10.1152/japplphysiol.00407.2017.
[5] S. Emaminejad, S. Pilehvar, A.J. Wilhelm, A.J. Wilhelm, K. King, Emerging wearable technologies for personalized health and performance monitoring. in: Micro- and Nanotechnology Sensors, Systems, and Applications X, 2018, https://doi.org/10.1117/12.2305693.
[6] Y. Yang, W. Gao, Wearable and flexible electronics for continuous molecular monitoring. Chem. Soc. Rev. (2018) https://doi.org/10.1039/c7cs00730b.
[7] J. Heikenfeld, Non-invasive analyte access and sensing through eccrine sweat: challenges and outlook circa 2016. Electroanalysis 28 (2016) 1242–1249, https://doi.org/10.1002/elan.201600018.
[8] A. Facchinetti, Continuous glucose monitoring sensors: past, present and future algorithmic challenges. Sensors 16 (2016) 2093, https://doi.org/10.3390/s16122093.

[9] Z. Sonner, E. Wilder, J. Heikenfeld, G. Kasting, F. Beyette, D. Swaile, et al., The microfluidics of the eccrine sweat gland, including biomarker partitioning, transport, and biosensing implications. Biomicrofluidics 9 (2015) 031301, https://doi.org/10.1063/1.4921039.

[10] A.J. Bandodkar, J. Wang, Non-invasive wearable electrochemical sensors: a review. Trends Biotechnol. 32 (2014) 363–371, https://doi.org/10.1016/j.tibtech.2014.04.005.

[11] M. Bariya, H.Y.Y. Nyein, A. Javey, Wearable sweat sensors. Nat. Electron. 1 (2018) 160–171, https://doi.org/10.1038/s41928-018-0043-y.

[12] T. Xiao, F. Wu, J. Hao, M. Zhang, P. Yu, L. Mao, In vivo analysis with electrochemical sensors and biosensors. Anal. Chem. 89 (2016) 300–313, https://doi.org/10.1021/acs.analchem.6b04308.

[13] Y. Liu, H. Wang, W. Zhao, M. Zhang, H. Qin, Y. Xie, Flexible, stretchable sensors for wearable health monitoring: sensing mechanisms, materials, fabrication strategies and features. Sensors 18 (2018) 645, https://doi.org/10.3390/s18020645.

[14] B.W. An, J.H. Shin, S.-Y. Kim, J. Kim, S. Ji, J. Park, et al., Smart sensor systems for wearable electronic devices. Polymers 9 (2017) 303, https://doi.org/10.3390/polym9080303.

[15] J. Heikenfeld, A. Jajack, J. Rogers, P. Gutruf, L. Tian, T. Pan, et al., Wearable sensors: modalities, challenges, and prospects. Lab Chip 18 (2018) 217–248, https://doi.org/10.1039/c7lc00914c.

[16] G. Matzeu, L. Florea, D. Diamond, Advances in wearable chemical sensor design for monitoring biological fluids. Sensors Actuators B Chem. 211 (2015) 403–418, https://doi.org/10.1016/j.snb.2015.01.077.

[17] É. Csősz, G. Emri, G. Kalló, G. Tsaprailis, J. Tőzsér, Highly abundant defense proteins in human sweat as revealed by targeted proteomics and label-free quantification mass spectrometry. J. Eur. Acad. Dermatol. Venereol. 29 (2015) 2024–2031, https://doi.org/10.1111/jdv.13221.

[18] S. Emaminejad, W. Gao, E. Wu, Z.A. Davies, H.Y.Y. Nyein, S. Challa, et al., Autonomous sweat extraction and analysis applied to cystic fibrosis and glucose monitoring using a fully integrated wearable platform. Proc. Natl. Acad. Sci. 114 (2017) 4625–4630, https://doi.org/10.1073/pnas.1701740114.

[19] A.N. Macedo, S. Mathiaparanam, L. Brick, K. Keenan, T. Gonska, L. Pedder, et al., The sweat metabolome of screen-positive cystic fibrosis infants: revealing mechanisms beyond impaired chloride transport. ACS Central Sci. 3 (2017) 904–913, https://doi.org/10.1021/acscentsci.7b00299.

[20] M.M. Reddy, M.J. Stutts, Status of fluid and electrolyte absorption in cystic fibrosis. Cold Spring Harb. Perspect. Med. 3 (2013) https://doi.org/10.1101/cshperspect.a009555.

[21] A. Vankeerberghen, H. Cuppens, J.-J. Cassiman, The cystic fibrosis transmembrane conductance regulator: an intriguing protein with pleiotropic functions. J. Cyst. Fibros. 1 (2002) 13–29, https://doi.org/10.1016/s1569-1993(01)00003-0.

[22] S.K. Hall, D.E. Stableforth, A. Green, Sweat sodium and chloride concentrations—essential criteria for the diagnosis of cystic fibrosis in adults. Ann. Clin. Biochem. 27 (1990) 318–320, https://doi.org/10.1177/000456329002700406.

[23] A.C. Gonçalves, F.A.L. Marson, R.M.H. Mendonça, C.S. Bertuzzo, I.A. Paschoal, J.D. Ribeiro, et al., Chloride and sodium ion concentrations in saliva and sweat as a method to diagnose cystic fibrosis. J. Pediatr. (2018) https://doi.org/10.1016/j.jped.2018.04.005.

[24] L.B. Baker, Sweating rate and sweat sodium concentration in athletes: a review of methodology and intra/interindividual variability. Sports Med. 47 (2017) 111–128, https://doi.org/10.1007/s40279-017-0691-5.

[25] L.B. Baker, K.A. Barnes, M.L. Anderson, D.H. Passe, J.R. Stofan, Normative data for regional sweat sodium concentration and whole-body sweating rate in athletes. J. Sports Sci. 34 (2015) 358–368, https://doi.org/10.1080/02640414.2015.1055291.

[26] W. Gao, S. Emaminejad, H.Y.Y. Nyein, S. Challa, K. Chen, A. Peck, et al., Fully integrated wearable sensor arrays for multiplexed in situ perspiration analysis. Nature 529 (2016) 509–514, https://doi.org/10.1038/nature16521.

[27] M. Villiger, R. Stoop, T. Vetsch, E. Hohenauer, M. Pini, P. Clarys, et al., Evaluation and review of body fluids saliva, sweat and tear compared to biochemical hydration assessment markers within blood and urine. Eur. J. Clin. Nutr. 72 (2017) 69–76, https://doi.org/10.1038/ejcn.2017.136.

[28] H.Y.Y. Nyein, W. Gao, Z. Shahpar, S. Emaminejad, S. Challa, K. Chen, et al., A wearable electrochemical platform for noninvasive simultaneous monitoring of Ca2 and pH. ACS Nano 10 (2016) 7216–7224, https://doi.org/10.1021/acsnano.6b04005.

[29] T. Senterre, I.A. Zahirah, C. Pieltain, V.D. Halleux, J. Rigo, Electrolyte and mineral homeostasis after optimizing early macronutrient intakes in VLBW infants on parenteral nutrition. J. Pediatr. Gastroenterol. Nutr. 61 (2015) 491–498, https://doi.org/10.1097/mpg.0000000000000854.

[30] M.J. Berridge, Calcium signalling in health and disease. Biochem. Biophys. Res. Commun. 485 (2017) 5, https://doi.org/10.1016/j.bbrc.2017.01.098.

[31] S. Jadoon, S. Karim, M.R. Akram, A.K. Khan, M.A. Zia, A.R. Siddiqi, et al., Recent developments in sweat analysis and its applications. Int. J. Anal. Chem. 2015 (2015) 1–7, https://doi.org/10.1155/2015/164974.

[32] G.N. Gowda, S. Zhang, H. Gu, V. Asiago, N. Shanaiah, D. Raftery, Metabolomics-based methods for early disease diagnostics. Expert. Rev. Mol. Diagn. 8 (2008) 617–633, https://doi.org/10.1586/14737159.8.5.617.

[33] C. Bommer, V. Sagalova, E. Heesemann, J. Manne-Goehler, R. Atun, T. Bärnighausen, et al., Global economic burden of diabetes in adults: projections from 2015 to 2030. Diabetes Care 41 (2018) 963–970, https://doi.org/10.2337/dc17-1962.

[34] Connolly, Simultaneous transdermal extraction of glucose and lactate from human subjects by reverse iontophoresis. Int. J. Nanomedicine (2008) 211, https://doi.org/10.2147/ijn.s1728.

[35] B. Levy, Lactate and shock state: the metabolic view. Curr. Opin. Crit. Care 12 (2006) 315–321, https://doi.org/10.1097/01.ccx.0000235208.77450.15.

[36] D.A. Maclean, J. Bangsbo, B. Saltin, Muscle interstitial glucose and lactate levels during dynamic exercise in humans determined by microdialysis. J. Appl. Physiol. 87 (1999) 1483–1490, https://doi.org/10.1152/jappl.1999.87.4.1483.

[37] M. Muller, A. Holmang, O.K. Andersson, H.G. Eichler, P. Lonnroth, Measurement of interstitial muscle glucose and lactate concentrations during an oral glucose tolerance test. Am. J. Physiol. Endocrinol. Metab. 271 (1996) https://doi.org/10.1152/ajpendo.1996.271.6.e1003.

[38] J.K. Kirk, J. Stegner, Self-monitoring of blood glucose: practical aspects. J. Diabetes Sci. Technol. 4 (2010) 435–439, https://doi.org/10.1177/193229681000400225.

[39] M.A. Birkett, The trier social stress test protocol for inducing psychological stress. J. Vis. Exp. (2011) https://doi.org/10.3791/3238.

[40] D. Schoofs, O.T. Wolf, Are salivary gonadal steroid concentrations influenced by acute psychosocial stress? A study using the Trier Social Stress Test (TSST), Int. J. Psychophysiol. 80 (2011) 36–43.

[41] S. Prasad, A.K. Tyagi, B.B. Aggarwal, Detection of inflammatory biomarkers in saliva and urine: potential in diagnosis, prevention, and treatment for chronic diseases. Exp. Biol. Med. 241 (2016) 783–799, https://doi.org/10.1177/1535370216638770.

[42] A.H. Marques, M.N. Silverman, E.M. Sternberg, Evaluation of stress systems by applying noninvasive methodologies: measurements of neuroimmune biomarkers in the sweat, heart rate variability and salivary cortisol. Neuroimmunomodulation 17 (2010) 205–208, https://doi.org/10.1159/000258725.

[43] T. Traustadóttir, P. Bosch, K. Matt, Gender differences in cardiovascular and hypothalamic-pituitary-adrenal axis responses to psychological stress in healthy older adult men and women. Stress 6 (2003) 133–140, https://doi.org/10.1080/1025389031000111302.

[44] N.D. Goncharova, Stress responsiveness of the hypothalamic–pituitary–adrenal axis: age-related features of the vasopressinergic regulation. Front. Endocrinol. 4 (2013) https://doi.org/10.3389/fendo.2013.00026.

[45] M. Jia, W.M. Chew, Y. Feinstein, P. Skeath, E.M. Sternberg, Quantification of cortisol in human eccrine sweat by liquid chromatography—tandem mass spectrometry. Analyst 141 (2016) 2053–2060, https://doi.org/10.1039/c5an02387d.

[46] T. Ganz, R.I. Lehrer, Antimicrobial proteins and peptides. in: Encyclopedia of Life Sciences, 2001, https://doi.org/10.1038/npg.els.0001212.

[47] M. Murakami, T. Ohtake, R.A. Dorschner, R.L. Gallo, B. Schittek, C. Garbe, Cathelicidin anti-microbial peptide expression in sweat, an innate defense system for the skin. J. Investig. Dermatol. 119 (2002) 1090–1095, https://doi.org/10.1046/j.1523-1747.2002.19507.x.

[48] M. Marcinkiewicz, S. Majewski, The role of antimicrobial peptides in chronic inflammatory skin diseases. Adv. Dermatol. Allergol. 1 (2016) 6–12, https://doi.org/10.5114/pdia.2015.48066.

[49] D. Porter, S. Weremowicz, K. Chin, P. Seth, A. Keshaviah, J. Lahti-Domenici, et al., A neural survival factor is a candidate oncogene in breast cancer. Proc. Natl. Acad. Sci. 100 (2003) 10931–10936, https://doi.org/10.1073/pnas.1932980100.

[50] M.D. Turner, B. Nedjai, T. Hurst, D.J. Pennington, Cytokines and chemokines: at the crossroads of cell signalling and inflammatory disease. Biochim. Biophys. Acta 1843 (2014) 2563–2582, https://doi.org/10.1016/j.bbamcr.2014.05.014.

[51] G. Cizza, A.H. Marques, F. Eskandari, I.C. Christie, S. Torvik, M.N. Silverman, et al., Elevated neuroimmune biomarkers in sweat patches and plasma of premenopausal women with major depressive disorder in remission: the POWER study. Biol. Psychiatry 64 (2008) 907–911, https://doi.org/10.1016/j.biopsych.2008.05.035.

[52] L. Soleimani, M.A. Oquendo, G.M. Sullivan, A.A. Mathe, J.J. Mann, Cerebrospinal fluid neuropeptide Y levels in major depression and reported childhood trauma. Int. J. Neuropsychopharmacol. 18 (2014) https://doi.org/10.1093/ijnp/pyu023.

[53] N.J. Ronkainen, H.B. Halsall, W.R. Heineman, Electrochemical biosensors. Chem. Soc. Rev. 39 (2010) 1747, https://doi.org/10.1039/b714449k.

[54] T. Guinovart, A.J. Bandodkar, J.R. Windmiller, F.J. Andrade, J. Wang, A potentiometric tattoo sensor for monitoring ammonium in sweat. Analyst 138 (2013) 7031, https://doi.org/10.1039/c3an01672b.

[55] A.J. Bandodkar, D. Molinnus, O. Mirza, T. Guinovart, J.R. Windmiller, G. Valdés-Ramírez, et al., Epidermal tattoo potentiometric sodium sensors with wireless signal transduction for continuous non-invasive sweat monitoring. Biosens. Bioelectron. 54 (2014) 603–609, https://doi.org/10.1016/j.bios.2013.11.039.

[56] D.-H. Choi, J.S. Kim, G.R. Cutting, P.C. Searson, Wearable potentiometric chloride sweat sensor: the critical role of the salt bridge. Anal. Chem. 88 (2016) 12241–12247, https://doi.org/10.1021/acs.analchem.6b03391.

[57] J. Park, J. Kim, S.-Y. Kim, W.H. Cheong, J. Jang, Y.-G. Park, et al., Soft, smart contact lenses with integrations of wireless circuits, glucose sensors, and displays. Sci. Adv. 4 (2018) https://doi.org/10.1126/sciadv.aap9841.

[58] H. Lee, C. Song, Y.S. Hong, M.S. Kim, H.R. Cho, T. Kang, et al., Wearable/disposable sweat-based glucose monitoring device with multistage transdermal drug delivery module. Sci. Adv. 3 (2017) https://doi.org/10.1126/sciadv.1601314.

[59] W. Jia, A.J. Bandodkar, G. Valdés-Ramírez, J.R. Windmiller, Z. Yang, J. Ramírez, et al., Electrochemical tattoo biosensors for real-time noninvasive lactate monitoring in human perspiration. Anal. Chem. 85 (2013) 6553–6560, https://doi.org/10.1021/ac401573r.

[60] J. Kim, G. Valdés-Ramírez, A.J. Bandodkar, W. Jia, A.G. Martinez, J. Ramírez, et al., Non-invasive mouthguard biosensor for continuous salivary monitoring of metabolites. Analyst 139 (2014) 1632–1636, https://doi.org/10.1039/c3an02359a.

[61] J. Kim, S. Imani, W.R.D. Araujo, J. Warchall, G. Valdés-Ramírez, T.R. Paixão, et al., Wearable salivary uric acid mouthguard biosensor with integrated wireless electronics. Biosens. Bioelectron. 74 (2015) 1061–1068, https://doi.org/10.1016/j.bios.2015.07.039.

[62] J. Kim, I. Jeerapan, S. Imani, T.N. Cho, A. Bandodkar, S. Cinti, et al., Noninvasive alcohol monitoring using a wearable tattoo-based iontophoretic-biosensing system. ACS Sens. 1 (2016) 1011–1019, https://doi.org/10.1021/acssensors.6b00356.

[63] Y.J. Hong, H. Lee, J. Kim, M. Lee, H.J. Choi, T. Hyeon, D. Kim, Multifunctional wearable system that integrates sweat-based sensing and vital-sign monitoring to estimate pre-/post-exercise glucose levels, Adv. Funct. Mater. (2018) 1805754.

[64] R.D. Munje, S. Muthukumar, B. Jagannath, S. Prasad, A new paradigm in sweat based wearable diagnostics biosensors using Room Temperature Ionic Liquids (RTILs). Sci. Rep. 7 (2017) https://doi.org/10.1038/s41598-017-02133-0.

[65] D. Kinnamon, R. Ghanta, K.-C. Lin, S. Muthukumar, S. Prasad, Portable biosensor for monitoring cortisol in low-volume perspired human sweat. Sci. Rep. 7 (2017) https://doi.org/10.1038/s41598-017-13684-7.

[66] Z. Hao, Z. Wang, Y. Li, Y. Zhu, X. Wang, C.G.D. Moraes, et al., Measurement of cytokine biomarkers using an aptamer-based affinity graphene nanosensor on a flexible substrate toward wearable applications. Nanoscale (2018) https://doi.org/10.1039/c8nr04315a.

[67] P.S. Sharma, A. Pietrzyk-Le, F. D'Souza, W. Kutner, Electrochemically synthesized polymers in molecular imprinting for chemical sensing. Anal. Bioanal. Chem. 402 (2012) 3177–3204, https://doi.org/10.1007/s00216-011-5696-6.100.

[68] B.T.S. Bui, K. Haupt, Molecularly imprinted polymers: synthetic receptors in bioanalysis. Anal. Bioanal. Chem. 398 (2010) 2481–2492, https://doi.org/10.1007/s00216-010-4158-x.

[69] S.A. Piletsky, A.P.F. Turner, Electrochemical sensors based on molecularly imprinted polymers, Electroanalysis 14 (2002) 317–323.

[70] O. Parlak, S.T. Keene, A. Marais, V.F. Curto, A. Salleo, Molecularly selective nanoporous membrane-based wearable organic electrochemical device for noninvasive cortisol sensing. Sci. Adv. 4 (2018) https://doi.org/10.1126/sciadv.aar2904.

[71] L. Hou, J. Hagen, X. Wang, I. Papautsky, R. Naik, N. Kelley-Loughnane, et al., Artificial microfluidic skin for in vitro perspiration simulation and testing. Lab Chip 13 (2013) 1868, https://doi.org/10.1039/c3lc41231h.

[72] A. Martín, J. Kim, J.F. Kurniawan, J.R. Sempionatto, J.R. Moreto, G. Tang, et al., Epidermal microfluidic electrochemical detection system: enhanced sweat sampling and metabolite detection. ACS Sens. 2 (2017) 1860–1868, https://doi.org/10.1021/acssensors.7b00729.

[73] A. Koh, D. Kang, Y. Xue, S. Lee, R.M. Pielak, J. Kim, et al., A soft, wearable microfluidic device for the capture, storage, and colorimetric sensing of sweat. Sci. Transl. Med. 8 (2016) https://doi.org/10.1126/scitranslmed.aaf2593.

[74] S. Xu, Y. Zhang, L. Jia, K.E. Mathewson, K.-I. Jang, J. Kim, et al., Soft microfluidic assemblies of sensors, circuits, and radios for the skin. Science 344 (2014) 70–74, https://doi.org/10.1126/science.1250169.

[75] S. Emaminejad, W. Gao, H.Y.Y. Nyein, S. Challa, R.W. Davis, A. Javey, Flexible systems for wearable physiological monitoring applications, in: Solid State Sensors, Actuators, and Microsystems Conference, (Hilton Head), 2016, pp. 108–109.

CHAPTER 3

Wearable biosensors and sample handling strategies

Onur Parlak[a,1], Vincenzo F. Curto[b,1], Edilberto Ojeda[c,d], Lourdes Basabe-Desmonts[d,e], Fernando Benito-Lopez[c], Alberto Salleo[a]

[a]Department of Materials Science and Engineering, Stanford University, Stanford, CA, United States
[b]Electrical Engineering Division, Department of Engineering, University of Cambridge, Cambridge, United Kingdom. [c]Analytical Microsystems & Materials for Lab-on-a-Chip (AMMa-LOAC) Group, Microfluidics Cluster UPV/EHU, Analytical Chemistry Department, University of the Basque Country UPV/EHU, Vitoria-Gasteiz, Spain [d]BIOMICs Research Group, Lascaray Ikergunea, Research Center, University of the Basque Country, Vitoria-Gasteiz, Spain [e]Ikerbasque, Basque Foundation for Science, Bilbao, Spain

Chapter Outline

3.1 Wearable biosensors

One of the most recent and important breakthroughs in the field of biosensor technology is the wearable biosensor [1]. The wearable biosensor has attracted considerable attention because of its potential to change classical medical diagnostics and continuous health monitoring concepts [2]. Wearable biosensor applications aim to change centralized hospital-based care system to

---

[1]These authors contributed equally.

Wearable Bioelectronics. https://doi.org/10.1016/B978-0-08-102407-2.00004-7

home-based personal medicine and reduce health-care cost and time for diagnosis. The understanding of traditional health-care diagnosis and related tools has started to evolve through an easy-to-use, and decentralized diagnosis perspective that offers concepts and devices including miniaturized, wearable, and implantable biosensors [3]. However, achieving these paradigm shifts requires significant progress and research in new materials, interfaces, circuit designs, data processing, and business models [4]. In this chapter, we aim to survey the recent trends of wearable biosensor technology and their implications for health applications. In the first section, we seek to piece together different types of wearable biosensors, highlight, and discuss early breakthroughs, key developments, and future of point-of-care diagnostics. In the second section, we highlight sample handling strategies for various wearable biosensors. Each section concludes with a discussion of prominent examples in corresponding branches and their implications.

Early research activities on wearable health monitoring have mainly focused on addressing demands in physical sensing [5]. These efforts have resulted in successful wearable physical sensors, such as temperature and pressure, for monitoring biophysical signals including heart rate, respiration rate, skin temperature, and brain activity [6]. However, these physical sensors require external complementary measures to diagnose diseases precisely. On the other hand, wearable biosensors are able to give direct information about specific disease biomarkers and metabolite changes in bodily fluids [7]. Although wearable biosensors present various technical challenges such as the acquisition of low sample volumes, biofouling, and biocompatibility, sweat, tears, and saliva have all been intensively explored. The most challenging and inherent problem of these systems is the lack of correlation between in vivo concentration of many metabolites with other bodily fluids including tear, saliva, and sweat (Fig. 3.1) [1]. Saliva-based biosensors offer reliable measurements of lactate, amylase and a few other proteins, but they usually fail to provide a precise determination of glucose concentration [8]. Another difficulty for saliva-based metabolite sensing is contamination from food or drink. Sweat shows a similarly poor correlation for many metabolites, despite being the target for a number of sensor approaches reported in the popular press [9]. Another interesting approach is tear-based biosensing whether using a contact lens as a sensing vehicle or mounting optical devices on glasses [10]. Nonetheless, blood still represents the most reliable human body fluid for clinical diagnostics. However, blood sampling is a rather intrusive method that is not preferred by the patients [11]. Therefore, other bodily fluids are still the focus of intense research and they are continuously explored as an alternative to blood for diagnostic purposes. In the following section, we try to highlight some key examples of all types of wearable biosensors. We also describe in detail challenges and possible methods to increase device performance.

3.1.1 Tear-based biosensors

Human tears are a complex physiological fluid composed of 98% of water and various proteins, metabolites, and electrolytes [12]. Many of these molecules offer potentially a suitable platform for diagnosis, especially for human metabolites. Even though tear-based

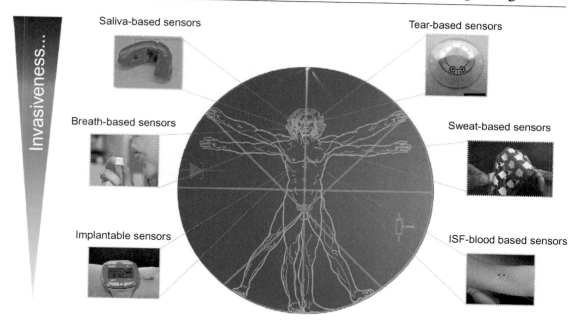

Fig. 3.1
Overview of the rapidly growing field of wearable biosensors [1].

bioelectronics has attracted much attention in the early 2000s, as evidenced by various media and press releases that have been published over the years describing smart wearable electronic devices, no commercial application of tear-based wearable biosensors has been accomplished yet [13]. One of the first successful examples of contact lens-based sensor was developed in 2009 [14]. In this study, Parviz et al. showed the very first on-body testing of a contact lens-based sensor on anesthetized rabbit eye (Fig. 3.2A and B) [14]. The first metabolite sensor was also developed by the same group by integrating a three-electrode amperometric sensor system consisting of a Pt working electrode coated on indium-thin oxide (ITO) surface where GOx was immobilized, and an Ag/AgCl reference electrode on poly(ethylene terephthalate) (PET) film. Improving further on the concept, researchers produced a reference electrode integrated into a three-electrode amperometric biosensor system on PET film using lithography, e-beam evaporation, and lift-off techniques. In addition to the glucose sensor, researchers produced a lactate biosensor by following the same fabrication methods on contact lenses. Similarly to enzyme-based electrochemical glucose biosensor, the authors measured the oxidation of H_2O_2 produced by the conversion of L-lactate to L-pyruvate in the presence of lactate oxidase (LOx) on a platinum electrode [15]. In another study, Mitsubayashi et al. developed a strategy which produces enzyme-based glucose biosensors by integrating a polydimethylsiloxane (PDMS) membrane with a contact lens. In this technique, Ag and Pt metals were sputtered onto a PDMS substrate, and Pt and Ag/AgCl counter and reference electrodes were integrated into the substrate. Then, flexible electrodes were bonded onto the surface of the contact lens using PDMS, and GOx was immobilized using a mixture of a copolymer of 2-methacryloyloxyethyl phosphorylcholine and 2-ethylhexylmethacrylate (PMEH) on the sensing region of the electrode. This integrated biosensor was successfully tested using a rabbit model (Fig. 3.2C and D) [16].

Recently, researchers also developed a multifunctional contact lens-based biosensor using an actual ocular contact lens [17]. The sensor was designed to monitor glucose within tears as well as intraocular pressure using the resistance and capacitance of the electronic device. The device was tested in vitro using la vie rabbit eye to demonstrate its reliability. They not only showed the fabrication of transparent, stretchable, and multifunctional sensors on wearable soft contact lenses for the wireless detection of glucose but also successfully measured intraocular pressure with high-sensitivity. The key components of the device were graphene and a hybrid with metal nanowires, providing sufficient transparency and stretchability that ensure reliability, comfort, and unobstructed vision when the soft contact lens was worn by users. Using these features, they were able to monitor glucose concentration in real-time. Also, they designed a wireless power system to run the device on-body without integrated power sources (Fig. 3.2E) [12, 15].

One of the technical challenges in wearable tear-based biosensors is to provide a suitable power source [4]. The main concerns of powering these devices are size, thickness, biocompatibility, and safety. Biofuel cells (BFCs) are considered one of the easiest and beneficial ways to power contact-lens-based devices due to their ability to generate power in situ and the simplicity of circuit design [12, 18, 19]. Tear fluid contains several metabolites including glucose, ascorbate, and pyruvate that can be used as biofuels for powering the sensor devices. One of the earliest and most prominent studies of tear-based BFC was developed by Shleev et al. [20]. In this study, authors fabricated nanostructured microelectrodes by coating gold nanoparticles onto gold nanowires. The gold nanoparticles were modified with *Corynascus thermophilus* CDH at the anodic side, and *Myrothecium verrucaria* bilirubin oxidase at the cathodic side. The assembled BFCs were tested on human tear, and the device showed $1\,\mu W/cm^2$ power density, and $20\,h$ operational activity [20]. Even though many successful studies have been reported, tear-based wearable biosensors have not yet been commercialized due to a number of technical challenges. The most important drawbacks of this method are lack of correlation with blood concentrations, sampling of analytes, detrimental side products, time-delay with respect to circulating blood levels, size, and transparency of the device. All these technical hurdles should be addressed before any successful implementation of this approach for commercial applications of tear-based wearable biosensors.

3.1.2 Saliva-based biosensors

Saliva is another important physiological fluid that contains various different compounds that diffuse from the blood via transcellular or paracellular paths. Saliva-based biosensor

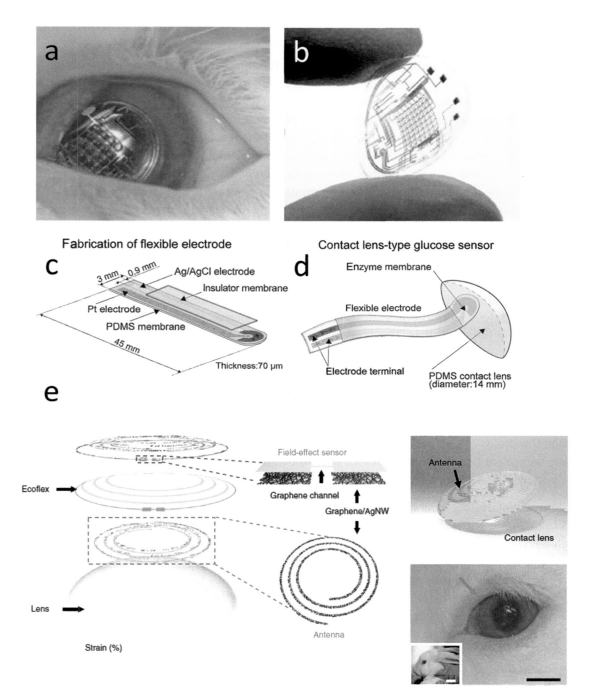

Fig. 3.2

Photographs of one of the first prototypes of contact lens containing metal circuit structures and illustration of animal trial on rabbit eye (A–B), fabrication method of the contact lens biosensor on flexible electrode (C) and bonding of electrode to the contact lens (D), schematic of the wearable contact lens sensor, integrating the glucose sensor and intraocular pressure sensor (*left*), and schematic illustration of the transparent glucose sensor on the contact lens with photographs of wireless sensor integrated onto the eyes of a live rabbit (*right*). Black and white scale bars, 1 and 5 cm, respectively (E).

approaches offer an alternative to blood analysis for continuous monitoring of important metabolites, hormones, and proteins [21]. In addition to recent progresses on in vitro salivary diagnostics, wearable salivary biosensing has been recently proposed. The early examples of salivary sensors date back to the late 1960s, where researchers monitored pH and biologically important electrolytes on tooth enamel [22]. One of the recent successful examples is a noninvasive mouthguard biosensor for continuous monitoring of uric acid, which is the end product of the metabolism of purine in the human body developed by Wang et al. [23]. In this study, the authors developed a screen-printed amperometric enzyme-based biosensor together with an integrated wireless transmitter. They printed a sensory system consisting of Prussian blue (PB) embedded in a carbon electrode on PET as a transducing element and electropolymerized o-phenylenediamine cross-linked with uricase as a biorecognition site. In this system, PB acts as an artificial peroxidase which helps to oxidize hydrogen peroxide and poly(o-phenylenediamine) is used as a protecting and immobilization layer for the uricase enzyme. Additionally, the authors also used a wireless amperometric circuit coupled with a Bluetooth low-energy communication system integrated on the mouthguard biosensor as shown in Fig. 3.3A [23]. The same research group also developed the first example of a wearable salivary metabolite biosensor based on the integration of printable enzymatic electrode on a mouthguard (Fig. 3.3B). This saliva-based enzymatic biosensor mainly was designed using LOx which was immobilized on electrode surface and used for low potential detection of the peroxide product. The research successfully demonstrated the real-time monitoring of lactate, which is important for the wearer's health, performance and stress level, and thus holds considerable promise for diverse biomedical and fitness applications. The advantages of this mouthguard sensor over in-dwelling type of devices are wearability, ease of operation, and renewability.

Another interesting wearable salivary biosensor was developed for continuous monitoring of bacteria on tooth enamel [24]. In this work, researchers developed an interesting technique that is transferable to fabricating similar devices for continuous monitoring of metabolites (Fig. 3.3C). In their study, the authors developed a graphene-modified silk tattoo biosensor. They fabricated interdigitated electrodes modified by peptide assembled graphene for selective binding of pathogenic bacteria, using an embedded inductive coil antenna for both wireless communication and powering the biosensor device. The whole structure was transferred to tooth enamel: the resulting device demonstrated strong biochemical sensing with a very low detection limit [24]. Similarly to tear-based biosensors, salivary wearable biosensors have not been commercialized yet due to important technical challenges such as contamination of the analytes by food, the variation in the rate of salivation in different patients, poor correlation with analyte concentration in the blood for some specific metabolites including glucose. If the other challenges can be overcome, saliva-based sensor systems can be used for lactate, and some other protein biomarkers [23].

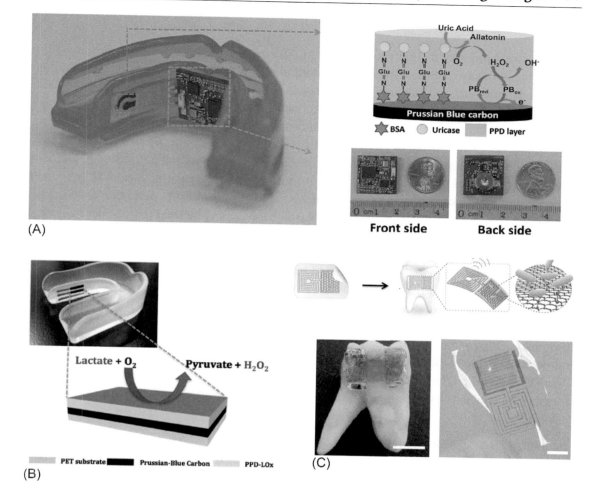

Fig. 3.3

A saliva-based mouthguard uric acid sensor and its various components with sensing principles (A), photograph of the mouthguard biosensor, with the integrated printable 3-electrode system, including the enzyme working electrode and schematic illustration of the PB working electrode coated with the PPD-LOx layer in the mouthguard biosensor for salivary lactate monitoring (B), graphene is printed onto bioresorbable silk and contacts are formed containing a wireless coil, biotransfer of the nanosensing architecture onto the surface of a tooth with magnified schematic of the sensing element, illustrating wireless readout, and example of binding of pathogenic bacteria by peptides self-assembled on the graphene nanotransducer (*top*), together with passive wireless telemetry system consisting of a planar meander line inductor and interdigitated capacitive electrodes integrated onto the graphene/silk film and graphene nanosensor biotransferred onto the surface of a human molar (*bottom*) (C).

3.1.3 Sweat-based biosensors

Human sweat provides a significant amount of information about patient's health status for wearable, noninvasive biosensing [25]. In addition to some important electrolytes including sodium, ammonium, and calcium, sweat contains different metabolites, aminoacids, proteins, and some small molecules and hormones allowing to monitor metabolic diseases, patient's intoxication levels or environmental contamination on the skin [26, 27]. Sweat-based wearable sensor systems have the ability to yield real-time information for health and fitness monitoring. Even though most of the research focuses on small number of physical or electrophysiological parameters, significant information about a patient's health status can be provided by biomarkers using a sweat-based wearable biosensor [28]. Wearable biosensors are mainly divided into two groups; textile/plastic based and epidermal (tattoo)-based systems [29]. Both designs have some advantages and disadvantages over their counterparts. For example, epidermal biosensors provide better contact with skin; however, they usually have a shorter life-time compared to textile-based biosensor systems. Epidermal-based sensor systems were developed first in 2009 by the Rogers' group for continuous monitoring of physical parameters [30]. Shortly after, Wang's group adapted this approach and combined it with biorecognition elements to fabricate the first printed tattoo-based electrochemical biosensor [31]. In their study, the authors fabricated a screen-printed electrode on temporary tattoo paper using carbon and Ag/AgCl as working and reference electrode, respectively. They then modified the working electrode with carbon nanotubes and a mediator molecule together with lactase oxidase for continuous monitoring of lactate level in sweat during exercise [32].

In another study, researcher recently published a wirelessly powered wearable patch-type sensor [33]. Even though the reported study is not directly related to metabolite sensing, the design and method established by Heikenfeld is worth mentioning, and more importantly, the same methodology can be easily adapted to sweat-based metabolite sensors [33]. In this study, the investigators fabricated electronic circuitry on an adhesive patch together with a radio frequency identification (RFID) chip that is used for potentiometric sensing of analytes in sweat, powering the device, and reading results wirelessly via an Android smartphone application (Fig. 3.4A and B) [33].

In another study, the same group introduced a wearable device that can measure sweat-lactate and electrophysiological parameters at the same time using an epidermal patch, which is composed of a screen-printed three electrode-based amperometric sensor and two carbon-based electrocardiogram electrodes (Fig. 3.4C and D) [34]. With this patch, the authors continuously monitored heart health and functions simultaneously with the L-lactate level in sweat following the same strategy of incorporating PB in a carbon electrode. The goal of the measurement was to provide reliable information about an individual's health and performance. Another significant progress of this work in comparison to early works

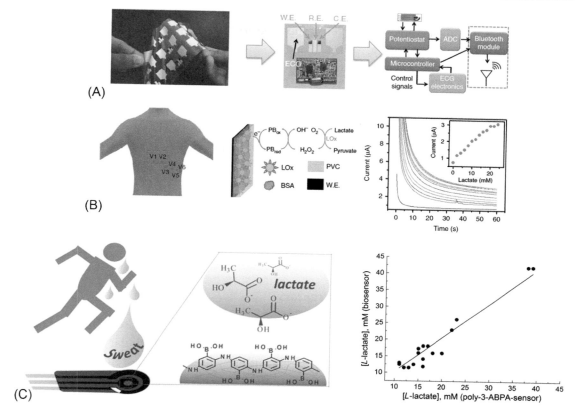

Fig. 3.4

Device photographs of sweat-based sensor on body and its sensor features (A–B), schematic representations of screen printed, block diagram of the circuit (C), enzymatic sensing mechanism and amperometric response of wearable sweat-based lactate biosensor (D), schematic illustration of nonenzymatic lactate sensor in human sweat and correlation diagram for lactate measurement in 17 sweat samples collected from seven healthy human subjects measured using poly(3-APBA) sensor and with the flow-injection system equipped with the biosensor (E).

was the ability to integrate all components of electronic circuitry including sensory part, microcontroller, wireless communication module and potentiostat in a single chip [34].

In another interesting study, Karyakin et al. developed a successful example of nonenzymatic sensor for lactate detection in human sweat [35]. They produced nonenzymatic impedimetric sensor based on screen-printed electrodes modified by electropolymerization of 3-aminophenylboronic acid (3-APBA) with imprinting of lactate. The developed sensor exhibited wide range of sensing between 3 and 100 mM with a detection limit of 1.5 mM. The response time was 2–3 min, with 6 months shelf life which is usually difficult to reach with enzyme-based sensors. They also tested the device on a real sample using 17 healthy subject.

The results were compared with enzyme-based lactate devices (Fig. 3.4E) [35]. Even though their device is not in wearable design yet, it shows great promise for wearable metabolite sensing for long-term monitoring.

Another important feature of wearable sweat-based systems is remote power transfer to the sensor device. Sweat contains essential metabolites that can be used as potential biofuels to power the wearable biosensor. The Wang group recently published a report on wearable sweat-based BFCs transferred to the skin with a temporary tattoo technique [36]. The authors use oxidation of the lactate present in sweat by immobilizing LOx to a carbon nanotube modified carbon electrode as a bioanode and use O_2 as a substrate for Pt black modified carbon electrode as a biocathode. Both electrodes were modified with chitosan to encapsulate the enzyme layer. The designed wearable BFCs exhibits high power density of 5–70 W/cm^2, which depends on lactate concentration in perspiration during exercise. This approach shows that in situ power generation can be used to fabricate self-powered biosensors using different range of metabolites [36].

3.1.4 Subcutaneous and implantable sensors

In recent years, there has been a growing interest in the development and use of subcutaneous devices in wearable settings to perform continuous monitoring of intercellular fluids [37, 38]. Commercially available subcutaneous devices are currently used to monitor glucose levels of diabetic patients, for example, the FreeStyle Libre from Abbott and the iPro Evaluation system from Medtronics [39]. Interstitial fluid (ISF) is the liquid that surrounds the cells and it is responsible for regulating and maintaining optimal organ homeostasis. Due to the essential body regulation function of ISF s, important ions, for example, Na$^+$, K$^+$, Cl$^-$, and metabolites, that is, glucose, lactate, are present in the ISF and wearable miniaturized devices can be used to perform real-time sensing of this important bodily fluid. Subcutaneous microdialysis probes and microneedles are the two main technologies that have been employed in this scenario [40]. Microdialysis makes use of coaxial microfluidic probes where a polymeric membrane with a selected cut-off pore size is put in direct contact with the tissue. Concentration gradients between the membrane and the surrounding tissue
are responsible for analyte diffusion to diffuse through the membrane inside the probe. In order to determine the concentration of the analytes of interest from the dialysate (liquid output from the probe), a certain volume of the dialysate can be collected inside sterile vials for downstream analysis, gaining access to averaged concentration values and low temporal resolution. Alternatively, online measurement can be also performed but bulky analytical tools, such as mass spectrometry, high performance liquid chromatography, etc., need to be employed. Thus, to date the use of microdialysis technology for the development of novel wearable devices has been limited by these two factors, that is, lack of real-time information and/or the bulkiness of the analytical tools that are conventionally coupled with

microdialysis [41]. To overcome the aforementioned limitations, Gowers et al. have proposed two possible alternatives [42, 43]. A delayed high temporal analysis of the dialysate was simply achieved through the use of tubing instead of vials to store the dialysate. By using this approach, the authors were able to measure levels of glucose and lactate from an implanted subcutaneous probe during a cycling routine. Using this configuration, the estimated time resolution was about 30 s. However, the main drawback of this approach is a substantial collection to analysis delay. A more interesting and innovative approach was developed through the use of a 3D printed microfluidics that can be integrated with Federal Drug Administration

(FDA)-approved microdialysis probes. The 3D printed microfluidics comprised of two side ports for the integration of two separate needle-based three electrode biosensors for real-time sensing of glucose and lactate in the dialysate. The needle-based biosensors were located inside 3D printed holders that can be easily plugged and unplugged from the main microfluidic device as needed. The device was also used to monitor lactate and glucose level of subcutaneous ISFs during approximately 1 h of cycling exercise. Although improvements on the wearability of this platform are still needed, the combination of the microdialysis probe with a 3D printed microfluidics provides an interesting approach to perform subcutaneous biosensing during physical exercise and further developments of this technology are expected.

Continuous glucose monitoring for diabetic patients has been one of the primary focuses in the development of portable sensors, where both integration of noninvasive detection and sampling techniques along with drug delivery tools have not been achieved yet. Microneedle technology consists of a micro-sized needle array that can be fabricated using rigid materials. For example, silicon or hard plastics, or through soft and biocompatible polymers [44]. Microneedles can be simultaneously used for intradermal sensing of ISFs as well as for the in situ delivery of drugs that can then reach the bloodstream [45]. To perform controlled delivery of drugs in a wearable fashion, several approaches have been used. Hyaluronic acid-based microneedles were integrated with stretch triggered micro-depot loaded with drug nanocapsules [44]. The wearable device consisted of a thin elastomeric material that can be worn on the skin and delivery of the nanocapsules was triggered by body motion. Alternative drug delivery mechanisms have been also shown, such as a finger-powered microfluidic device to induce motion of the drug solution toward the microneedle array. Bendable microneedles can also be connected to a microfluidic network to be used as the pumping system of a liquid drug formulation. In the latter device, the authors also demonstrated the fabrication of a dry adhesive system consisting of PDMS micropillars as well as of a triboelectric energy harvester that can be potentially used to power wearable devices. However, these systems can be only used to deliver drugs upon application of external stimuli, such as pressure and lateral deformation. Lee et al. have recently proposed a more interesting approach to control the delivery of diabetic drugs when using temperature-responsive microneedles. In their most recent report, a wearable patch and a disposable strip sweat sensor were integrated with a glucose, pH, humidity, and temperature sensors in order to control the actuation of the microneedles. By correlating the measured signals from these sensors, a feedback loop was used to thermally actuate the microneedles using a patch-based three-channel thermal actuator. The device was successfully tested with diabetic mice, showing decreasing level of glucose in blood upon thermal actuation and delivery of a drug from the microneedles connected to the feedback loop.

ISF is a type of body fluid which provides precise information on patient health status. The main advantage of ISF-based approach over other wearable sensor systems is that metabolite concentrations in the ISF can be easily correlated with blood analyte levels. This technique essentially employs minimally invasive method such as reverse iontophoresis, which enables small volumes of ISF to be extracted through the skin [27]. Even though there has been no commercial success in noninvasive wearable metabolite sensing using saliva, tears and sweat, limited commercial success has been achieved with ISF-based biosensors. One of the earlier and well-known examples is the GlucoWatch Biographer (Cygnus, Inc.). Even though this device initially attracted considerable attention in the market, it was quickly withdrawn due to the significant inaccuracy reason from sampling errors, skin irritation problems, and frequent calibration needs [39]. Nevertheless, Abbott launched FreeStyeLibre as a new wearable continuous glucose monitoring device in Europe in October 2016. This newly launched wearable biosensor follows the skin-ISF sensing approach similarly to previously designed continuous monitoring devices; additionally, initial reviews show that this new device provides better comfort and it has an easier user interface. FreeStyle Liber contains a small sensory part (0.2 in. in length) that directly connects to a plastic patch and can be easily placed on the upper arm. The sensor can be used for 14 days and does not require any finger-stick calibration. Another novelty in this device is that is transfers data wirelessly *via* a near infra-red identification tag by simply holding the reader close to the sensor device. Furthermore, the sensor is able to send real-time glucose concentration to an external reader. The reader also provides a report on its screen that can be downloaded to any user interface.

As one of the recent and successful examples of implantable biosensor, researchers have recently described the application of an implantable biochip for intravenous glucose biosensor in rat blood [46]. The fabricated microelectrode modified with a carbon-based composite consists of flexible carbon fibers (FCFs), neutral red as a mediator and glucose oxidase as an enzyme layer. The researchers fabricated FCF-based microelectrodes by pretreating carbon cloth with concentrated nitric acid and by separating single fibers using microscopy tweezers. Around 100 mm in size flexible biochips were prepared using a millimeter-long poly(propylene) catheter to fabricate both working and counter electrodes. In the next step, microfabricated electrodes were inserted in the thoracic region of a living rat for in vivo measurements. The capability of in vivo glucose detection was tested by simulating the diabetic conditions by injecting glucose to rat blood [46].

While academic studies reach some initial level, considerable success has been achieved in industrial research and the implantable biosensor market started to appear in the market in the last 10 years [3]. In 2005, Medtronic (USA) launched the first implantable continuous glucose monitoring device for personal use. The self-implanted sensor follows the amperometric sensing approach based on the oxidation of H_2O_2 produced by the oxidation glucose in the presence of glucose oxidase. The biosensor device was initially designed to use for 3 days periods and collected data every 5 min. One year later, another US company, Dexcom, announced a new glucose biosensor having longer use life (7 days). Despite their commercial and medical successes, there are still several technical restrictions in all these devices. For instance, The US FDA still stipulates that the finger stick blood test must be performed while using these self-implantable biosensors. Furthermore, the current status of implantable biosensors is such that there is still work to do to achieve biocompatibility, reliability, and powering issues to fabricate fully implantable, long life-time (6–12 months) biosensor devices [39].

Recently, Senseonics, formerly known as Sensors for Science and Medicine introduced an excellent approach for a fully implantable continuous glucose monitoring system that last up to 29 days in vivo when implanted in the upper arm [47]. The sensory element uses anthracene-derived diboronic acid chemistry, which was developed by James et al. [48]. They used very novel technique to prevent the breakdown of boronic acid-based recognition site which is coupled to a fluorescent transduction molecule. The authors also used an additional Pt layer to decompose H_2O_2 produced during the inflammatory response. The whole device is powered via an RF power harvesting approach through inductive coupling with an external induction coil, which helps to design a battery-free sensor platform.

3.2 Sample handling strategies

In the previous sections of this chapter, we have discussed some of the most recent developments in the field of wearable biosensors, showing the tremendous potentials and future trends of this fast-growing research area. However, despite the clear advantages of this technology, only a limited number of these sensors reach the commercialization stage due to major challenges when going beyond the proof-of-concept. One of the main challenges remains the integration of highly sensitive biosensors within these wearable platforms to achieve long term (from days to months), stable, and reliable operation of the sensors. Moreover, platform wearability and conformability to the body contours are important factors to consider in order to minimize discomfort for the wearer.

Effective sampling strategies of the target bodily fluid is another crucial requirement in these platforms, as the sample needs to be collected and delivered to the sensor active area where the sensing mechanism takes place. In this scenario, recent advances in microfluidic technology, in particular for point-of-care diagnosis, have enabled the development of novel sensor integration strategies and architectures that can also open up new opportunities in the realm of wearable biosensors [49]. Microfluidics is the technology that aims to develop micrometer-sized channels to finely control the transport of fluids, that is, liquids or gases, within the microchannels to create lab-on-a-chip devices [50]. Microfluidics aims to use very small amounts of sample volume to generate the same quality of response compared to traditional analytical methods. Microfluidic devices can be fabricated using a wide range of substrates, rigid materials such as silicon and glass as well as flexible and cheap plastic as PDMS, poly(methyl methacrylate) (PMMA), polycarbonate (PC), and cyclo-olefin polymers (COP) [51]. The latter material category is preferred for the realization of wearable platforms given their flexibility. The use of microfluidics or miniaturized fluid-handling strategies has the advantage of reducing the required sample volume, thus the total device size can also be reduced [52]. In addition to this, direct collection and delivery of the bodily fluid inside the micro-fluidics has the potential to reduce to the minimum the risk of sample contaminations during the collection stage as well as from the surrounding environment, leading to an enhance output signal accuracy and sensitivity. Due to all the aforementioned advantages, in the last years the use of microfluidics on the development of wearable devices has become increasingly popular and we believe that this area will witness a rapid expansion in the near future. In the following sections, we are going to introduce some of the most recent advances on the integration of biosensors in microfluidic wearable devices to perform real-time monitoring of the human health.

3.2.1 Sampling strategies of sweat

Skin perspiration is the process through which sweat is produced in the sweat glands and secreted on the skin surface. Generation of sweat in the secretory coil of sweat glands is caused by the difference in osmolality between the secretory coil lumen and the cell plasma. Several sweat collection strategies have been proposed over the years, with some of these techniques commonly used in clinical practices. The most common sweat collection technique involves the use of flexible patches made out of a polyurethane/adhesive layer. These patches do not alter the skin perspiration properties, as water vapor can still go through the plastic layer while retaining the nonvolatile components for downstream analysis. When low concentration analytes need to be collected from sweat, patches have been used continuously up to 7 days [53]. Alternatively, sweat secretion can be stimulated using pilocarpine iontophoresis, where sweat is collected inside of a macroduct sweat collection system consisting of a coiled tubing. During electrical delivery of pilocarpine, secreted sweat is stored inside the tubing and collected through a syringe. To date, pilocarpine iontophoresis sweat stimulation is used clinically for the diagnosis of cystic fibrosis through the measurement of sodium-ion concentrations in sweat. In the literature other sweat collection methods can be also found, such as capsules made of flexible adhesive membranes using Parafilm [54] and the whole body wash down technique, where body sweat loss is simply measured by weighing the subject before and after exercise and the concentration of the analytes of interest is determined from the whole fluid loss during the training period [55]. In spite of the effectiveness of the collection techniques, one of their main limitations is a substantial sampling to analysis delay (which can be from several hours to days in the case of the patches), limiting the access to real-time information of the body condition during sweat secretion. The use of wearable microfluidics has the potential to overpass these limiting factors, providing the required tools for more efficient sweat sampling and analysis strategies. Standard fabrication of microfluidic devices involves the bonding of a microstructured PDMS slab, obtained via replica molding, with glass, silicon or other chemically compatible substrates [56, 57]. These microfluidic devices need to be connected to tubing and pumps to operate and support liquid motions inside the microchannels. It is clear how the use of standard microfluidic tools, that is, pumps, tubing, and rigid substrates, is not compatible for the realization of wearable microfluidics and alternative solutions need to be pursued for the operation of worn microfluidics. As sweat is naturally secreted to the skin surface, it is possible to obtain sweat pumping inside micro-channel networks with zero-power consumption. To achieve this result, several approaches have been described, making us of highly conformal PMDS devices [58] hydrophilic/hydrophobic fabric [59] and in situ osmotic pumping systems [60].

PDMS is a highly stretchable silicone-based material and a good candidate for the fabrication of highly conformal microfluidics. Choi et al. have recently demonstrated easy-to-use flexible PDMS wearable microfluidics that can be employed to estimate the secretory fluidic pressure generated by the sweat glands on the skin surface [58]. The wearable PDMS microfluidics was fabricated in three separate layers, the adhesive layer in contact with the skin, a mid-layer made of PDMS containing the microfluidic structures and a terminal capping layer to define the outlet of the microfluidics. The total thickness of the device was less than 1 mm. As a mean to estimate the secretory fluidic pressure of sweat, the microfluidic layer includes 12 capillary burst valves (CBV) of different dimensions, from 120 to 10 μm in width to achieve different bursting pressure (from 2 to 13 kPa) due to their difference in geometry. Colorimetric estimation of the secretory sweat pressure was achieved by placing the 12 CBVs within 12 independent microfluidic channels, hence each micro-channel presented a different bursting pressure. The PDMS sweat patch was also tested in vivo on different exercise routines with the patch positioned on several body locations. The same research group had also shown the use of similar conformable wearable microfluidics devices to measure different sweat analytes; these systems will be described in more detail in the following section. Another example of a PDMS-based microfluidics for wearable application has been given by Shay et al. with a hydrogel-enabled osmotic in situ micropump. Differently from before, osmotic pressure was used as the driving force to achieve liquid flow inside a micro-channel [60]. The hydrogel was loaded with sodium chloride and glycerol at a concentration higher than the one present in the human sweat and difference in the salt concentrations induces liquid motion in the microchannel. Interestingly, the presence of the hydrogel inside the microfluidics did not affect the glucose concentration of the pumped liquid. Although the development of the osmotic micropump in a wearable fashion has to be yet demonstrated, it is believed that this can be easily achieved due to the soft nature of both PDMS and hydrogels.

Another interesting approach for the realization of zero-power consumption wearable microfluidics is through the use of hydrophilic textile where the wicking properties of the yarns is used to drive the fluid in the microfluidic networks. Thread-based microfluidic devices were first proposed by Reches et al. [61] as an easy route for the fabrication of colorimetric biomedical assays, in a similar way to the paper microfluidic technology [62]. Fabrication of textile-based wearable microfluidics can be performed by selective hydrophobic/hydrophilic pattering technique [63] and stereo-stitching [59]. For the former, Yang et al. made use of a fabric-based digital droplet microfluidic to measure sweat flow rate. The microfluidics structured was made by laser cutting and the microfluidics consisted of three main components: (1) fluid collection network, (2) a microfluidic junction for droplet formation and removal, and (3) two-electrode integrated circuitry for estimation of the flow rate. One of the key components of this system was the microfluidics junction, responsible for generating discrete droplets of fixed volume by collecting the liquid flowing through the microfluidic network. Estimation of the flow rate was then performed by measuring the electrolyte resistance across two silver-plated nylon threads, which were embedded in the hydrophilic fabric. Xing et al. had also proposed stereo-stitching of hydrophilic cotton yarns threads on superhydrophobic textile to create an interfacial microfluidics transport through the cotton fibers [59]. Interestingly, the difference in the surface tension between the liquid/hydrophilic and the liquid/hydrophobic fabrics induced a pressure gradient along the flow path that facilitates the liquid motion in addition to the wicking properties of the yearns. The authors also showed the fabrication of interfacial microfluidic device that can be used for collection and removal of sweat from the skin surface. However, the device was not tested in vivo but only with an artificial skin model. Another benefit of using a superhydrophilic material for fabric-based wearable microfluidics is the high gas permittivity of the fabric even in high humidity environment. When comparing wearable PDMS microfluidics with fabric microfluidics, one of the main advantages for the latter is the possibility to achieve a more straightforward integration of these devices with clothing, for the realization of smart garments. However, further developments of this technology are still needed especially on alternative fabrication routes that can guarantee high reproducibility and easy integration of microfluidics networks and sensors within clothing. Yarn weaving for the generation of hydrophilic/hydrophobic patterns as well as integration of electric active functional threads can possibly provide valid solutions to these challenges [64].

To conclude, it is also worth mentioning in this section a novel use of microfluidics for the fabrication of artificial skin models [65]. The most recent example of in vitro microfluidic skin model by Hou et al. was developed by mimicking both the skin pore density, hydrophobicity, wetting hysteresis, and skin texture [65]. An essential feature of this device was the use of a 0.2-mm track etched PC membrane that provides uniform sweat rate among the fabricated sweat pores. The use of these systems can be particularly advantageous for future in vitro testing of fluid transport in wearable microfluidic devices as well as to perform calibration of the sensors integrated inside those platforms. In addition to this, artificial skin model can also reduce the number of human and animal lab tests of wearable devices during development and testing phases.

3.2.2 Sampling strategies of other bodily fluids

Similarly, to sweat wearable sensors, adequate sampling strategies are required in order to perform real-time analysis of other bodily fluids. On the one hand, saliva and tears can be easily collected from the oral cavity and the eye, respectively, without the need of complex fluid-handling systems due to their abundance in normal conditions. On the other hand, the presence of mucus, food residuals, and blood in saliva has to be taken into account as these can interfere with the operation of the biosensors. Access to ISFs requires the use of semi-invasive technologies such as microdialysis probe or microneedles. An additional feature of the microneedle technology is the possibility to perform transdermal drug delivery, such as insulin that can easily reach the blood stream [66, 67]. However, one of the main drawbacks of this approach is possible clogging of needles during their operation when implanted under the epidermis, resulting in changes of their fluid dynamics and response time of the biosensor.

3.3 Microfluidic-based wearable devices

3.3.1 Colorimetric sensors

An ideal detection system for real-time analysis of sweat has to be simple, fast, and low cost. Colorimetric sensing systems offer rapid detection of analytes as a change in color of a specific chemistry occurs when expose to the analyte. Depending on the interaction of the analyte with the sensing molecules, colorimetric sensors can be able to detect single molecules (glucose, lactate, etc.), ions (H^+, Na^+, K^+, Cl^-), proteins, or even pathogens [68]. Colorimetric detection can be performed using standard spectrophotometry tools as well as high-definition cameras that are now integrated with smartphones.

Colorimetric sensors can be integrated with textile materials and used as textile-based fluid-handling platforms to collect and analysis sweat for real-time analysis, avoiding the use of mechanical micropumps. Morris et al. [69] have shown a first example of these devices through the combination of polyester/lycra textiles, where the fluid transport characteristic is influenced by the density and the ratio of the two materials. The fabric microfluidic was also functionalized with pH dyes sensors to obtain an on-fabric pH sensor with great fluid transport characteristics. An alternative approach was also described by Curto et al., where a flexible PMMA microfluidic device was developed, integrating a cotton thread to facilitate sweat transport inside the microchannel where sweat was driven toward the sensing area to measure real-time changes of sweat's pH [52]. This device was equipped with an LED-based detection system and a wireless module for data acquisition. Caldara et al. has also described the use of cotton textile modified with organic silicate to measure the pH of sweat, which is continuously monitored in situ with a wireless electronic sensor [70]. The use of paper for the realization of wearable sensors has been also investigated due to the excellent wicking and lightweight properties of paper as well as the easy functionalization of this substrate with chromophores. An excellent example has been proposed by Mu et al. for the realization of a paper skin patch able to detect sweat anions (lactate, bicarbonate, chloride) for a potential use in the screening of patients at risk of suffering of cystic fibrosis[71]. This easy-to-use paper-based skin patch was incorporated on an adhesive skin patch for seamless skin contact. Colorimetric detection can be performed with a mobile-phone camera, providing a valid alternative to the bulky and expensive devices commonly used for the diagnosis of cystic fibrosis. In addition to this, paper-based sensors have also found application for the colorimetric determination of pH levels in sweat and saliva as a tool to estimate dehydration levels during exercise and to prevent enamel decalcification, respectively [72]. The developed sensor platform consists of a 3D printed accessory that can be fitted to the backside of a smartphone covering both the smartphone camera and the LED. After exposure of the paper strip to the bodily fluid, the pH sensitive paper is inserted in the smartphone accessory and colorimetric determination of the pH is performed with a custom-made smartphone application.

Several other colorimetric sensors using flexible plastic-based microfluidic devices were also developed. One example of this type of device was demonstrated by Curto et al. with a PMMA microfluidic wearable sensor to collect and guide sweat to the active area to measure pH. Four different ionic liquid polymer gels (ionogels) were functionalized with four different pH dyes that present different pK_a in order to cover the full spectrum of the sweat pH [73]. The sensor was designed in order to create a pH colorimetric barcode. The four ionogels were photopolymerized at the inlet of the microfluidics and placed in direct contact with the skin in order to minimize the delay between sweat production and sensor response. Analyzed sweat was then collected on a highly absorbing fabric placed at the end of four independent channels. Colorimetric detection was also used by Matzeu et al. to study the sweat rate during exercise [74]. By combining a commercially available system (Macroducts) with video analysis, an estimation of the sweat flow rate over time was performed on several cycling trials showing the effectiveness of this simple and low-cost method. Future development of mobile phone applications for this system can provide a more straightforward way to estimate sweat rate in real time. PDMS-based microfluidic systems have also been proven as effective platforms to collect, store, and analyze sweat samples. Choi et al. have developed a thin, soft device able to conform to the skin, which allows the collection of sweat in micro reservoirs through a network of microchannels that integrates valves that open at different pressures [58]. A further development of a similar platform was also achieved by the integration of colorimetric sensors for sweat metabolites on the PDMS chip along with near-field communication (NFC) electronics [75]. Colorimetric analysis of sweat was performed by embedding functionalized filter paper within the microfluidic network for quantitative measurements of sweat rate, total sweat loss, pH, and concentration of chloride, glucose, and lactate. Estimation of the color change of the embedded paper was performed by digital image capture and analysis using a smartphone application. Interestingly, the NFC electronics integrated in the wearable patch was used to initiate the image capture and analysis software by simply placing the smartphone in close proximity to the sweat patch. However, one of the main limitations of this device is the impossibility to provide information of time-dependent changes in the biomarkers concentration. Future integration of enzyme-based sensors or functionalization of the microfluidic walls instead of the paper can give access to real-time feedbacks.

3.3.2 Electrochemical sensors

Electrochemical biosensing represents an appealing alternative to colorimetric sensors due to the greater sensitivity and selectivity of this technique for a large numbers of metabolites, such as glucose, lactate, sodium, and potassium [76–78]. The enhanced sensitivity and low detection limit of electrochemical biosensors has been possible due to recent advances in materials science with the development of novel materials such as conducting polymers, molecular imprinted polymers, organic, and inorganic nanoparticles [52].

Integration of electrochemical sensors with pilocarpine iontophoresis sweat harvesting techniques provides an alternative route for sweat analysis when the use microfluidic is not possible. In fact, this technique is more suitable for sweat analysis of individuals at rest where natural secretion of sweat does not occur and sweat stimulation is required. Temporary tattoos incorporating screen printed electrodes and cryogels were used to developed an ethanol biosensor [79]. Following sweat stimulation, a three electrode electrochemical biosensor using alcohol-oxidase enzyme was used for the amperometric determination of alcohol in sweat. Remarkably, in the same work the tattoo was integrated with a flexible integrated circuit with Bluetooth data communication capability. Sonner et al. used a similar approach to perform on-skin electrochemical measurements of sodium ions and sweat resistance with an iontophoretic device [80]. Carbon-based electrodes were printed and integrated on a PET substrate to provide mechanical stability to the whole platform. However, in this device the use of pressure to minimize the gap between the sensor and the skin was required and further improvements are required.

One of the first examples of a wearable electrochemical sensors for real-time sweat analysis was shown by Schazmann et al. with the development of a sweat sensor belt integrating a sodium selective electrode and a fabric-based pumping system to collect and guide the sweat toward the electrode active area [81]. However, this device made use of a glass sodium selective electrode and glass is not the most suitable substrate for wearable application. Matzeu et al. followed a different approach by integrating screen-printed electrodes with PMMA and a double-sided adhesive for the fabrication of a more compact and flexible sensor to measure sodium in sweat [82]. The electrodes were then incorporated in a microfluidic platform and a compact electronic read-out system was developed to perform real-time monitoring of sodium in sweat using wireless communication. A similar device was then further developed into a more compact design through the use of a passive pump microfluidic using highly absorbent fabric to collect and drive the liquid through the microchannels [83].

Novel sweat sensors that combine flexible epidermal microfluidic collection devices, electrochemical sensors, and a flexible electronic board have also been demonstrated. Martin et al. developed a skin-mounted device that integrates a flexible microfluidic and electrochemical sensing technology to detect lactate and glucose in sweat samples [84]. The wearable PDMS microfluidic consisted of a large reservoir for the electrochemical sensing of sweat and several inlets from which the sweat can be collected. Using four different inlets a total time of 8 min was required to fill the sensing chamber instead of the 30 min needed when using a single inlet, substantially decreasing the collection to analysis delay. The device was then tested during cycling activities while measuring levels of lactate and glucose in sweat. A different approach was employed by Anastasova et al. on the development of a PMMA-based microfluidic platform for sweat sensing [8]. In this case the microchannel of the flexible PMMA microfluidic was embedded with a fast-wicking paper to control the sweat flow inside the microdevice. Several sensors were placed inside the microchannels in order to measure pH, lactate, and sodium in sweat during running and cycling exercise routines. A very promising platform was recently proposed by Gao et al. with a fully integrated biosensing platform where the sensors in direct contact with the skin. In this novel sensor, simultaneous and selectively electrochemical measurement of glucose, lactate, sodium, and potassium in sweat, and skin temperature were successfully performed using an integrated flexible circuit capable of transmitting real-time data to a mobile phone via Bluetooth [85]. The sensors and a flexible circuit board were integrated into a silicone band which can be worn around the head or wrist during a physical activity. Interestingly, in this study the authors were able to test this platform on a large number of athletes and identifying trends in the time course variation of the sweat analytes related to changes in the physical state of the wearers.

3.4 Conclusion

The application of fully autonomous portable biosensors to measure body analytes for early detection of health issues is still in its infancy. Despite of the invasiveness of the collection techniques, blood is still the most used bodily fluid for patient health screening tests. As an emerging trend, much more interest has been given to the testing and use of other bodily fluids that are naturally secreted from the human body and are more accessible when compared to blood. In this regard, scientists have been working on novel strategies and technologies in order to establish direct correlation between analyte levels in blood and other biological fluids. Among the several biological fluids present in the body, there has been a great interest in the use of sweat, tears, and saliva due to the noninvasive techniques that can be employed for their collection and analysis.

Recent improvements in sensor miniaturization as well as microfluidic systems have made possible tremendous advances in the biosensor sensitivity and reproducibility, integration as well as portability. In the future, the development of novel sensor device architectures will heavily rely on the parallel development and interaction of all of these components rather than of the single ones. Concerning the detection techniques, electrochemical sensors are the most employed due to their typical higher sensitivity. However, colorimetric techniques bring the advantage of being easier to assess and analyze by bare eyes or more accurately through the use of mobile phone cameras. Microfluidics will also play an important role in the future and we have already shown examples of several wearable microfluidic devices with an enhanced performance. Delivery of the collected samples, for example, sweat, ISF, tears, etc., to the active area of the sensors as well as minimization of the collected sample volume are some of the improvements that microfluidics can bring to the wearable biosensor technology. Nevertheless, we believe there is considerable potential for future progress in these fields, and we await further creative experimentation and approaches to reveal the true efficacy of this interdisciplinary research. Given the size and importance of the biosensor market, paradigm-changing technologies are quick to grab the headlines. If all these recent trends reach commercial success, it would signal a major shift in the health-care industry and patients' life.

References

[1] A.M. Pappa, O. Parlak, G. Scheiblin, P. Mailley, A. Salleo, R.M. Owens, Organic electronics for point-of-care metabolite monitoring, Trends Biotechnol. 36 (1) (2018) 45–59.

[2] S. Choi, H. Lee, R. Ghaffari, T. Hyeon, D.H. Kim, Recent advances in flexible and stretchable bio-electronic devices integrated with nanomaterials, Adv. Mater. 28 (22) (2016) 4203–4218.

[3] A.P.F. Turner, Biosensors: sense and sensibility, Chem. Soc. Rev. 42 (8) (2013) 3184.

[4] A.N. Sekretaryova, M. Eriksson, A.P.F. Turner, Bioelectrocatalytic systems for health applications, Biotechnol. Adv. 34 (2016) 177–197.

[5] J. Heikenfeld, Bioanalytical devices: technological leap for sweat sensing, Nature 529 (7587) (2016) 475–476.

[6] Y. Yang, W. Gao, Wearable and flexible electronics for continuous molecular monitoring, Chem. Soc. Rev. 48 (6) (2019).

[7] J. Kim, A.S. Campbell, B.E.F. de Ávila, J. Wang, Wearable biosensors for healthcare monitoring, Nat. Biotechnol. 37 (2019) 389–406.

[8] S. Anastasova, et al., A wearable multisensing patch for continuous sweat monitoring, Biosens. Bioelectron. 93 (2017) 139–145.

[9] A.J. Bandodkar, J. Wang, Non-invasive wearable electrochemical sensors: a review, Trends Biotechnol. 32 (7) (2014) 363–371.

[10] J. Kim, et al., Wearable smart sensor systems integrated on soft contact lenses for wireless ocular diagnostics, Nat. Commun. 8 (2017) 14997.

[11] Y. Khan, A.E. Ostfeld, C.M. Lochner, A. Pierre, A.C. Arias, Monitoring of vital signs with flexible and wearable medical devices, Adv. Mater. 28 (2016) 4373–4395.

[12] D. Pankratov, E. González-Arribas, Z. Blum, S. Shleev, Tear based bioelectronics, Electroanalysis 28 (6) (2016) 1250–1266.

[13] A. Pantelopoulos, N.G. Bourbakis, A survey on wearable sensor-based systems for health monitoring and prognosis, IEEE Trans. Syst. Man Cybern. Part C Appl. Rev. 40 (1) (2010) 1–12.

[14] A.J. Shum, M. Cowan, I. Lähdesmäki, A. Lingley, B. Otis, B.A. Parviz, Functional modular contact lens, in: Biosensing II, 2009.

[15] N. Thomas, I. Lähdesmäki, B.A. Parviz, A contact lens with an integrated lactate sensor, Sensors Actuators B Chem. 162 (2012) 128–134.

[16] M.X. Chu, et al., Soft contact lens biosensor for in situ monitoring of tear glucose as non-invasive blood sugar assessment, Talanta 83 (2011) 960–965.

[17] D. Bruen, C. Delaney, L. Florea, D. Diamond, Glucose sensing for diabetes monitoring: recent developments, Sensors 17 (8) (2017) 1–21.

[18] D. Pankratov, Z. Blum, D.B. Suyatin, V.O. Popov, S. Shleev, Self-charging electrochemical biocapacitor, ChemElectroChem 1 (2) (2014) 343–346.

[19] D. Pankratov, Z. Blum, S. Shleev, Hybrid electric power biodevices, ChemElectroChem 1 (11) (2014) 1798–1807.

[20] M. Falk, et al., Biofuel cell as a power source for electronic contact lenses, Biosens. Bioelectron. 37 (2012) 38–45.

[21] J.R. Windmiller, J. Wang, Wearable electrochemical sensors and biosensors: a review, Electroanalysis 25 (2013) 29–46.

[22] H. Graf, H.R. Mühlemann, Oral telemetry of fluoride ion activity, Arch. Oral Biol. 14 (1969) 259–263.

[23] J. Kim, et al., Wearable salivary uric acid mouthguard biosensor with integrated wireless electronics, Biosens. Bioelectron. 74 (2015) 1061–1068.

[24] M.S. Mannoor, et al., Graphene-based wireless bacteria detection on tooth enamel, Nat. Commun. 3 (2012) 763.

[25] J. Heikenfeld, Non-invasive analyte access and sensing through eccrine sweat: challenges and outlook circa 2016, Electroanalysis 28 (2016) 1242–1249.

[26] O. Parlak, S.T. Keene, A. Marais, V.F. Curto, A. Salleo, Molecularly selective nanoporous membrane-based wearable organic electrochemical device for noninvasive cortisol sensing, Sci. Adv. 4 (2018).

[27] A.J. Bandodkar, et al., Tattoo-based potentiometric ion-selective sensors for epidermal pH monitoring, Analyst 138 (1) (2013) 123–128.

[28] J. Heikenfeld, Technological leap for sweat sensing, Nature 529 (2016) 475–476.

[29] M.D. Steinberg, P. Kassal, I.M. Steinberg, System architectures in wearable electrochemical sensors, Electroanalysis 28 (6) (2016) 1149–1169.

[30] D.H. Kim, et al., Epidermal electronics, Science 333 (2011) 838–843.

[31] J.R. Windmiller, A.J. Bandodkar, G. Valdés-Ramírez, S. Parkhomovsky, A.G. Martinez, J. Wang, Electrochemical sensing based on printable temporary transfer tattoos, Chem. Commun. 48 (54) (2012) 6794.

[32] W. Jia, et al., Electrochemical tattoo biosensors for real-time noninvasive lactate monitoring in human perspiration, Anal. Chem. 85 (14) (2013) 6553–6560.

[33] D.P. Rose, et al., Adhesive RFID sensor patch for monitoring of sweat electrolytes, IEEE Trans. Biomed. Eng. 62 (2015) 1457–1465.

[34] S. Imani, et al., A wearable chemical–electrophysiological hybrid biosensing system for real-time health and fitness monitoring, Nat. Commun. 7 (May) (2016) 11650.

[35] N.V. Zaryanov, V.N. Nikitina, E.V. Karpova, E.E. Karyakina, A.A. Karyakin, Nonenzymatic sensor for lactate detection in human sweat, Anal. Chem. 89 (2017) 11198–11202.

[36] W. Jia, G. Valdés-Ramírez, A.J. Bandodkar, J.R. Windmiller, J. Wang, Epidermal biofuel cells: energy harvesting from human perspiration, Angew. Chem. Int. Ed. 52 (28) (2013) 7233–7236.

[37] N. Kakehi, T. Yamazaki, W. Tsugawa, K. Sode, A novel wireless glucose sensor employing direct electron transfer principle based enzyme fuel cell, Biosens. Bioelectron. 22 (9–10) (2007) 2250–2255.

[38] A.K. Yetisen, J.L. Martinez-Hurtado, B. Ünal, A. Khademhosseini, H. Butt, Wearables in medicine, Adv. Mater. (2018) e1706910.

[39] R. Gifford, Continuous glucose monitoring: 40 years, what we've learned and what's next, ChemPhysChem 14 (2013) 2032–2044.

[40] A. Poscia, D. Messeri, D. Moscone, F. Ricci, F. Valgimigli, A novel continuous subcutaneous lactate monitoring system, Biosens. Bioelectron. 20 (2005) 2244–2250.

[41] A. Poscia, et al., A microdialysis technique for continuous subcutaneous glucose monitoring in diabetic patients (part 1), Biosens. Bioelectron. 18 (2003) 891–898.

[42] S.A. Gowers, et al., 3D printed microfluidic device with integrated biosensors for online analysis of subcutaneous human microdialysate, Anal. Chem. 87 (2015) 7763–7770.

[43] I.C. Samper, et al., 3D printed microfluidic device for online detection of neurochemical changes with high temporal resolution in human brain microdialysate, Lab Chip 19 (2019) 2038–2048.

[44] H. Lee, et al., Wearable/disposable sweat-based glucose monitoring device with multistage transdermal drug delivery module, Sci. Adv. 3 (3) (2017) e1601314.

[45] R. Guy, Diagnostic devices: managing diabetes through the skin, Nat. Nanotechnol. 11 (6) (2016) 493–494.

[46] R.M. Iost, F.C.P.F. Sales, M.V.A. Martins, M.C. Almeida, F.N. Crespilho, Glucose biochip based on flexible carbon fiber electrodes: in vivo diabetes evaluation in rats, ChemElectroChem 2 (2015) 518–521.

[47] A.E. Colvin, H. Jiang, Increased in vivo stability and functional lifetime of an implantable glucose sensor through platinum catalysis, J. Biomed. Mater. Res. A 101 (2013) 1274–1282.

[48] T.D. James, K.R.A.S. Sandanayake, S. Shinkai, A glucose-selective molecular fluorescence sensor, Angew. Chem. Int. Ed. 33 (1994) 2207–2209.

[49] F. Benito-Lopez, M. Antoñana-Díez, V.F. Curto, D. Diamond, V. Castro-López, Modular microfluidic valve structures based on reversible thermoresponsive ionogel actuators, Lab Chip 14 (2014) 3530.

[50] E.K. Sackmann, A.L. Fulton, D.J. Beebe, The present and future role of microfluidics in biomedical research, Nature 507 (2014) 181–189.

[51] C.W. Tsao, Polymer microfluidics: simple, low-cost fabrication process bridging academic lab research to commercialized production, Micromachines 7 (2016).

[52] V.F. Curto, S. Coyle, R. Byrne, N. Angelov, D. Diamond, F. Benito-Lopez, Concept and development of an autonomous wearable micro-fluidic platform for real time pH sweat analysis, Sensors Actuators B Chem. 175 (2012) 263–270.

[53] H.J. Liberty, B.D. Johnson, N. Fortner, Detecting cocaine use through sweat testing: multilevel modeling of sweat patch length-of-wear data, J. Anal. Toxicol. 28 (2004) 667–673.

[54] G.R. Brisson, P. Boisvert, F. Péronnet, H. Perrault, D. Boisvert, J.S. Lafond, A simple and disposable sweat collector, Eur. J. Appl. Physiol. Occup. Physiol. 63 (1991) 269–272.

[55] S.M. Shirreffs, R.J. Maughan, Whole body sweat collection in humans: an improved method with preliminary data on electrolyte content, J. Appl. Physiol. 82 (2017) 336–341.

[56] D.C. Duffy, J.C. McDonald, O.J.A. Schueller, G.M. Whitesides, Rapid prototyping of microfluidic systems in poly(dimethylsiloxane), Anal. Chem. 70 (1998) 4974–4984.

[57] F.K. Balagaddé, L. You, C.L. Hansen, F.H. Arnold, S.R. Quake, Microbiology: long-term monitoring of bacteria undergoing programmed population control in a microchemostat, Science 309 (2005) 137–140.

[58] J. Choi, et al., Soft, skin-mounted microfluidic systems for measuring secretory fluidic pressures generated at the surface of the skin by eccrine sweat glands, Lab Chip 17 (2017) 2572–2580.

[59] S. Xing, J. Jiang, T. Pan, Interfacial microfluidic transport on micropatterned superhydrophobic textile, Lab Chip 13 (10) (2013) 1937.

[60] T. Shay, M.D. Dickey, O.D. Velev, Hydrogel-enabled osmotic pumping for microfluidics: towards wearable human-device interfaces, Lab Chip 17 (2017) 710–716.

[61] M. Reches, K.A. Mirica, R. Dasgupta, M.D. Dickey, M.J. Butte, G.M. Whitesides, Thread as a matrix for biomedical assays, ACS Appl. Mater. Interfaces 2 (2010) 1722–1728.

[62] A.W. Martinez, S.T. Phillips, G.M. Whitesides, E. Carrilho, Diagnostics for the developing world: microfluidic paper-based analytical devices, Anal. Chem. 82 (2010) 3–10.

[63] Y. Yang, S. Xing, Z. Fang, R. Li, H. Koo, T. Pan, Wearable microfluidics: fabric-based digital droplet flowmetry for perspiration analysis, Lab Chip 17 (2017) 926–935.

[64] P. Mostafalu, M. Akbari, K.A. Alberti, Q. Xu, A. Khademhosseini, S.R. Sonkusale, A toolkit of thread-based microfluidics, sensors, and electronics for 3D tissue embedding for medical diagnostics, Microsyst. Nanoeng. 2 (2016) 16039.

[65] L. Hou, et al., Artificial microfluidic skin for in vitro perspiration simulation and testing, Lab Chip 13 (2013) 1868–1875.

[66] L. Ventrelli, L. Marsilio Strambini, G. Barillaro, Microneedles for transdermal biosensing: current picture and future direction, Adv. Healthc. Mater. 4 (2015) 2606–2640.

[67] M. Venugopal, et al., Clinical evaluation of a novel interstitial fluid sensor system for remote continuous alcohol monitoring, IEEE Sensors J. 8 (2008) 71–80.

[68] J.A. Adkins, K. Boehle, C. Friend, B. Chamberlain, B. Bisha, C.S. Henry, Colorimetric and electrochemical bacteria detection using printed paper- and transparency-based analytic devices, Anal. Chem. 89 (2017) 3613–3621.

[69] D. Morris, S. Coyle, Y. Wu, K.T. Lau, G. Wallace, D. Diamond, Bio-sensing textile based patch with integrated optical detection system for sweat monitoring, Sensors Actuators B Chem. 139 (2009) 231–236.

[70] M. Caldara, C. Colleoni, E. Guido, V. Re, G. Rosace, Optical monitoring of sweat pH by a textile fabric wearable sensor based on covalently bonded litmus-3-glycidoxypropyltrimethoxysilane coating, Sensors Actuators B Chem. 222 (2016) 213–220.

[71] X. Mu, et al., A paper-based skin patch for the diagnostic screening of cystic fibrosis, Chem. Commun. 51 (2015) 6365–6368.

[72] V. Oncescu, D. O'Dell, D. Erickson, Smartphone based health accessory for colorimetric detection of biomarkers in sweat and saliva, Lab Chip 13 (2013) 3232–3238.

[73] V.F. Curto, et al., Real-time sweat pH monitoring based on a wearable chemical barcode micro-fluidic platform incorporating ionic liquids, Sensors Actuators B Chem. 171-172 (2012) 1327–1334.

[74] G. Matzeu, C. Fay, A. Vaillant, S. Coyle, D. Diamond, A wearable device for monitoring sweat rates via image analysis, IEEE Trans. Biomed. Eng. 63 (2016) 1672–1680.

[75] A. Koh, et al., A soft, wearable microfluidic device for the capture, storage, and colorimetric sensing of sweat, Sci. Transl. Med. 8 (2016).

[76] F. Xiao, L. Wang, H. Duan, Nanomaterial based electrochemical sensors for in vitro detection of small molecule metabolites, Biotechnol. Adv. 34 (2016) 234–249.

[77] W. Jiang, D. Tian, L. Zhang, Q. Guo, Y. Cui, M. Yang, Dual signal amplification strategy for amperometric aptasensing using hydroxyapatite nanoparticles. Application to the sensitive detection of the cancer biomarker platelet-derived growth factor BB, Microchim. Acta 184 (2017) 4375–4381.

[78] X. Huang, Y. Liu, B. Yung, Y. Xiong, X. Chen, Nanotechnology-enhanced no-wash biosensors for in vitro diagnostics of cancer, ACS Nano 11 (2017) 5238–5293.

[79] J. Kim, et al., Noninvasive alcohol monitoring using a wearable tattoo-based iontophoretic-biosensing system, ACS Sens. 1 (2016) 1011–1019.

[80] Z. Sonner, E. Wilder, T. Gaillard, G. Kasting, J. Heikenfeld, Integrated sudomotor axon reflex sweat stimulation for continuous sweat analyte analysis with individuals at rest, Lab Chip 17 (2017) 2550–2560.

[81] B. Schazmann, et al., A wearable electrochemical sensor for the real-time measurement of sweat sodium concentration, Anal. Methods 2 (2010) 342–348.

[82] G. Matzeu, et al., An integrated sensing and wireless communications platform for sensing sodium in sweat, Anal. Methods 8 (2016) 64–71.

[83] T. Glennon, et al., 'SWEATCH': a wearable platform for harvesting and analysing sweat sodium content, Electroanalysis 28 (2016) 1283–1289.

[84] A. Martín, et al., Epidermal microfluidic electrochemical detection system: enhanced sweat sampling and metabolite detection, ACS Sens. 2 (2017) 1860–1868.

[85] W. Gao, et al., Fully integrated wearable sensor arrays for multiplexed in situ perspiration analysis, Nature 529 (7587) (2016) 509–514.

CHAPTER 4

Powering wearable bioelectronic devices

Alina Sekretaryova

Researcher, Department of Chemistry, Uppsala University, Uppsala, Sweden

Chapter outline

4.1 Introduction

Bioelectronics is defined as a field, exploiting "biology in conjunction with electronics in a wider context encompassing, for example, biological fuel cells, bionics, and biomaterials for information processing, information storage, electronic components, and actuators. A key aspect is the interface between biological materials and micro- and nano-electronics" [1]. The date of the invention of the wearable pacemaker, which relies on electronic technology applied to biology, in 1957 [2] is, thus, can be considered as a "birthday" of wearable bioelectronics. Wearable bioelectronics received revived attention starting from the beginning of the 21st century due to the progress in computer technology and the evolvement of the Internet of Things (IoT) devices. Over the last years, a wide variety of wearable devices, such as smartwatches, wristbands, activity trackers, smart jewelry, and skin patches, has appeared on the market [3]. And according to the recent market reports, the wearable technology market will grow with an expected 3 times increase by 2022 compared to 2016. At the same time, an enormous research effort is devoted to the development of the next-generation wearable devices with multiple functionalities able to detect numerous chemical and physical parameters of the human body [4].

Wearable Bioelectronics. https://doi.org/10.1016/B978-0-08-102407-2.00005-9

Wearable bioelectronic devices, able to perform measurements of multiple parameters and quickly transmit/receive data, demand integration of efficient wearable energy sources. The primary requirements such as small size, lightweight, and autonomous operation, imposed on wearable devices by wearer comfort limit suitable power sources. Most of the commercially available wearable devices use batteries as a power supply. Existing energy storage devices, however, are often too bulky, heavy, and rigid for continuous comfortable wearing, and currently, represent the main constraint of wearable technology [5]. The high power consumption of multifunctional wearables requires energy storage devices with higher energy densities, confined in smaller volumes, which can provide longer autonomous operation times without frequent replacement or recharging. Flexibility and/or stretchability of wearable devices essential for the wearer's convenience demand flexibility of a power supply or its special design allowing accommodating a rigid structure into a supple device.

Researchers are working in various directions to overcome issues facing powering technology for wearable applications. The studies focus mainly on improvement of existing energy storage/supply devices in terms of energy densities and flexibility, on the investigation of new energy-harvesting technologies, on development of integrated powering schemes based on a combination of energy-harvesting approaches and energy storage devices towards self-charging power systems [6] and on the employment of wireless power transfer (WPT). In the following text, we overview recent developments in power approaches for wearable bioelectronic devices. In Section 4.2, we start with a discussion of the existing power technology utilized in commercially available wearable devices and its limitations. We further consider strategies to improve energy densities and duration of autonomous operation of power storage/supply devices. Finally, we survey flexible batteries and chemical capacitors used in wearable devices. In Section 4.3, we examine energy-harvesting technologies that can potentially provide a "perpetual" power supply and thus are highly desirable for powering of wearable bioelectronic devices. We discuss main power sources available for energy harvesting by wearable devices, including chemical and physical energy of the human body and radiant energy provided by the sun, and power densities that can be generated with energy harvesters powered by these sources in comparison with power requirements of wearable devices presented on the market. In Section 4.4, we overview WPT strategies and their applications in wearable bioelectronic devices. Finally, in Section 4.5 we underline current problems and limitations of various powering approaches and strategies for their improvement, as well as general trends in powering technology for wearable bioelectronic devices.

4.2 Wearable energy storage/supply devices

Utilization of energy storage/supply devices, batteries, and supercapacitors, remains the most commonly applied powering strategy for wearable devices. While batteries and capacitors have many similarities, they differ significantly in the energy storage and conversion principle. Batteries convert chemical energy of a redox reaction taking place on an anode and a cathode to electrical energy. Potential energy in a capacitor is stored in an electric field. Currently, chemical energy storage technologies are more effective compared to potential energy storage systems, leading to higher energy densities of batteries and electrochemical capacitors (ECs) relative to conventional capacitors (Fig. 4.1). However, capacitors have an advantage of shorter charge and discharge times, generating higher power densities. ECs have relatively high power densities and higher energy densities compared to batteries and conventional capacitors, respectively [7].

To satisfy the needs of wearable devices, energy densities of batteries and capacitors and power densities of batteries should be further improved. While commercially available wearables are mainly powered by batteries, the recent trend of wearable bioelectronics towards increased complexity and multifunctionality will require more efficient technologies able to provide significantly higher energy densities confined in smaller volumes while retaining high power densities (the trend is shown as an arrow in Fig. 4.1). In this section, we discuss recent progress in energy storage/supply devices aiming to match the increasing demands of wearable bioelectronics.

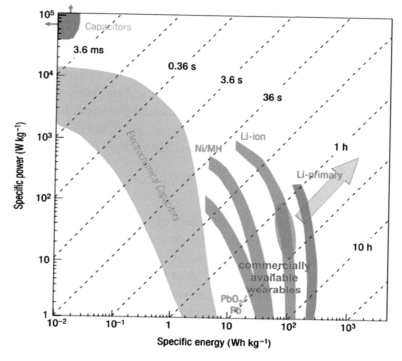

Fig. 4.1
A Ragon plot showing the performance comparison of various energy storage/supply devices with requirements of currently available wearable devices [3]. *Reproduced with modifications from P. Simon, Y. Gogotsi, Materials for electrochemical capacitors. Nat. Mater. 7 (2008) 845. Copyright ©2008, Springer Nature.*

4.2.1 Batteries

4.2.1.1 Limitations of conventional lithium batteries for wearable bioelectronics

Lithium-ion batteries (LIBs), despite their limitations which will be discussed further, are one of the most popular types of power supplies for wearable electronic devices due to their high energy densities, low self-discharge rates, and high working voltages [8]. A typical LIB consists of a cathode, an anode, and an electrolyte in between them (Fig. 4.2). During discharge, Li^+ ions are moving from a negative electrode, anode, to a positive electrode, cathode, through an electrolyte, while electrons in an external circuit are flowing in the opposite direction producing energy. During charging the movement of ions is reversed by applying electric energy. A cathode in conventional LIBs is made from lithium metal oxides, such as $LiCoO_2$, $LiFePO_4$, and $LiMn_2O_4$, while carbon materials such as graphite are used as an anode. These materials in the form of a slurry are coated on the surface of a rigid copper or aluminum foil, which acts as an electrode. Lithium salts dissolved in an organic solvent or Li-containing polymers are usually used as an electrolyte [8, 9].

Applications in wearable electronics impose a number of requirements on conventional LIBs, such as lightweight and compactness while retaining high power densities. Conventional small-size batteries can maintain low-power wearable devices, but their compelled use in more power-demanding commercially available wearables such as fitness bands and smartwatches resulted in products that should be constantly recharged. The current trend of wearable technology towards the incorporation of chemical and biosensors together with physical sensors in one device [10] introduces one more prerequisite for LIBs. Chemical sensors and biosensors need to be in direct contact with liquid samples of the human body, which will be measured by a wearable device, thus, demanding flexibility of the device and all its parts including a power source.

4.2.1.2 Strategies to increase battery durability

A possible solution to the problem of short battery life of LIBs is to develop batteries with higher storage capacity. Battery material design on a nanoscale is a common strategy to boost charge capacity. There are a number of recent reviews available on the utilization of nanomaterials for energy storage [11–13]. Most frequently used nanomaterials include nanofibers [14] and nanowires (NWs) [15], carbon-based nanomaterials, such as graphene [16] and carbon nanotubes (CNTs) [17, 18] and nanoparticles [19]. Another approach is to expand redox chemistries between charge-carrier ions and a host material beyond the conventional intercalation mechanism. Materials based on the intercalation of charge ions for energy storage have a limited number of crystallographic sites available for ion storing. So, new chemistries for energy storage attract the significant attention of scientists resulting in growth of so-called post-lithium-ion batteries (post-LIBs) research [20]. Studies are

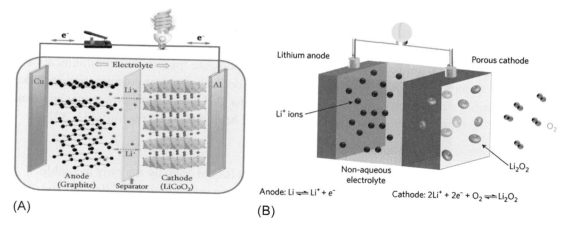

Fig. 4.2

Conventional and post-LIBs. (A) A scheme of a conventional rechargeable LIB. (B) Example of a post-LIB based on Li_2O_2 cathode. *Part (A) reprinted with permission from C. Liu, Z.G. Neale, G. Cao, Understanding electrochemical potentials of cathode materials in rechargeable batteries. Mater. Today 19 (2016) 109–123. Copyright ©2015 The Authors. Published by Elsevier Ltd and (B) reprinted with permission from D. Aurbach, B.D. McCloskey, L.F. Nazar, P.G. Bruce, Advances in understanding mechanisms underpinning lithium–air batteries. Nat. Energy 1 (2016) 16128. Copyright ©2016, Springer Nature.*

implemented in a few directions: investigations of silicon as an anode material, of layered nickel-rich or manganese-rich cathode materials, of lithium-metal anodes, of lithium-sulfur batteries, of metal-oxygen battery systems, and of sodium-ion batteries. A wide range of post-LIBs promising for wearable electronics is discussed in several excellent reviews on the topic [20–23].

A battery developed by Li's group at Kansas State University is a remarkable example of a combination of these two approaches. The authors reported a high-performance hybrid lithium-ion anode material based on silicon rather than graphite for Li intercalation that provided higher capacity limits, shorter charging periods, and significantly longer battery lifetimes [14, 24]. Coaxially coated silicon shells on vertically aligned carbon nanofiber cores and vertically aligned carbon nanofiber coated with lithium cobalt oxide were used as an anode and a cathode, respectively. This invention resulted in a number of patents [25, 26] and a formation of a spin-off company Catalyst Power Technologies Inc. Imprint Energy is another high-tech company, originating from research at Berkley University [27, 28], which targets the wearables market with miniaturized post-LIBs zinc-carbon batteries that work similarly to LIBs but use zinc instead of lithium. By printing multiple layers of ultra-thin film, Imprint can create highly flexible batteries that could power ultra-thin medical sensors and smart bandages.

Another solution to the problem of short battery life in wearables is to reduce the power consumption of electronics. Since wireless communication is typically the most power-demanding activity in wearable bioelectronics, many researchers are trying to develop systems with lower power requirements of the part responsible for wireless communication. Approaches to increase battery durability through the decreased power consumption include development of effective data compression mechanisms [29] and various power management strategies [30]. Many reviews covering this topic have been published recently [31, 32].

4.2.1.3 Flexible/stretchable batteries

The current progress of soft truly wearable electronics is held back by the only available bulky and rigid powering sources, which triggers intensive investigations of flexible and stretchable wearable batteries [33–35]. An ideal wearable battery should maintain safe and stable operation under mechanical deformations and not cause discomfort to a user. Such batteries can be implemented using deterministic or random composite architectures [36]. The random composite design is based on the incorporation of highly conductive fillers, such as carbon nanomaterials and metallic NWs, into a stretchable matrix. Deterministic composites use intrinsically rigid materials, which are transformed into elastic structures by the specific engineering [36]. For example, Yan et al. reported a stretchable silver-zinc battery based on silver nanowires (AgNWs) embedded into an elastomeric polydimethylsiloxane (PDMS) substrate [15]. An AgNW/PDMS structure was used as a cathode and a stretchable anode was fabricated by electroplating zinc on an AgNW/PDMS substrate. Roger's group developed a stretchable battery that consisted of disks of rigid lithium batteries electrically connected in parallel by deformable electrical interconnects (Fig. 4.3A) [37].

Development of wearable fiber-shaped batteries has emerged recently as a new direction in battery research. In contrast to conventional batteries, fiber-shaped devices are highly resistive to deformations and can be woven into textiles with porous structures, allowing the fabrication of breathable power supplies. Fiber-shaped batteries are generally constructed by twisting two fiber electrodes [8], forming helically coaxial or parallel structures [33]. For example, Kwon et al. designed a cable-type flexible battery with a helically coaxial structure comprised of several Ni-Sn anode strands coiled into a hollow spiral (helical) core and surrounded by a tubular outer $LiCoO_2$ cathode [19]. While being highly flexible and exhibiting stable discharge characteristics, the battery under bending was too large to be further woven and demonstrated the low capacity of $1\,mA\,h\,cm^{-1}$. Peng and coworkers developed a wire-shaped LIB with better performances made from two parallelly aligned multi-walled CNT/lithium oxide composite yarns as an anode and a cathode [38]. The battery had remarkable energy densities of $27\,Wh\,kg^{-1}$ or $17.7\,mWh\,cm^{-3}$ and power densities of $880\,W\,kg^{-1}$ or $0.56\,W\,cm^{-3}$. The aforementioned fiber-shaped batteries possess a deterministic architecture, which makes them endurable to bending, tying, and twisting. However, their structures could be damaged under stretching limiting their application for wearable bioelectronic devices. Elastic fiber-shaped batteries with the random composite design have

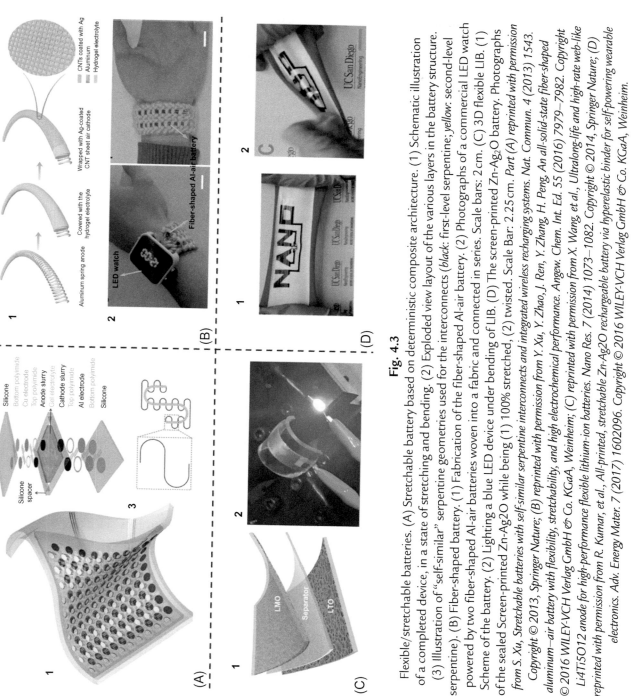

Fig. 4.3

Flexible/stretchable batteries. (A) Stretchable battery based on deterministic composite architecture. (1) Schematic illustration of a completed device, in a state of stretching and bending. (2) Exploded view layout of the various layers in the battery structure. (3) Illustration of "self-similar" serpentine geometries used for the interconnects (*black*: first-level serpentine; *yellow*: second-level serpentine). (B) Fiber-shaped battery. (1) Fabrication of the fiber-shaped Al-air battery. (2) Photographs of a commercial LED watch powered by two fiber-shaped Al-air batteries woven into a fabric and connected in series. Scale bars: 2 cm. (C) 3D flexible LIB. (1) Scheme of the battery. (2) Lighting a blue LED device under bending of LIB. (D) The screen-printed Zn-Ag$_2$O battery. Photographs of the sealed Screen-printed Zn-Ag$_2$O battery while being (1) 100% stretched, (2) twisted. Scale Bar: 2.25 cm. Part (A) reprinted with permission from S. Xu, Stretchable batteries with self-similar serpentine interconnects and integrated wireless recharging systems. *Nat. Commun.* 4 (2013) 1543. Copyright © 2013, Springer Nature; (B) reprinted with permission from Y. Xu, Y. Zhao, J. Ren, Y. Zhang, H. Peng, An all-solid-state fiber-shaped aluminum—air battery with flexibility, stretchability, and high electrochemical performance. *Angew. Chem. Int. Ed.* 55 (2016) 7979–7982. Copyright © 2016 WILEY-VCH Verlag GmbH & Co. KGaA, Weinheim; (C) reprinted with permission from X. Wang, et al., Ultralong-life and high-rate web-like Li$_4$Ti$_5$O$_{12}$ anode for high-performance flexible lithium-ion batteries. *Nano Res.* 7 (2014) 1073–1082. Copyright © 2014, Springer Nature; (D) reprinted with permission from R. Kumar, et al., All-printed, stretchable Zn-Ag$_2$O rechargeable battery via hyperelastic binder for self-powering wearable electronics. *Adv. Energy Mater.* 7 (2017) 1602096. Copyright © 2016 WILEY-VCH Verlag GmbH & Co. KGaA, Weinheim.

been also developed. Zhang et al. developed a "super-stretchable" battery by winding aligned CNT fibers incorporated with active lithium oxides, on an elastomer substrate, followed by coating with a thin layer of a gel electrolyte [17]. The specific capacity of $91.3\,mA\,h\,g^{-1}$ was achieved and could be maintained up to 88% after stretching by 600%.

Fiber-shaped LIBs can be further woven into textiles, which was demonstrated for fiber-shaped batteries developed by Peng and coworkers [38, 39] (Fig. 4.3B) and by Zhang et al. [17] Research on LIB textiles is still in its infancy, and many factors, such as washability, comfort, and safety should be carefully considered before this technology can be used for powering wearable electronics [40].

Another important type of flexible batteries that can be advantageous for wearable bioelectronics are 3D flexible LIBs. An example is a flexible LIB, developed by Shen and coworkers, with 3D web-like $Li_4Ti_5O_{12}$ (LTO) nanorods attached to a flexible stainless steel foil as the cathode and $LiMn_2O_4$ (LMO) nanorods on a Ti foil as the anode (Fig. 4.3C) [41]. The assembled battery showed good mechanical flexibility and high stability under deformation.

All described flexible batteries are, in general, not economically efficient since they rely on expansive fabrication procedures. Printed non-rechargeable batteries—an emerging market with main applications in wearable electronics, which is expected to have a value of 1.2 billion by 2020 [36]. Cost-effective stretchable batteries can be effectively produced using printing inks based on random composites. The earlier-mentioned Imprint Energy manufactures 3D-printed zinc rechargeable batteries. The technology developed by the company allows the production of slim and flexible batteries of various shapes. Wang and coworkers reported a highly stretchable zinc-silver oxide all-printed battery (Fig. 4.3D) [36]. The battery was printed on hyperplastic (~1300% elongation) polystyrene-block-polyisoprene-block-polystyrene. The resulted battery demonstrated a reversible capacity density of $2.5\,mA\,h\,cm^{-2}$ even after multiple iterations of 100% stretching.

4.2.2 Electrochemical capacitors

ECs (or supercapacitors) are promising power sources for wearable bioelectronics since they possess fast charge/discharge rates, high power densities and, what is more important, long cycle lives (thousands to millions of cycles compared to hundreds for rechargeable batteries) [7].

4.2.2.1 Charge storage mechanism

Based on the energy storage mechanism, ECs are further divided into several types: electrochemical double-layer capacitors (EDLCs), pseudocapacitors, and hybrid capacitors. In EDLCs, electrical energy is stored by double-layer capacitance, while pseudocapacitors store electrical energy by surface Faradaic processes, that is, electron charge transfer reactions between an electrode and an electrolyte. A hybrid capacitor is a combination of an EDLC or a pseudocapacitor and a battery [7] (Fig. 4.4).

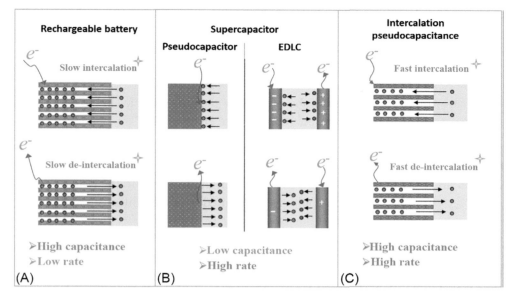

Fig. 4.4
A scheme of different charge storage mechanisms: (A) rechargeable battery, (B) supercapacitor, and (C) intercalation pseudocapacitance. *Reproduced with modifications from Y. Wang, Y. Song, Y. Xia, Electrochemical capacitors: mechanism, materials, systems, characterization and applications. Chem. Soc. Rev. 45 (2016) 5925–5950. Copyright © 2016, Royal Society of Chemistry.*

Rechargeable batteries and pseudocapacitors both use redox reactions to store charges. However, processes taking place in batteries and pseudocapacitors differ significantly in their electrochemistry [42]. Redox reactions in batteries are controlled by cation diffusion within the active material, and the observed current response for this process can be described as follows [43]:

$$i = nFACD^{1/2}v^{1/2}\left(\frac{\alpha n\pi F}{RT}\right)^{1/2}$$
(4.1)

where n is the number of electrons involved in the electrode reaction, F is the Faraday constant, A is the surface area of the electrode, C is a surface concentration of the active material, D is the diffusion coefficient, v is the potential sweep rate, α is the transfer coefficient, R is the gas constant, and T is the temperature. As can be seen from Eq. (4.1), the current response of the battery depends on the square root of the potential sweep rate. The electrode process of a pseudocapacitor is not diffusion controlled, since electroactive species are electro-adsorbed on the electrode material, and the current should vary linearly with the potential sweep rate according to [43]:

$$i = C_d Av$$
(4.2)

where C_d is the capacitance of a pseudocapacitor.

Batteries and pseudocapacitors can be distinguished by cyclic voltammetry (CV). While batteries show clear redox peaks on CVs, pseudocapacitors exhibit rectangular CV shapes. This difference originates from the charge storage mechanism. In pseudocapacitors, the electrode potential of the electroabsorbed redox species is a continuous logarithmic function of the extent of sorption, resulting in rectangular-shaped CVs. In batteries, the electrode potential is determined by the free Gibbs energies of the redox species in the system, resulting in peaks on CVs at potentials, corresponding to these energies [42].

Intercalation pseudocapacitance is a new type of charge storage mechanism and is a hybrid mechanism between those of a pseudocapacitor and a battery (Fig. 4.4). The charge, in this case, is stored by the intercalation/de-intercalation of cations to the bulk of the active material. In general, this process should not be limited by cation diffusion and current should linearly depend on the potential sweep rate, as described in Eq. (4.2). However, for many reported electrode materials possessing intercalation pseudocapacitance, the current dependence on the potential sweep rate cannot be described by Eq. (4.2), and the current is proportional to v^b, where b is <1. Thus, these materials demonstrate a hybrid storage mechanism, where the current can be described as a combination [44]:

$$i = k_1 v + k_2 v^{1/2}$$

(4.3)

where $k_1 v$ represents the capacitive storage mechanism as in a pseudocapacitor and $k_2 v^{1/2}$ represents the diffusion-controlled insertion mechanism as in a battery.

The intercalation pseudocapacitance mechanism unites the main advantage of batteries, high energy densities, due to charge storage in the bulk of the electrode material, and advantages of supercapacitors, high power densities, and long cycle lives due to a lack of diffusion limitations [42]. Thus, materials based on the intercalation mechanism can be of high importance for the powering of wearable bioelectronics. However, powering devices for wearables using this mechanism have not been reported yet.

4.2.2.2 Flexible electrochemical capacitors

As in the case of wearable batteries, flexible ECs are the most suitable capacitors to fit the requirements of wearable electronics. Flexible ECs usually consist of two electrodes, an aqueous or solid electrolyte, and a separator layer. ECs can be asymmetric, assembled from two different electrodes, or symmetric, made of two identical electrodes. Flexible ECs could be classified based on their microstructures into three groups: fiber-like, three-dimensional porous, and paper-like ECs [7]. Mechanical and electrochemical properties of flexible ECs, as well as their further subclassification within each type, are described in detail in the recent review [7]. Here, we consider most interesting examples of flexible ECs for wearable applications.

Meng et al. designed an all-graphene core-sheath fiber with a graphene flake core covered with a sheath of a 3D porous network-like graphene structure [45]. The flexible all-solid state EC was assembled from two intertwined fibers solidified in a sulfuric acid-polyvinyl alcohol gel electrolyte. The resulted EC exhibited high flexibility being able to be bent, knotted, and shaped into a stretchable spring-like structure. It could be also woven into textiles for wearable applications. However, the areal capacitance of the EC was not very high (1.2–1.7 mF cm^{-2}), which is too low for powering wearable electronics. Fiber-like ECs based on an activated carbon fiber (CF) cloth modified with CNTs and MnO$_2$ were recently developed (Fig. 4.5A) [46]. The final composite electrode had the capacitance of 640 mF cm^{-2}, the energy density of 11.1 µW h cm^{-2}, and the power density of 8028 µW cm^{-2}, which is much higher than the previously reported values for flexible ECs. The composite flexible electrode

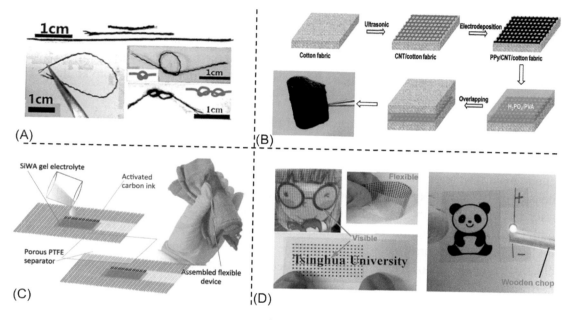

Fig. 4.5

Flexible electrochemical capacitors. (A) Photos of flexible fiber-shaped ECs. (B) Schematic illustration for the preparation and the photograph of the flexible fabric-based EC. (C) Schematic of EC fabricated by screen printing onto a knitted carbon cloth. To the right is an assembled device demonstrating the flexibility as it is bent almost in half. PTFE: Porous membrane separator, SiWA: a solid polymer electrolyte. (D) Photographs of screen-printed paper-like electrodes demonstrating good optical transparency and mechanical flexibility and of the "panda" asymmetric EC lighting up a red light emitting diode. *Part (A) reprinted with permission from L. Dong, et al., Flexible electrodes and supercapacitors for wearable energy storage: a review by category. J. Mater. Chem. A 4 (2016) 4659–4685. Copyright © 2016, Royal Society of Chemistry; (B) reproduced with modifications from S Huang, et al., Electrodeposition of polypyrrole on carbon nanotube-coated cotton fabrics for all-solid flexible supercapacitor electrodes. RSC Adv. 6 (2016) 13359–13364. Copyright © 2016, Royal Society of Chemistry; (C) reprinted with permission from K. Jost, et al., Knitted and screen printed carbon-fiber supercapacitors for applications in wearable electronics. Energy Environ. Sci. 6 (2013) 2698–2705. Copyright © 2013, Royal Society of Chemistry; (D) reproduced with modifications from S. Shi, et al., Flexible asymmetric supercapacitors based on ultrathin two-dimensional nanosheets with outstanding electrochemical performance and aesthetic property. Sci. Rep. 3 (2013). Copyright © 2013, Springer Nature.*

could be bent and knotted with a retention of 91% of the capacitance after 100 repetitive bending.

3D porous structures based on textiles, such as cotton cloths, polyester microfibers twills, and CF fabrics, loaded with active materials can be used for the fabrication of power-supplying garments for wearable bioelectronics [40]. For example, Huang et al. loaded cotton fabrics with CNTs modified with electrochemically deposited polypyrrole to fabricate all-solid, flexible ECs (Fig. 4.5B) [47]. The EC had a specific capacitance of $201.99\,F\,g^{-1}$ at $1.8\,A\,g^{-1}$. Due to the cotton-based substrate, the supercapacitor is comfortable when worn and when in contact with the skin. Its flexibility, low-cost, and wearability make this supercapacitor a good candidate as an energy-storage device for wearable bioelectronics. Direct printing of an active material onto textiles represents another promising technology for the cost-effective fabrication of flexible ECs. Dion and coworkers reported the fabrication of a textile EDLC that was made by the screen printing of an activated carbon paint onto a custom knitted CF cloth and utilized a solid polymer electrolyte (SiWA) (Fig. 4.5C) [48].

Printing can be also used for the fabrication of paper-like flexible ECs. Shi et al. reported flexible asymmetric ECs made of ultrathin two-dimensional MnO_2 and graphene nanosheets screen-printed on the indium tin oxide-polyethylene terephthalate substrate as cathode and anode materials, respectively (Fig. 4.5D) [49]. The screen-printed EC showed a high energy density up to $97.2\,Wh\,kg^{-1}$, a specific capacitance of up to $175\,F\,g^{-1}$, which reduced by <3% after 10,000 charging cycles. Fan and coworkers demonstrated an all-solid-state planar EC with interdigitated metal finger arrays inkjet printed on a flexible substrate [50]. Following inkjet printing, the hierarchical nickel/manganese dioxide nanocoral structures were electrochemically deposited on the interdigitated finger arrays to enhance pseudocapacitive performance. The EC exhibited the highest specific power of $39.6\,W\,cm^{-3}$ and the specific energy of $11.1\,mWh\,cm^{-3}$.

4.3 Wearable energy-harvesting devices

An energy harvesting (or an energy scavenging) device is a "green" power generator that uses energy available in the ambient, such as electromagnetic energy, temperature gradients, wind, water flows, etc. to power electronics. Energy sources available for powering of wearable bioelectronics can be divided into four main types: mechanical, thermal, radiant, and biochemical (Fig. 4.6) [51]. These energy sources are able to generate different power densities and the use of one or another source is determined by the power consumption of the wearable device. Typically, wearable sensors require power densities ranging from several µW to several mW [52]. So, theoretically, energy harvesters can provide sufficient power densities for the constant use of wearable bioelectronics without additional power supplies; however, practical considerations are needed to demonstrate feasibility of this approach.

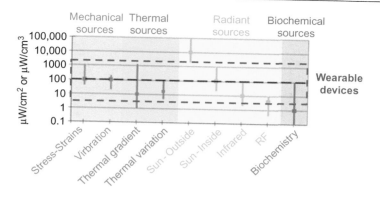

Fig. 4.6

Energy sources available for energy harvesting devices with their typical power outputs. The power output range required for the powering of commercially available wearable devices [3] is highlighted. *Source: CEA-Leti.*

In this section, energy harvesting devices utilizing the energy of the human body and radiant sources will be considered. Human energy is available in physical and chemical forms. Physical sources include thermal and kinetic energy of the human body. Thermoelectric generators (TEGs) convert the human body's heat into electricity. Kinetic energy is generated from the movement of the human body, such as muscle movements, motions of joints, and center-of-gravity (COG) motion of the upper body [52]. Chemical energy can be harvested from body fluids, such as interstitial fluids, sweat, saliva, or tears using biofuel cells (BFCs).

4.3.1 Biofuel cells

A BFC is an electrochemical cell that converts the chemical energy of a biological catalytic reaction into electricity by oxidizing a fuel at an anode and reducing an oxidant at a cathode (Fig. 4.7A) [53–55]. Depending on a catalyst used for the fuel oxidation, BFCs can be divided to microbial BFCs and enzymatic BFCs. Microbial BFCs utilize whole cells or organelles as catalysts. In enzymatic BFCs, enzymes are used as a catalyst for fuel oxidation. Cells in which the reaction at only one electrode is catalyzed by an enzyme and the other is a noble metal catalyst are also categorized as enzymatic BFCs [54]. Both microbial and enzymatic BFCs can be potentially used as a power supply for wearable electronics.

4.3.1.1 Figure-of-Merit for BFCs

There are a number of parameters that should be considered when using BFCs as a power source for wearable bioelectronics. One of the main characteristics of a BFC is the power output, which depends on the current detected at different cell voltages (Fig. 4.7B–D). One side of this dependence is the so-called open circuit potential (OCP), which is an indicator

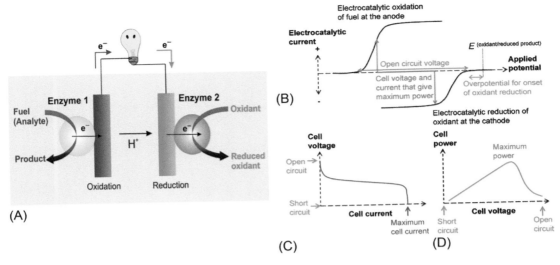

Fig. 4.7

The working principle of a biofuel cell and factors determining its performance. (A) An illustration of a BFC. Voltage and current response for a pair of fuel cell electrodes tested separately (B) or operating together in a BFC (C and D). Features that determine BFC performance are highlighted. *(A) Reprinted with permission from A. N. Sekretaryova, Facilitating Electron Transfer in Bioelectrocatalytic Systems. PhD Theses, Linköping University Electronic Press, Linköping, 2016, Copyright © 2016 The Author. Published by Linkoping University Electronic Press. (B–D) Reprinted with permission from J.A. Cracknell, K.A. Vincent, F.A. Armstrong, Enzymes as working or inspirational electrocatalysts for fuel cells and electrolysis, Chem. Rev. 108 (2008) 2439–2461, Copyright © 2008 American Chemical Society.*

of the maximum voltage that can be supplied by the BFC. It is determined as a difference between the formal redox potentials of the fuel/product and oxidant/reduced oxidant couples. On the other side, there is the short circuit current, which occurs when the anode and the cathode are electrically connected without any voltage being applied. The current generated by a BFC is determined by the slowest electrocatalytic reaction, either the reaction taking place on the cathode or the reaction on the anode. The maximum electrocatalytic current that can be achieved at the anode or the cathode depends on the density of catalytically active sites and the rate of catalysis per active site. A useful power density that can be used for powering electronic devices lies usually at the current and voltage values between the OCP and the short circuit potential [54].

The power density generated by a BFC is a key parameter determining its potential applicability for powering wearable devices. While microbial BFCs have a number of advantages compared to enzymatic BFCs such as higher stability and capability to completely oxidize fuels due to multiple enzymes present in cells, they, in general, have much lower power densities than enzymatic BFCs, which limits their use in wearable bioelectronics [5].

4.3.1.2 Noninvasive body fluid-based BFCs

Body fluids available for noninvasive sampling contain a number of metabolites such as lactate, glucose, pyruvate, and ethanol that can be oxidized by appropriate enzymes in the anodic reaction and, thus, act as a fuel for a BFC. The cathode reaction is usually based on oxygen-reducing enzymes, multicopper oxidases: laccases or bilirubin oxidases, which reduce oxygen to water in a four-electron reaction. The typical reaction taking place in a BFC using glucose as a fuel can be described as follows [19]:

$$\text{anode}: C_6H_{12}O_6 + 2OH^- \rightarrow C_6H_{12}O_7 + H_2O + 2e^-, \tag{4.4}$$

$$\text{cathode}: 1/2\,O_2 + H_2O + 2e^- \rightarrow 2OH^-, \tag{4.5}$$

$$\text{overall}: C_6H_{12}O_6 + 1/2\,O_2 \rightarrow C_6H_{12}O_7, \tag{4.6}$$

$$\Delta G^0 = 0.251 \times 10^6 \text{ Jmol}^{-1}, \tag{4.7}$$

$$U^0 = 1.30 \text{ V} \tag{4.8}$$

where ΔG^0 is the standard free energy and U^0 is the theoretical cell voltage.

Human sweat can be used as an efficient fuel for a BFC. Lactate concentration in sweat lies in the range between 3.7 and 50 mM [56], which is significantly higher than the concentrations of other metabolites and is sufficient to produce power densities required for a wearable operation. Sweat-based wearable BFCs reported in the literature have two different architectures: epidermal, that is, BFCs worn directly on the skin, and BFCs embedded into textiles [5]. Wang and coworkers designed an epidermal BFC which uses sweat lactate as a fuel [57]. The BFC was constructed from two carbon electrodes screen-printed onto a tattoo paper. The anode was first modified with carboxy-functionalized CNTs and tetrathiafulvalene as an enzyme mediator, then a mixture of lactate oxidase, an enzyme-oxidizing lactate to pyruvate with high selectivity, and albumin was drop-cast onto the surface of the anode, followed by a chitosan solution. The cathode was modified with platinum black, an oxygen reduction catalyst, and covered by a Nafion membrane. Mediated enzymatic oxidation of lactate at the anode and oxygen reduction at the cathode in real time resulted in power densities in the range of 5–70 μW cm^{-2} depending on the individual [10]. The same group later demonstrated the incorporation of the lactate-based BFC with the above-described structure into textiles [58]. This time, the BFCs were printed onto detachable care labels that can be applied to clothing and apparels. To demonstrate BFCs operation in real time, the labels were attached to a headband and a wristband, and using a DC/DC converter, were used to power an LED or a digital watch. Low power densities of the developed wearable BFCs and their limited stretchability restrain their real-life applications for powering wearable bioelectronics. Bandodkar et al. tried to overcome these issues by designing a soft, stretchable electronic-skin-based BFC that demonstrated a power density of nearly 1.2 mW cm^2, which is the highest power density achieved by a wearable BFC to date [59]. The high power density was achieved due to the special BFC design: a lithographically patterned stretchable electronic framework was combined with a screen-printed, 3D carbon-nanotube-based bioanode and cathode array arranged in a stretchable "island-bridge" structure, similar to those reported earlier for batteries (Fig. 4.8A) [37]. The designed BFC was able to power a Bluetooth Low Energy radio, however, only under in vitro conditions.

Tears contain a number of analytes that can be used to power wearable BFCs [60]. Shleev's group demonstrated the integration of a glucose-powered BFC into a contact lens as a power source for the biosensing device operating in tears [61]. The reported BFC consisted of gold microwires covered with gold nanoparticles, which were functionalized by cellobiose dehydrogenase, an enzyme able to oxidize glucose to gluconolactone, and bilirubin oxidase, an enzyme from the multicopper oxidases family catalyzing four-electron oxygen reduction to water, as the anodic and cathodic counterparts, respectively (Fig. 4.8B). The BFCs generated the maximum power density of $1\,\mu W\,cm^{-2}$ and showed more than 20 h of operational half-life. The same group later reported a similar gold nanoparticles/gold-microwires-based BFC powered by ascorbate in tears [62]. While the cathode retained the same architecture, the anode was modified with an efficient catalyst for ascorbate oxidation—the tetrathiafulvalene/

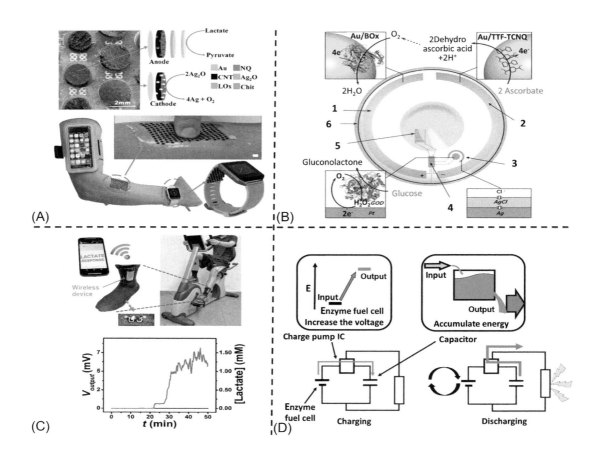

tetracyanoquinodimethane (TTF-TCNQ) complex. When operating in tears, the BFC generated the maximal power densities of $3.1\,\mu W\,cm^{-2}$ at $0.25\,V$ and $0.72\,\mu W\,cm^{-2}$ at $0.4\,V$, with the stable current density output of over $0.55\,\mu A\,cm^{-2}$ at $0.4\,V$ for 6 h of continuous operation.

Recently, saliva-powered BFCs have been reported. Shleev's group tested the operation of the aforementioned gold nanowires-based BFC powered by glucose [61] in human saliva [63]. The BFC had the OCP of $560\,mV$ and the power density of $0.1\,\mu W\,cm^{-2}$ at a cell voltage of $0.5\,V$. Approximately a twofold increase in the power density was observed in saliva collected after meal ingestion. Bollella et al. demonstrated a proof-of-concept glucose/oxygen enzymatic BFCs operating in human saliva [64]. A graphene working electrode, modified with gold nanoparticles, poly(vinyl alcohol) *N*-methyl-4(4-formylstyryl)pyridinium methosulfate acetal, and cellobiose dehydrogenase, and a graphite counter electrode modified with laccase and gold nanoparticles, localized on the same screen printed electrode was used as an anode and a cathode, respectively. The BFC operated in human saliva delivered the maximal power output of $1.10\,\mu W\,cm^{-2}$.

Fig. 4.8

Wearable biofuel cells (A, B) and biofuel cells-based self-powered biosensors (C, D). (A) Optical image showing the close-up view of the anode and cathode of the BFC with a schematic illustration of the working principle and an example of possible wearable application of the soft, stretchable electronic-skin-based BFC. (B) The scheme of a bionic contact lens-based BFC consisting of (1) a biocathode, modified with AuNPs and bilirubin oxidase, (2) an anode, modified with AuNPs and the TTF-TCNQ complex, (3) a glucose biosensor, (4) an interface chip, (5) a simple display, and (6) an antenna. (C) The lactate self-powered biosensor on the sock applied to a volunteer's foot and a real-time lactate response obtained from the on-body test during the cycling exercise. The subject maintained a constant cycling rate for 50 min. (D) Schematic diagram and analytical operation principle of the BioCapacitor—an integrated self-powered biosensor. Resulting from the charge pump circuit, the closed-circuit voltage charges the capacitor until its potential reaches $1.8\,V$. Then, the charge pump circuit switch discharges the capacitor and a current flow, which generates a light pulse in the LED. *Part (A) reprinted with permission from A.J. Bandodkar, A. et al. Soft, stretchable, high power density electronic skin-based biofuel cells for scavenging energy from human sweat. Energy Environ. Sci. 10 (2017) 1581–1589. Copyright © 2017, Royal Society of Chemistry; (B) reprinted with permission from M. Falk, V. Andoralov, M. Silow, M.D. Toscano, S. Shleev, Miniature biofuel cell as a potential power source for glucose-sensing contact lenses. Anal. Chem. 85 (2013) 6342–6348. Copyright © 2013, American Chemical Society; (C) reprinted with permission from I. Jeerapan, J.R. Sempionatto, A. Pavinatto, J.-M. You, J. Wang, Stretchable biofuel cells as wearable textile-based self-powered sensors. J. Mater. Chem. A 4 (2016) 18342–18353. Copyright © 2016, Royal Society of Chemistry; (D) reprinted with permission from K. Sode, T. Yamazaki, I. Lee, T. Hanashi, W. Tsugawa, BioCapacitor: a novel principle for biosensors. Biosens. Bioelectron. 76 (2016), 20–28. Copyright © 2015 The Authors. Published by Elsevier B.V.*

4.3.1.3 Self-powered biosensors

BFCs can act not only as an energy supply but also as an analytical device in the so-called self-powered biosensors. While any biosensor combined with an energy harvesting device can be called a self-powered biosensor, historically the term "self-powered biosensor" refers to a type of BFC with the power output, the OCP or a generated current proportional to the concentration of the analyte/fuel. In such a configuration, the sensor itself provides the power for the sensing device. The main advantages of self-powered biosensors are their plain design of just two electrodes and conjugation of energy generation and electroanalysis in one simple device. These features make them particularly attractive for applications in battery-free, low-cost, integrated wearable biosensing systems [10]. While BFCs have been known for a long time, with early works dating back to 1911 and 1931, followed by more detailed studies since 1964 [65], resumed attention to self-powered biosensors as a promising powering technology for bioelectronics began from a publication by Willner and coworkers reporting a membraneless enzymatic BFC operating as an analytical device [66, 67].

In the device designed by Willner's group, the anode and the cathode of the cell were modified with monolayers of glucose oxidase, an enzyme specifically oxidizing glucose to gluconolactone, and a cytochrome c/cytochrome oxidase couple, a biocatalyst reducing oxygen, respectively. The BFC operated in a 1-mM-glucose containing air-saturated buffer generated a maximum power density of $5\,\mu W\,cm^{-2}$ [66]. They further demonstrated application of the system for the self-powered detection of glucose, where the OCP of the developed BFC was proportional to the analyte concentration [67]. Wang and coworkers used a similar approach to design a minimally invasive microneedle BFC harvesting energy from the wearer's interstitial fluid and providing the power output proportional to the glucose concentration [68]. Although the microneedle-based glucose self-powered biosensor has potential as a wearable device for patients with diabetes, biofouling of electrodes and potential risks of invasive operation limit applicability of invasive BFCs for wearable electronics. The same group demonstrated noninvasive glucose and lactate self-powered biosensors operating in sweat [69]. The self-powered biosensors were fabricated by the screen printing of stretchable nanomaterial-based inks on textiles (Fig. 4.8C). Glucose or lactate BFCs were constructed by the immobilization of glucose or lactate oxidase, respectively, onto the printed CNTs-based anode and used printed silver as the cathode. Power signals of both BFCs incorporated into a sock were proportional to the sweat fuel concentrations.

In our group, we introduced the concept of a single enzyme-based self-powered biosensor with both anode and cathode modified with the same enzyme performing biocatalytic conversion of the fuel [70]. Such a configuration overcomes the problem of having two biocatalysts with different optimum operational conditions, which should be combined in a common sample with a specific pH, temperature and ionic concentration. As an example, we demonstrated application of the system for the self-powered detection of free cholesterol in whole plasma. The system can be adapted for operation in noninvasively available body fluids. The OCP, power density, and generated current of the cholesterol self-powered biosensor were proportional to the concentrations of the analyte, but the generated current was used as the analytical signal for the detection of cholesterol in the plasma since it provided better analytical performances. The maximum power density generated by the cell was $11 \, \mu W \, cm^{-2}$ [10]. Katz and coworkers applied a similar approach and designed a sweat-operated BFC based on the biocatalytic conversion of lactate on both anode and cathode, although still using two enzymes, lactate dehydrogenase, and lactate oxidase, respectively [71]. The self-powered lactate biosensor powered by human sweat combined with a DC/DC converter produced power sufficient to activate an electronic watch. The converter has allowed increasing the output voltage of the BFC (ca. 0.5 V) to the operational voltage of the electronic watch (ca. 3 V). However, on body operation of the system was not demonstrated.

Self-powered, logic-gate biocatalytic sensing systems represent one of the latest trends in bioelectronic technology. BFCs-based logic-gate biosensing devices combine biocomputing elements with the sensing process for the creation of potentially "smart" electroanalytical systems, which are able to detect multiple analytes in a complex matrix using a single transducer, by applying Boolean logic operations [72]. The first logic gate made of a self-powered enzymatic biosensor was reported by Dong's group [73]. The system consisted of a glucose oxidase-based anode and a bilirubin oxidase-based cathode. Both enzymes were co-immobilized with mediators in a biopolymer, chitosan. The ON state (high power output) for the system was achieved in air-saturated solutions, too high or too low levels of O_2 led to an OFF state (low power output). Such O_2-controlled switchable BFCs could be used as a diagnostic system to monitor the O_2 content in body fluids and make a logic decision whether the level of dissolved O_2 in the body fluid is within acceptable limits or not [10]. Logic-gate sensing systems are attractive for wearable applications since they combine "smart" sensing and power generation with an effective power managing strategy in one device. There are some reports in the literature describing attempts to integrate self-powered biosensors with read-out systems, allowing naked-eye detection and thus being completely autonomous and applicable for wearable applications. Sode's group reported an integrated, wireless, self-powered system referred to as a "BioCapacitor," which was based on an enzymatic BFC combined with a capacitor functioning as a transducer and a LED (Fig. 4.8D) [74]. As a model system, a BFC composed of glucose dehydrogenase as the anodic biocatalytic system for the oxidation of glucose, and Pt/C as the cathodic catalyst for oxygen reduction, was used. The power generated during oxidation of glucose charged the capacitor connected to the LED via a charge pump circuit. The charging rate of the capacitor was proportional to the concentration of the analyte. The charged capacitor was discharged through the LED, making it blink with a frequency indicative of the fuel concentration. Besides being an integrated system available for naked-eye, autonomous detection, the BioCapacitor overcomes the problem of low power densities of BFCs. Miyake et al. reported similar devices for glucose [75] and fructose sensing [76].

4.3.2 Human body physical energy harvesters

A person's daily physical activity can be used to power wearable electronics. Fig. 4.9A [77] demonstrates available power associated with this activity. Typical sources of physical energy use thermal or kinetic energy of the human body. Thermoelectric and pyroelectric generators convert human body's heat into electricity. Kinetic energy is generated from the movement of the human body, such as muscle movements, motions of joints and COG motion of the upper body [52]. Mechanical kinetic energy can

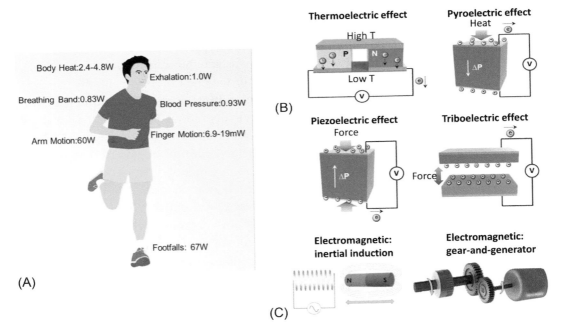

Fig. 4.9

Schematic illustrations of a person's everyday activity and human body physical energy harvesters. (A) Available power from a person's everyday activity. (B) Thermal energy harvesting based on the thermoelectric effect and the pyroelectric effect. (C) Kinetic energy harvesting based on the piezoelectric effect, the triboelectric effect inertial induction and gear-and-generator-type electromagnetic energy harvesting. *(A) Reprinted with permission from W. Zeng, et al., Fiber-based wearable electronics: a review of materials, fabrication, devices, and applications, Adv. Mater. 26 (2014) 5310–5336, © 2014 Wiley-Vch Verlag GmbH & Co. KGaA, Weinheim. (C) Reproduced with modifications from J.-H. Lee, et al., All-in-one energy harvesting and storage devices, J. Mater. Chem. A 4 (2016) 7983–7999, Copyright © 2016, Royal Society of Chemistry; Reprinted from Y.-M. Choi, M.G. Lee, Y. Jeon, Wearable biomechanical energy harvesting technologies, Energies 10 (2017) 1483.*

be scavenged using piezoelectric, electrostatic or electromagnetic energy harvesting principles (Fig. 4.9B and C) [78].

4.3.2.1 Thermal energy harvesters

The human body constantly generates more than 100 W of heat as a result of metabolic processes [79]. Part of this heat is dissipated as a heat flow that can be converted into electricity based on the pyroelectric or thermoelectric effects. In the case of the pyroelectric effect, voltage is generated by the temperature fluctuations in a pyroelectric material. Devices based on the pyroelectric effect are called pyroelectric generators (Fig. 4.9B). Energy conversion efficiency in pyroelectric generators is restricted by the fast temperature fluctuations, and at this stage of development, they are insufficient for the powering of wearable devices. A TEG harvests body heat through direct contact with the human body and its operation is based on the thermoelectric or Seebeck effect: generation of voltage in a thermoelectric element when there is a temperature gradient between its sides (Fig. 4.9B). The generated voltage, V, is directly proportional to the temperature gradient:

$$V = \alpha \, \Delta T_{TEG} \tag{4.9}$$

where α is the Seebeck coefficient of the thermoelectric material and ΔT_{TEG} is the temperature difference between two sides of the generator. A thermoelectric element is formed by p- and n-type semiconductors. Upon heat flow from the hot side to the cold side, holes, and electrons in p- and n-type semiconductors, respectively, also move. Movement of charges converts thermal energy into electrical energy. The power output of the TEG is determined by the temperature gradient, but it is not the difference between the body and ambient temperatures (ΔT). Instead, it depends on the temperature of the the device surface exposed to the ambient temperature and skin temperature [80]:

$$\Delta T_{TEG} = \frac{R_{TEG}}{R_{air} + R_{TEG} + R_{body}} \times \Delta T \tag{4.10}$$

where R_{TEG}, R_{air}, and R_{body} are thermal resistivities of the thermoelectric material, air and the human body in the location of the TEG, respectively. Since resistivities of ambient air and the human body are usually higher than the TEG resistivity, the temperature gradient determining the power output becomes lower than the measured temperature difference between the human body and the air. The thermal resistance can be optimized to match the ambient and maximize the power output [79]:

$$R_{TEG} = \frac{\left(R_{body} + R_{si}\right) R_{et}}{2\left(R_{body} + R_{si}\right) + R_{et}} \tag{4.11}$$

where R_{si} is the thermal resistance of a heat sink, that is, the thermal resistance due to convection and radiation on the outer side of a TEG, R_{et} is the thermal resistance of a TEG without a thermoelectric material. These equations impose the requirement of a semi-emptiness for electrical efficiency of a TEG, where the thermoelectric elements occupy a small part of the device volume and the rest is occupied by air or a material with lower thermal conductivity than air. To increase the power output of TEGs, typically, a large number of thermoelectric elements are connected electrically in series and thermally in parallel [81].

The efficiency of thermoelectric devices is determined also by thermoelectric material's figure of merit, ZT, which can be expressed as follows: [78]

$$ZT = \frac{\sigma S^2 T}{k_e + k_l} \tag{4.12}$$

where σ is the electrical conductivity, S is the Seebeck coefficient, T is the mean operating temperature, and k is the thermal conductivity. The subscripts e and l on k signify the electronic and lattice contributions, respectively. A higher value of the ZT corresponds to the higher efficiency of a TEG. The practically available after thermoelectrical conversion power typically lies in the range of $10–30\,\mu W\,cm^{-2}$ on the 24 h average [79].

The first TEG-powered wearable electronic device, a wireless pulse oximeter, was demonstrated in 2006 (Fig. 4.10A) [82, 83]. A watch-sized TEG providing the minimal power output of $100\,\mu W$ at night and powers in the range of $100–600\,\mu W$ during the day was used in this device to power noninvasive measurements of the oxygen content in arterial blood. Commercially available battery-powered pulse oximeters require more than $10\,mW$ power; so, the power consumption of electronics was reduced by a factor of 10^3 before it could be powered by a human heat. The same group later fabricated a self-powered electroencephalography (EEG) system [84]. As in the previous example, first, the power consumption of EEG was significantly reduced using a low-power biopotential readout application-specific integrated circuit and only after that it was integrated with a body heat-powered TEG. The resulting power required for EEG operation was $0.8\,mW$; so, the large size TEG consisting of 10 sections with the size of $1.6 \times 4\,cm^2$ on a stretchable headband was designed. At $22°C$, the TEG powered by human heat generated the power of $30\,\mu W\,cm^{-2}$. Even a higher power generation at lower ambient temperatures can bring discomfort to a wearer since the TEG in contact with the skin becomes too cold. To solve this problem, the device could be worn on top of the system which will limit a heat flow and make it comfortable. Since these early publications by Leonov and coworkers many groups employed wearable TEGs for the powering of bioelectronics [81, 85]. For example, Lay-Ekuakille et al. demonstrated a TEG able to generate power sufficient to supply a hearing aid using human body's heat [86]. Lossec et al. developed a TEG placed on the human body and connected to a DC/DC converter to boost the surface power density of the system [87]. The system

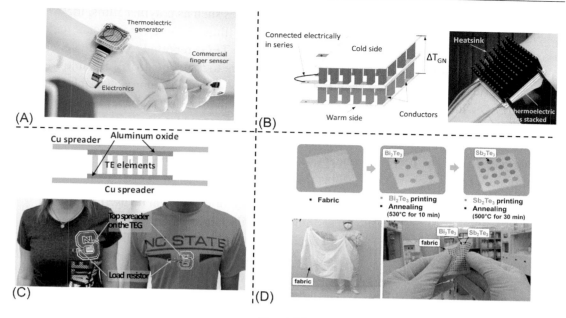

Fig. 4.10

Example of wearable thermoelectric generators. (A) A photograph of the first TEG-powered wearable electronic device, a wireless pulse oximeter. (B) TEG consisted of stacked thermoelectric modules. An illustration showing greater recovery per unit area through the stacking of several thermoelectric modules and the TEG operated on a human arm. (C) A scheme and photographs of the fabric-integrated flexible TEG. TE: thermoelectric material. (D) A schematic illustration of the fabrication process and a photograph of the TEG screen printed on a glass fabric. *Part (A) reprinted with permission from V. Leonov, R.J.M. Vullers. Wearable electronics self-powered by using human body heat: the state of the art and the perspective. J. Renew. Sustain. Energy 1 (2009) 062701. Rights managed by AIP Publishing LLC; (B) reprinted from M. Lossec, B., Multon, H.B., Ahmed, C. Goupil. Thermoelectric generator placed on the human body: system modeling and energy conversion improvements. Eur. Phys. J. Appl. Phys. 52 (2010). © EDP Sciences, 2010; (C) reprinted with permission from M. Hyland, H., Hunter, J., Liu, E., Veety, D. Vashaee. Wearable thermoelectric generators for human body heat harvesting. Appl. Energy 182, 518–524 (2016). © 2016 Elsevier Ltd. All rights reserved; (D) reproduced with modifications from S. Jin Kim, J. Hyung We, B. Jin Cho. A wearable thermoelectric generator fabricated on a glass fabric. Energy Environ. Sci. 7, 1959–1965 (2014). Copyright © 2014, Royal Society of Chemistry.*

consisted of three stacked thermoelectric modules combined with a heat sink generated the power of around $7\,\mu W\,cm^{-2}$ when the wearer was stationary, and $30\,\mu W\,cm^{-2}$ when the wearer was walking at a speed of $1.4\,m\,s^{-1}$ (Fig. 4.10B).

For wearable applications, flexible TEGs might be more advantageous than the above-described rigid TEGs. While only a small amount of the heat flow can be harvested in a wearer-friendly, unobtrusive rigid device, a conformal to the body TEG would increase the surface area available for heat collection without discomfort to a wearer and reduce the thermal contact resistance. Various flexible substrates such as polymer films, including polyethylene (PE), PDMS, polyimide (PI), and Kapton films are used for fabrication of flexible TEGs [88–90]. The performance of the flexible TEGs reported to date, in general, are far below the performance of rigid TEGs, mainly due to lower quality of flexible thermoelectric materials. Suarez et al. have recently reported a new approach to fabricate a flexible TEG with improved performances using a rigid thermoelectric material embedded in a stretchable elastomer [91]. The rigid parts were connected by GaIn liquid metal interconnects, which provided the low interconnect resistance and stretchability with self-healing properties. The proof-of-concept device generated power in the range of $1.48–6.0\,\mu W$ for stationary and full air velocity, respectively at $24°C$.

Flexible TEGs can be embedded into or fabricated on fabrics that can be used for "smart" clothing. For example, Li and coworkers reported a silk fabric-based wearable TEG [92]. Nanostructured Bi_2Te_3 and Sb_2Te_3 were deposited on both sides of the silk fabric to form thermoelectric columns of n-type and p-type materials, respectively. A prototype device with a 4×8-cm area consisted of 12 pairs of the thermoelectric columns connected by silver foils generated the power of 15 nW at a 35-K temperature difference. While the form of the device is favorable for wearable applications, the power output is too low to supply sufficient power for wearable bioelectronics. Hyland et al. developed a fabric-integrated TEG with much better power characteristics [93]. The thermoelectric elements were constructed from n- and p-type bismuth telluride and sandwiched by two aluminum oxide ceramic headers with a heat spreader layer glued to the bottom of the device (Fig. 4.10C). The device integrated into a T-shirt generated power densities of ca. $8\,\mu W/cm^2$ at a walking speed.

Printing techniques can be used to directly print TEGs on fabrics. Kim et al. described a fabrication process of a textile-based flexible TEG with a high power output fabricated by screen printing on a glass fabric (Fig. 4.10D) [94]. A prototype device consisted of eight thermocouples (an n-type Bi_2Te_3 film and a p-type Sb_2Te_3 film and generated a power density of $3.8\,mW\,cm^{-2}$ at a 50-K temperature gradient. The same group later reported flexible screen-printed TEGs with even higher power outputs increased by 80% by means of engineering of the contact resistance and its formation process [95].

4.3.2.2 Kinetic energy harvesters

The human body's motions can be classified into two categories: continuous motions, such as respiration and blood flow, and discontinuous motions, such as muscles movements and motions of joints [96]. Mechanical kinetic energy of the human body can be harvested through piezoelectric, electrostatic, or electromagnetic mechanisms (Fig. 4.9C). Piezoelectric energy harvesting is based on the piezoelectric effect, a phenomenon discovered in 1880 by the French physicists Jacques and Pierre Curie, in which certain materials generate a proportional electrical polarization under applied mechanical stress [96]. Various materials, including crystals, ceramics, polymers, etc. have been used to generate energy based on the piezoelectric effect [52]. Electrostatic energy harvesting is realized through the triboelectric effect or electrostatic induction. The triboelectric effect is a phenomenon of electrical charging of a certain material when it brought into frictional contact with another material. Displacement of these two charged materials relative to each other generates an electric current through an electrode connecting them. Electrostatic induction is based on a redistribution of electrical charges in certain materials (electrets) in the electrical field. Electromagnetic energy harvesting is based on Faraday's law of induction, saying that the relative motion between a coil and a permanent magnet will produce a time-varying magnetic flux and therefore generate a voltage [52].

Wearable piezoelectric generators (PEGs) use the piezoelectric effect to generate electricity from the mechanical energy produced by the human body's motions. Under mechanical stress the crystal structure of the material is deformed, leading to electrical charge movement. The polarization charge density due to the electrical moment is proportional to the applied mechanical stress as follows [78]:

$$\rho = d\text{X} \tag{4.13}$$

where ρ is the polarization charge density, d is the piezoelectric coefficient, and X is the applied stress. The charge density creates an electric field and potential, according to: [78]

$$\nabla E = \frac{\rho}{\varepsilon} \tag{4.14}$$

where ∇E is the divergence of the electric field, ρ is the charge density, and ε is the permittivity. Thus, a device constructed from a piezoelectric material, electrodes and an external circuit can generate an electrical current in the external circuit due to the electrical potential induced by the piezoelectric effect [78]. PEGs typically have low power outputs in the range of mW, and poor efficiency in a low-frequency regime but they can be miniaturized and can generate electricity even when the applied mechanical stress is small [52, 97], thus, being promising for powering wearable low-power bioelectronics. To maximize the power output based on the piezoelectric effect, a PEG should be placed in the part of the human body that is subjected to a large compressive or tensile force. Thus, wearable PEGs scavenging energy from the movements of the knees, center of gravity, and feet have been reported [52]. Different inorganic and organic materials, such as $BaTiO_3$ [98], ZnO [99, 100], lead zirconate titanate (PZT) [98], poly(vinylidene) (PVDF) [101], and composite polymers [102] have been utilized for wearable PEGs. Recently, many attempts have been made to fabricate flexible and stretchable PEGs which are especially desirable for wearable applications. The use of ZnO NWs to design flexible piezoelectric nanogenerators was first reported in 2006 [100] and since then it is one of the most studied inorganic materials for biointegrated, flexible PEGs. The reported ZnO wires-based PEG for energy harvesting on the human body consisted of a single ZnO NW laterally bonded by a silver paste onto a Kapton PI film [102]. The semiconducting properties of the ZnO wire with metal electrodes on its ends result in the formation of the Schottky barrier in the wire under a tensile strain, creating the piezo-potential in the wire and driving a flow of electrons to an external load circuit [103]. The PEG based on a vertically aligned ZnO NWs array has demonstrated a record high level of the peak open-circuit voltage and the current of 58 V and 134 μA, respectively, with the maximum power density of 0.78 W cm^{-3} [99]. Inorganic semiconducting materials are brittle and typically have limited strain levels and low fatigue life. Polymer-based PEGs on the other hand, generally have higher flexibility, longer fatigue life, and lower weights. For example, Zeng et al. reported an all-fiber-based flexible PEG with a PVDF-NaNbO$_3$ nanofiber as the top electrode and an elastic knitted fabric electrode made from segmented polyurethane and silver-coated polyamide multifilament yarns as the bottom electrode [101]. The PEG produced the peak open-circuit voltage of 3.4 V and the peak current of 4.4 μA under conditions of the normal human walking motion and retained its performance after 1,000,000 compression cycles. Skorobogatiy and coworkers designed piezoelectric fibers consisted of a soft hollow polycarbonate core surrounded by a spiral multilayer cladding made of alternating layers of a piezoelectric nanocomposite (polyvinylidene enhanced with BaTiO$_3$, PZT, or CNTs) and a conductive polymer (carbon-filled PE), served as two electrodes (Fig. 4.11A) [98]. The fibers exhibited a high output voltage of up to 6 V under moderate bending.

Electrostatic generators (ESGs) transform electrostatic energy into electricity via electrostatic induction. Typically, ESG consists of two conductive plates isolated from each other by air, vacuum, or a dielectric material and which can move relative to each other. ESGs can be fabricated by silicon micromachining fabrication techniques and, thus, can be easily integrated with microelectronic circuits [96]. Several works on the applications of ESGs to power wearable or implantable bioelectronics have been reported recently [104]. However, the main disadvantage of EGs is that they require an additional voltage source for operation since the plates need to be charged for the conversion process to start, resulting in low amounts of energy produced.

Triboelectric nanogenerators (TENGs) harvest electrostatic energy via the triboelectric effect. The first flexible TENG was reported by Wang and coworkers in 2012 [105]. Since then, energy harvesting through the triboelectric effect became a popular area of research due to its potential applications in self-powered wearable bioelectronics, and much higher efficiencies of TENGs compared to ESGs. A TENG typically consists of two dissimilar polymers placed between metal electrodes. Under applied external force, opposite charges are induced on two polymers in contact due to friction, forming an interface dipole layer, which is called a triboelectric potential layer. The formation of this layer leads to the inner potential layer between metal electrodes, which results in an electrostatically induced free

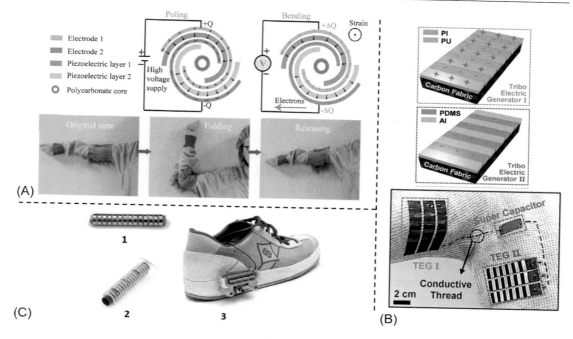

Fig. 4.11

Example of kinetic energy harvesters. (A) A schematic illustration of the operational principle of the piezoelectric fibers and photographs of the textile-embedded fiber-based PEG operated on the body. (B) A schematic illustration and a photograph of the TENG fabricated on a conductive carbon fabric. PI: polyimide, PU: polyurethane, PDMS: polydimethylsiloxane, Al: aluminum. (C) Wearable inertial induction-based harvester. (1) A magnet stack mounted with nuts. (2) Multiple coils placed on a plastic channel. (3) Harvester attached externally to the shoe in order to perform treadmill runs. An accelerometer is attached to the bottom of the harvester to synchronously record the accelerations. *Part (A) reprinted with permission from X. Lu, H., Qu, M. Skorobogatiy. Piezoelectric micro- and nanostructured fibers fabricated from thermoplastic nanocomposites using a fiber drawing technique: comparative study and potential applications. ACS Nano 11 (2017) 2103–2114. Copyright © 2017, American Chemical Society; (B) reprinted with permission from S. Jung, J. Lee, T. Hyeon, M. Lee, D.-H. Kim. Fabric-based integrated energy devices for wearable activity monitors. Adv. Mater. 26 (2014) 6329–6334. © 2014 WILEY-VCH Verlag GmbH & Co. KGaA, Weinheim; (C) reprinted with permission from K. Ylli, et al. Energy harvesting from human motion: exploiting swing and shock excitations. Smart Mater. Struct. 24 (2015) 025029. Copyright © 2014, IOP Publishing.*

charges flow across the external load between the two electrodes. The generated potential can be calculated using: [78]

$$V = -\frac{\rho d}{\varepsilon_0} \tag{4.15}$$

where ρ is the triboelectric charge density, ε_0 is the vacuum permittivity, and d is the distance between layers. The generated current can be determined as follows: [78]

$$I = C\frac{\partial V}{\partial t} + V\frac{\partial C}{\partial t} \tag{4.16}$$

where C is the capacitance of the system and V is the voltage across the two electrodes. The first term in Eq. (4.16) depicts the potential change between the top and bottom electrodes due to the triboelectric charges. The second term shows changes in the capacitance of the PEG as a result of distance changes due to mechanical deformations. The efficiency of TENGs depends on the triboelectric material, the surface condition, the contact speed, and the contact area used for charging [52]. An instantaneous energy conversion efficiency of wearable TENGs can reach up to 70%, but the average efficiency is only 10.6% due to the low frequency of human body's motions. The power output of wearable TENGs is in the mW level, which is sufficient to power wearable devices. A foot strike is the most commonly used energy source for conversion by wearable TENGs [52]. For example, Haque et al. fabricated a soft triboelectric-based shoe insole consisted of PDMS and polyurethane placed between two conductive electrodes. The TENG in the shoe insole generated the power output of 0.25 mW at walking with a frequency of 0.9±0.2 Hz [106]. As mentioned above, usually two electrodes and two polymer layers are used to construct TENGs, however, the human skin can act as a triboelectric layer allowing to design single-electrode-based devices, which can decrease production costs and the size of the wearable device. So, Lee and coworkers designed a TENG using the human skin as one of the electrodes and a PDMS layer laid on PI coated with a thin gold film as a second electrode [107]. When placed on the index finger the TENG generated the maximum power output of ~30 µW/cm^2 (a maximum voltage of 70 V and a current area density of 2.7 µA/cm^2 at a load resistance of 5 MΩ) and were able to power LEDs. TENGs can be integrated into fabrics making the device more comfortable for wearable applications. Jung et al. integrated TENGs fabricated on a conductive carbon fabric onto an armpit region of clothing to maximize friction (Fig. 4.11B) [108]. The first TENG consisted of polyurethane and PI alternatingly patterned onto the carbon fabric and was placed on the inner side of the arm. The second TENG fabricated similarly from PDMS and aluminum was positioned on the body in the armpit region. Such design allowed to harvest energy from both vertical and horizontal frictions generated between the arm and the torso, producing an average output power density of ~0.18 µW/cm^2 in running conditions.

Electromagnetic energy harvesters can be divided into two groups based on the method of energy harvesting: inertial induction type and gear-and-generator-type harvesters. In gear-and-generator-type harvesters, the human motion is amplified by a gear train and used to run a rotary electric generator. This method is a classical power generation technique, which allows generating significantly higher power, in order of watts at the normal walking speed, compared to other generators [52]. While this technique is attractive for charging of mobile devices, such as laptops, cell phones, and radios, at the moment it cannot be used for comfortable powering of wearable devices due to the high weight of essential mechanical elements required to operate the generator. A detailed overview of this type of generators is available in the literature [52].

Inertial induction-type harvesters are operated by the current electromagnetically induced through the relative movement of a permanent magnet or a coil. The generated power is typically in the range of a few mW with a low output voltage that often requires a complex power conversion circuit. The generated power output depends on magnetic field strength, motion velocity of the coil relative to the magnet, and the number of turns of the coil [52]. To provide the maximum possible relative motion velocity generators are usually placed on feet [109, 110] or arms [111]. The oscillations induced by the human motions are sustained by mechanical [110] or magnetic springs [109, 111]. Harvesters based on inertial induction are still rather bulky (Fig. 4.11C) compared to PEGs and TENGs and produce lower power densities.

4.3.3 Photovoltaic cells

Besides chemical, thermal, and kinetic energies of the human body, solar energy is an important form of ambient energy available for powering wearable bioelectronics. Photovoltaic (PV) cells (or solar cells, or solar batteries) convert radiant energy of the sun to electrical energy based on the PV effect, a phenomenon of creation of a voltage and an electric current in certain materials upon exposure to light. A PV cell usually consists of two dissimilar materials, p-type and n-type semiconductors, brought into contact and connected to two electrodes. Illumination with light produces pairs of positive and negative charges which flow in opposite directions, electrons move from the p-type to the n-type semiconductor, holes move from the n-type to the p-type semiconductor, creating a potential difference between electrodes and forcing an electron flow in the connected external load (Fig. 4.12A) [112]. The conversion efficiency (η) of a PV cell is determined as a ratio of the usable energy produced by the cell to solar energy shone on the device and determined through the exposure of the cell to the constant, standard level of light while maintaining the constant cell temperature, and measuring the current and voltage that are produced for different load resistances. The efficiency is determined as follows: [113]

$$\eta(\%) = \frac{P_{max}}{P_{in}} = \frac{V_{oc} \times J_{sc} \times FF}{P_{in}} a \times 100 \tag{4.17}$$

where V_{oc} is the OCP, J_{sc} is the short-circuit current, and FF is the fill factor. The fill factor is a parameter that determines the maximum power of a PV. FF can be determined as follows: [113]

$$FF = \frac{P_{max}}{V_{oc} \times J_{sc}} = \frac{V_{max} \times J_{max}}{V_{oc} \times J_{sc}} \tag{4.18}$$

where P_{max} is the maximum power from the solar cell, calculated as the product of the maximum voltage, V_{max}, and the maximum current, J_{max}. PV cells can be classified based on

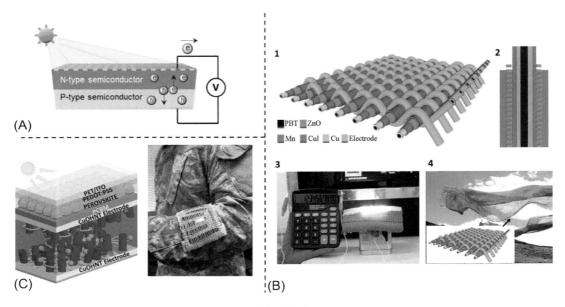

Fig. 4.12

Wearable photovoltaic cells. (A) A schematic illustration of the operational principle of a photovoltaic cell. (B) All-solid photovoltaic textile. Schematic illustrations of (1) the photovoltaic textile and (2) the structure of photoanode. (3) Demonstration of the photovoltaic textile to power a digital calculator under natural solar irradiation. (4) The application of photovoltaic textile as a flexible, ultrathin, and wearable power source. (C) A schematic illustration and a photograph of the ribbon-like flexible wearable device that integrates a perovskite solar cell and a supercapacitor. *Part (A) reprinted with permission from J.-H. Lee, et al. All-in-one energy harvesting and storage devices. J. Mater. Chem. A 4 (2016) 7983–7999. Copyright © 2016, Royal Society of Chemistry; (B) reprinted with permission from N. Zhang, et al. A wearable all-solid photovoltaic textile. Adv. Mater. 28 (2016) 263–269. © 2015 Wiley-vCH Verlag GmbH & Co. KGaA, Weinheim; (C) reprinted with permission from C. Li, et al. Wearable energy-smart ribbons for synchronous energy harvest and storage. Nat. Commun. 7 (2016). Copyright © 2016, Springer Nature.*

the semiconducting material to: silicon-based solar cells, dye-sensitized solar cells (DSSCs), organic solar cells, including organic unit molecules and polymers, quantum dot solar cells, and perovskite solar cells [78].

PV cells can be integrated into textiles to design flexible and stretchable power sources for wearable electronics [34, 112]. For example, Zhang et al. developed the all-solid PV textile made of wire-shaped photoanodes and counter electrodes woven in an interlaced manner [114]. The photoanode was prepared by growing a layer of ZnO nanoarrays on an Mn-plated polymer wire coated with a copper layer. The layer of CuI was deposited onto ZnO as the hole-transfer material. The counter electrode was made of copper-coated polymer wires. The device generated the OCP of 4.6 V and the short-circuit current of 0.16 mA and had the energy conversion efficiency of 1.3%. The PV cell has the potential to be used for powering of wearable devices, however, it has not been demonstrated by the authors.

PV cells are often combined with capacitors or batteries to produce integrated devices [78, 115, 116]. PV cells can be directly combined with energy storage devices without any electrical circuit because of their DC behavior [78]. The performance of the integrated device is dictated by the PV conversion efficiency and the energy storage capacity and is characterized by multiplying the power conversion and the energy storage efficiencies. Energy storage devices have been integrated with silicon-based PV cells, polymer PV cells, DSSCs [117–119], perovskite solar cells [120, 121] for wearable applications. For example, Thomas and coworkers fabricated a ribbon-like flexible proof-of-principle device that integrates a perovskite solar cell and a supercapacitor [121]. Electrons generated by the PV cell are directly transferred and stored on the reverse side of its electrode which works as a supercapacitor. Under simulated solar light the supercapacitor holds the energy density of $1.15\,mWh\,cm^3$ and the power density of $243\,mW\,cm^3$. The ribbons could be woven into fabric for wearable applications. The authors, however, did not test the integrated device on the human body. To the best of our knowledge integrated devices operating on the human body have been not reported yet.

4.4 Wireless power transfer

While independent bioelectronic devices are more comfortable in wearable applications, present power limitations of wearable energy storage devices and energy harvesters compel researches to consider additional power options based on WPT to power wearable bioelectronics. Wireless data transfer for long distances via electromagnetic waves has been known and applied for radio, television, and communication systems from the beginning of the 20th century. However, the methods of WPT are much less developed due to technological limitations resulted from a more demanding design required for power compared to data transfer [122].

WPT systems could be divided into two main categories: systems based on radiative methods and systems based on non-radiative methods. The non-radiative or near-field power transfer could be performed via inductive or capacitive power transfer (CPT) mechanisms [123]. CPT is based on power transfer by electric fields through capacitive coupling between a transmitter and a receiver, acting as two separated capacitor plates. CPT at the moment cannot be used to power wearable bioelectronic devices since the maximum achieved distance of WPT based on this mechanism is only 360 mm [124]. Inductive power transfer (IPT) is based on Faraday's law of magnetic induction and was first reported in 1914 by Tesla [125]. A current flow through the source coil produces a magnetic flux which induces a current flow in the load coil. The compensating capacitor cancels out the leakage inductance of the winding, providing wireless energy conversion between two coils without significant radiation. Currently, IPT could be performed at the distances up to 2 m [126]. Non-radiative power transfer could be performed between non-resonated or resonated objects. Non-radiative WPT between resonated objects can be realized for longer distances and has higher efficiency compared to power transfer between non-resonating objects due to the better coupling between resonated objects [122]. IPT between resonated objects was introduced in

2007 [126] and can be described by the "strongly resonance couple mode" theory [122]. This method allows WPT to distances of 2 m with 40% efficiency.

In radiative or far-field power transfer techniques power is transferred by electromagnetic radiation, like radio waves, microwaves, or lasers for distances in the order of hundreds of meters to kilometers. The wirelessly powered device should have an antenna to capture electromagnetic waves and a power conversion circuit that can extract enough DC power from the incident electromagnetic waves to power the device (Fig. 4.13).

WPT by an inductive coupling mechanism [127, 128], microwave [129], and radio-frequency [130–132] waves for wearable and implantable bioelectronics have been reported. For example, Rogers and coworkers reported an ultraminiaturized flexible device for WPT based on inductive coupling [127]. The device consists of copper coils with the dual-coil layout made of copper traces with nine turns (18 μm thick) to provide high coupling and resonance frequencies near 14 MHz. The devices incorporate PI coatings above and below each layer to physically encapsulate the copper traces and place them near the neutral mechanical plane to minimize bending induced strains (Fig. 4.14A). Multiple devices with different purposes can be integrated with the miniaturized WPT device. The device can be placed on nails and used, for example, to unlock the phone. Fig. 4.14A demonstrates the WPT device mounted on finger nails used to power LEDs, placed on the skin for temperature sensing, placed on teeth. The device can function in the mouth or under water and can be used for powering of chemical sensors in biofluids. The same group also demonstrated the soft, elastic WPT device based on the radio frequency (RF) power transfer mechanism (Fig. 4.14B) [133]. The wireless systems had a laminated construction that facilitated optimization of analogue performance, with the ability for robust operation under significant levels of mechanical deformation.

The device consisted of an impedance matcher connected to a loop antenna and a voltage doubler connected by the soft-contact lamination technique (Fig. 4.14B-1). Each component incorporated stacked ultrathin layers of metals, polymers, and semiconducting materials (Fig. 4.14B-3) in open-mesh serpentine layouts, providing flexibility. Wireless operation of a small-scale LED in full epidermal platforms placed on the skin of the arm and positioned at distances of several meters from a transmitter and of several centimeters from a standard cell phone, both with and without device deformation has been shown (Fig. 4.14B-6,7).

4.5 Problems and future perspectives

While significant progress has been made in powering technology for wearable applications, there are still many remaining problems that should be solved before wearable bioelectronics become the reality of everyday life. All powering approaches discussed in this chapter face some serious hurdles when applied for wearables. This impediment can be resolved either by further technological improvements of powering systems or by the development of integrated power systems combining several approaches.

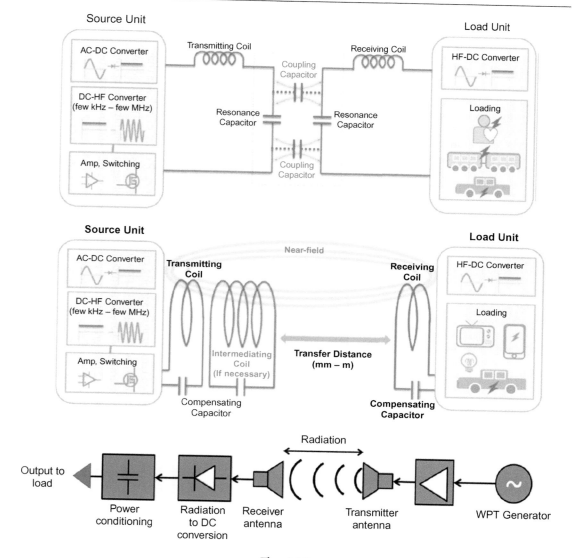

Fig. 4.13

Wireless power transfer mechanisms. (A) Capacitive power transfer. (B) Inductive power transfer. Reprinted with permission from Ref. [123]. © 2017 Elsevier B.V. All rights reserved. (C) Radiative power transfer.

Small-size rechargeable batteries, the most widely used energy source for commercially available wearables cannot provide energy densities sufficient for a long autonomous operation of wearable devices. Battery-powered wearables require constant recharging, making them troublesome for a wearer [3]. Another disadvantage of energy storage devices is their high operating voltages relative to lower operating voltages of emerging wearable bioelectronics [9], which require the integration of additional converters making the device

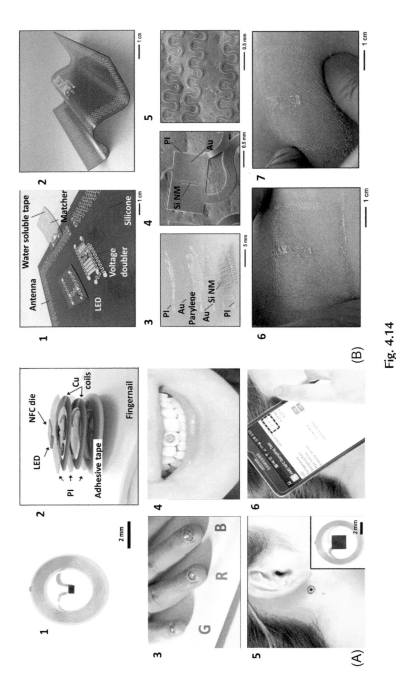

Fig. 4.14

Wireless power transfer. (A) The ultraminiaturized flexible device for WPT based on inductive coupling. (1) A Picture of the device. (2) Exploded-view schematic illustration of each layer of a device mounted on a fingernail. (3) Picture of a set of devices with integrated LEDs mounted on the fingernails. (4) Pictures of the device on a tooth. (5,6) Pictures of a device mounted on the skin behind the ear, with integrated temperature sensing capabilities. Inset: Picture of a device that enables temperature sensing. (B) The WPT device based on radio frequency power transfer mechanism. (1) The diagram that illustrates the modularization approach to device assembly, where sequential lamination of separately fabricated thin film components yields an integrated, functional system. (2) Diagram of a completed system on a thin silicone substrate. (3) Exploded view illustration of a voltage doubler. (4) Colorized scanning electron microscopy (SEM) image of a silicon nanomembrane RF diode, integrated as part of a voltage doubler resting on a skin replica. (5) Colored SEM image of parallel plate capacitors in serpentine geometries on a skin replica. (6, 7) Pictures of an epidermal RF system integrated on the skin under uniaxial stretch and while twisted, respectively. *Part (A) reprinted with permission from J. Kim, et al. Miniaturized flexible electronic systems with wireless power and near-field communication capabilities. Adv. Funct. Mater. 25 (2015) 4761–4767. © 2015 Wiley-vCH Verlag GmbH & Co. KGaA, Weinheim; (B) reprinted with permission from X. Huang, et al. Epidermal radio frequency electronics for wireless power transfer. Microsyst. Nanoeng. 2 (2016) 16052. Copyright © 2016, Springer Nature.*

bulkier. The majority of scientific efforts have been devoted recently to further improvements in the material design that can bring significant improvements in energy densities [11, 12, 134]. Although the new material design can be intuitive, chemistry-driven theoretical considerations should not be neglected. Elaboration of new chemistries for energy storage can possibly increase the energy storage capabilities of energy storage devices, as well as allow solving the problem of high voltages through the use of low-voltage active chemistries [20, 22]. The integration of energy storage/supply devices with energy harvesting functions can resolve recharging issue leading to convenient for a user self-powered systems. Various combinations of energy storage and energy harvesting technologies have been demonstrated [6, 78, 115]. Solar cells and TEGs can be connected directly with energy storage devices without any electrical circuit due to their DC behavior [81, 116]. To connect PEGs or TENGs to energy storage devices additional rectification diodes are required [135, 136]. For effective charging of an energy storage device, a constant voltage and current with the appropriate values are required, which often could not be provided by an energy harvester due to its irregular and unstable power output. To build an effective hybrid system, an optimized circuit including a capacitor filter, an AC/DC or a DC/DC converter should be designed [78]. Further development of hybrid systems should be directed towards a more effective design of the device, which minimizes energy losses and improves overall energy performance.

Major issues of BFCs are low generated power densities and low stability of enzyme-based BFCs [5, 137]. Low power densities are a result of the low OCPs and the low current densities. The current densities can be increased in different ways: by improvements in enzyme immobilization techniques to increase the density of an active catalyst per area [138], by better electronic coupling between enzymes and electrodes [138, 139], by utilization of nanostructured electrodes with a high surface area [140, 141], by the use of engineered enzymes with smaller sizes providing higher volumetric catalytic activity [137], and by implementation of enzyme cascades allowing full oxidation of fuels to carbon dioxide [142, 143]. Both the output voltage and the current densities can be increased when using stacks of devices combined in various series and parallel combinations. The application of DC/DC converters allows increasing the voltage output of BFCs [5]. The low stability of BFCs is a more complicated problem, which significantly limits their feasible use in most wearable applications. The low stability of BFCs results from the low stability of enzymes, mediator leakages, and limited availability of a fresh fuel. Standard operating conditions of wearable devices (varying temperatures, humidity, varying concentrations of electrolytes, and changes in pH) can easily denature enzymes. Considerable effort should be directed towards stability improvement of biocatalysts in wearable BFCs through the combination of biotechnology strategies, such enzyme engineering, and materials engineering strategies to improve the chemical microenvironment for enzymes immobilized on the electrode surfaces [144, 145]. The problem of mediator instability can be solved either by improving mediator immobilization strategies or by designing mediatorless systems based on the direct electron communication between the biocatalyst and the electrode [5, 6]. The problem of constant fuel supply might be solved by combining BFCs with ECs. Such hybrid systems can provide stable power output independent of the availability of fresh fuel and allow significantly improved power densities [146].

The physical energy harvesters overviewed in this chapter endure disparate challenges depending on underlying energy harvesting mechanisms. The performance of TEGs strongly depends on the temperature changes in the environment of the human body. The temperature difference between different body sites and inner environment rarely exceed 20°C and body temperature variations over 24 h do not exceed 5°C [81, 93]. These limited variations restrain energy that can be generated by TEGs. To overcome this problem, materials with higher energy conversion coefficients at room temperatures or thinner systems that can yield large temperature gradients at the thermoelectric material should be developed. The attachment of TEGs to the body may cause discomfort to a wearer due to heat exchange between the human skin and the device. Further improvement of the device configuration design is thus required for the comfortable use of TEGs. The main problem of mechanical energy harvesters is the difference between the frequency range of the human motions (1–10 Hz) and that of the energy harvesting device that significantly lowers energy conversion efficiency [147]. While there are devices that claim to be operational at low frequencies compatible with the human body's motions, irregularities of body movement are rarely considered. For powering of wearable devices, adaptive mechanical generators that can efficiently harvest energy from the low-frequency irregular body motions should be developed. Additional problems for ESGs lies in the fabrication of small-size devices able to significantly change its capacitance. So, new dielectric materials and/or new methods to change device capacitance should be developed. Currently, PEGs and TENGs are the most promising energy harvesting approaches for the powering of wearable devices that are expected to advance further with developments in nanotechnology [6, 103]. Thus, PEGs generate relatively high power outputs and have an operation frequency close to that of human motion [148]. Further advancement of piezoelectric materials will allow bringing PEGs even close to the real-life application in wearable technologies. TENGs produce relatively high power density due to undesirable high voltages (10–1000 V) and extremely low currents. Nevertheless, performances of TENGs are continuously improving [149].

In order to achieve satisfactory power densities in PV devices for wearable applications, they should have an as large a surface area as possible that is best achieved by designing of PV textiles [112, 113]. One of the main problems of designing such textiles is the integration of PVCs and a textile. The first challenge of such an integration is contrasting properties of conductivity and flexibility [112]. Metallic structures are highly conductive but generally not flexible, while polymers are highly flexible but lack conductivity. The design of systems that use carbon nanomaterials integrated into polymers to increase conductivity could provide a solution to this problem. The application of PVCs for wearable devices inserts additional requirements regarding operating conditions, washability, comfort, and aesthetic appeal of the textile [112]. Flexible PV materials desired for wearable devices have, in general, lower conversion efficiencies compared to Si-based PVCs. Although the required voltage can be provided by coupling cells in series, the current is proportional to cell area and many small cells would be needed to provide enough current. Moreover, it should be considered that wearable PVCs operate under much lower light intensity compared to standard PV panels due to extensive and changeable shadowing for flexible PV whose shape is continuously changing with the movement. To provide a stable power output, a PVC needs to be functionally integrated with a device for storing electricity, such as a battery or a supercapacitor [116, 121].

As was mentioned earlier, the problem of recharging for energy storage devices can be solved by integration with energy harvesting devices. At the same time, this combination solves the problem of fluctuating power output of energy harvesting systems. Hybridization can be extended even further by a combination of several energy harvesting technologies and an energy storage system in one device [78]. Today, none of the individual energy harvesting mechanisms are sufficient to provide enough power output for wearable applications. The integration of two or more energy conversion mechanisms in one prototype is auspicious since some physical mechanisms are naturally compatible with each other and can provide a synergistic effect. Hybrid cells have been designed for harvesting mechanical and solar energy [150, 151], mechanical and thermal energy [152], thermal and solar energy [153, 154], and mechanical, thermal, and solar energy [155, 156]. The major challenge for hybrid energy-harvesting devices is then the design of integrated device configuration to include a certain combination of energy-harvesting mechanisms. Solar cells and TEGs generate DC current, while PEGs and TENGs generate AC electricity; so, rectification diodes should be integrated to convert an AC signal to a DC signal [78]. In addition, impedance matching depending on materials and operation frequencies using a resistive load to the PEGs and TENGs is crucial to produce a maximum power output [78]. To build more efficient hybrid systems the interaction between different mechanisms in the same device should be explored.

The main limitation of WPT systems is the distance to which power can be efficiently transferred. A long distance between the primary and secondary coils in the system increases the magnetizing current and the leakage magnetic flux lowering efficiency. The possible solution to this problem lies in improving the architecture design [122]. Operating frequency is another important factor that should be considered. A higher frequency of the power signal results in the higher overall efficiency of the system. The frequency of the power signal is restricted by a semiconductor used for capacitor construction. It is also affected by radiative loss and magnetization currents. Further advances in semiconducting technology might provide a solution to this problem, as well as reduce the cost of WPT systems [123].

References

[1] C. Léger, et al., Enzyme electrokinetics: using protein film voltammetry to investigate redox enzymes and their mechanisms, Biochemistry (Mosc) 42 (2003) 8653–8662.

[2] O. Aquilina, A brief history of cardiac pacing, Images Paediatr. Cardiol. 8 (2006) 17–81.

[3] S. Seneviratne, et al., A survey of wearable devices and challenges, IEEE Commun. Surv. Tutor. 19 (2017) 2573–2620.

[4] A. de Poulpiquet, et al., Mechanism of chloride inhibition of bilirubin oxidases and its dependence on potential and pH, ACS Catal. 7 (2017) 3916–3923.

[5] A.J. Bandodkar, J. Wang, Wearable biofuel cells: a review, Electroanalysis 28 (2016) 1188–1200.

[6] X. Pu, W. Hu, Z.L. Wang, Toward wearable self-charging power systems: the integration of energy-harvesting and storage devices, Small 14 (2018) 1702817.

[7] L. Dong, et al., Flexible electrodes and supercapacitors for wearable energy storage: a review by category, J. Mater. Chem. A 4 (2016) 4659–4685.

[8] Y. Zhang, Y. Zhao, J. Ren, W. Weng, H. Peng, Advances in wearable fiber-shaped lithium-ion batteries, Adv. Mater. 28 (2016) 4524–4531.

[9] J.-M. Tarascon, M. Armand, Issues and challenges facing rechargeable lithium batteries. in: Materials for Sustainable Energy, Macmillan Publishers Ltd, UK, 2010, pp. 171–179. https://doi.org/10.1142/9789814317665_0024.

[10] A.N. Sekretaryova, M. Eriksson, A.P.F. Turner, Bioelectrocatalytic systems for health applications, Biotechnol. Adv. 34 (2016) 177–197.

[11] Y. Liu, G. Zhou, K. Liu, Y. Cui, Design of complex nanomaterials for energy storage: past success and future opportunity, Acc. Chem. Res. 50 (2017) 2895–2905.

[12] Y. Sun, N. Liu, Y. Cui, Promises and challenges of nanomaterials for lithium-based rechargeable batteries, Nat. Energy 1 (2016) 16071.

[13] L. Ji, Z. Lin, M. Alcoutlabi, X. Zhang, Recent developments in nanostructured anode materials for rechargeable lithium-ion batteries, Energy Environ. Sci. 4 (2011) 2682–2699.

[14] S.A. Klankowski, et al., A high-performance lithium-ion battery anode based on the core–shell heterostructure of silicon-coated vertically aligned carbon nanofibers, J. Mater. Chem. A 1 (2013) 1055–1064.

[15] C. Yan, et al., Stretchable silver-zinc batteries based on embedded nanowire elastic conductors, Adv. Energy Mater. 4 (2014) 1301396.

[16] L. David, R. Bhandavat, U. Barrera, G. Singh, Silicon oxycarbide glass-graphene composite paper electrode for long-cycle lithium-ion batteries, Nat. Commun. 7 (2016) 10998.

[17] Y. Zhang, et al., Super-stretchy lithium-ion battery based on carbon nanotube fiber, J. Mater. Chem. A 2 (2014) 11054–11059.

[18] Y. Zhang, et al., Flexible and stretchable lithium-ion batteries and supercapacitors based on electrically conducting carbon nanotube fiber springs, Angew. Chem. Int. Ed. 53 (2014) 14564–14568.

[19] Y.H. Kwon, et al., Cable-type flexible lithium ion battery based on hollow multi-helix electrodes, Adv. Mater. 24 (2012) 5192–5197.

[20] J.W. Choi, D. Aurbach, Promise and reality of post-lithium-ion batteries with high energy densities, Nat. Rev. Mater. 1 (2016) 16013.

[21] D. Aurbach, B.D. McCloskey, L.F. Nazar, P.G. Bruce, Advances in understanding mechanisms underpinning lithium–air batteries, Nat. Energy 1 (2016) 16128.

[22] F. Wang, et al., Nanostructured positive electrode materials for post-lithium ion batteries, Energy Environ. Sci. 9 (2016) 3570–3611.

[23] W. Xu, et al., Lithium metal anodes for rechargeable batteries, Energy Environ. Sci. 7 (2014) 513–537.

[24] S.A. Klankowski, et al., Anomalous capacity increase at high-rates in lithium-ion battery anodes based on silicon-coated vertically aligned carbon nanofibers, J. Power Sources 276 (2015) 73–79.

[25] Rojeski, R. A., Klankowski, S., Li, J. Lithium-Ion Battery Anode Including Core-Shell Heterostructure of Silicon Coated Vertically Aligned Carbon Nanofibers. US Patent 9362549, 2016.

[26] Rojeski, R. A., Klankowski, S., Li, J. Energy Storage Devices. US Patent 9412998, 2016.

[27] C.C. Ho, J.W. Evans, P.K. Wright, Direct write dispenser printing of a zinc microbattery with an ionic liquid gel electrolyte, J. Micromech. Microeng. 20 (2010) 104009.

[28] C.C. Ho, K. Murata, D.A. Steingart, J.W. Evans, P.K. Wright, A super ink jet printed zinc–silver 3D microbattery, J. Micromech. Microeng. 19 (2009) 094013.

[29] M. Hooshmand, D. Zordan, D.D. Testa, E. Grisan, M. Rossi, Boosting the battery life of wearables for health monitoring through the compression of biosignals, IEEE Internet Things J. 4 (2017) 1647–1662.

[30] M. Magno, et al., Energy-efficient context aware power management with asynchronous protocol for body sensor network, Mob. Netw. Appl. 22 (2017) 814–824.

[31] R. Pérez-Torres, C. Torres-Huitzil, H. Galeana-Zapién, Power management techniques in smartphone-based mobility sensing systems: a survey, Pervasive Mob. Comput. 31 (2016) 1–21.

[32] M.A. Razzaque, S. Dobson, Energy-efficient sensing in wireless sensor networks using compressed sensing, Sensors 14 (2014) 2822–2859.

[33] K.K. Fu, J. Cheng, T. Li, L. Hu, Flexible batteries: from mechanics to devices, ACS Energy Lett. 1 (2016) 1065–1079.

[34] A.M. Zamarayeva, et al., Flexible and stretchable power sources for wearable electronics, Sci. Adv. 3 (2017) e1602051.

[35] G. Zhou, F. Li, H.-M. Cheng, Progress in flexible lithium batteries and future prospects, Energy Environ. Sci. 7 (2014) 1307–1338.

[36] R. Kumar, et al., All-printed, stretchable $Zn-Ag_2O$ rechargeable battery via hyperelastic binder for self-powering wearable electronics, Adv. Energy Mater. 7 (2017) 1602096.

[37] S. Xu, et al., Stretchable batteries with self-similar serpentine interconnects and integrated wireless recharging systems, Nat. Commun. 4 (2013) 1543.

[38] J. Ren, et al., Elastic and wearable wire-shaped lithium-ion battery with high electrochemical performance, Angew. Chem. 126 (2014) 7998–8003.

[39] Y. Xu, Y. Zhao, J. Ren, Y. Zhang, H. Peng, An all-solid-state fiber-shaped aluminum–air battery with flexibility, stretchability, and high electrochemical performance, Angew. Chem. Int. Ed. 55 (2016) 7979–7982.

[40] K. Jost, G. Dion, Y. Gogotsi, Textile energy storage in perspective, J. Mater. Chem. A 2 (2014) 10776–10787.

[41] X. Wang, et al., Ultralong-life and high-rate web-like $Li_4Ti_5O_{12}$ anode for high-performance flexible lithium-ion batteries, Nano Res. 7 (2014) 1073–1082.

[42] Y. Wang, Y. Song, Y. Xia, Electrochemical capacitors: mechanism, materials, systems, characterization and applications, Chem. Soc. Rev. 45 (2016) 5925–5950.

[43] A.J. Bard, L.R. Faulkner, J. Leddy, C.G. Zoski, Electrochemical Methods: Fundamentals and Applications, vol. 2, Wiley, New York, 1980.

[44] T. Brezesinski, J. Wang, S.H. Tolbert, B. Dunn, Ordered mesoporous α-MoO_3 with iso-oriented nanocrystalline walls for thin-film pseudocapacitors, Nat. Mater. 9 (2010) 146.

[45] Y. Meng, et al., All-graphene core-sheath microfibers for all-solid-state, stretchable fibriform supercapacitors and wearable electronic textiles, Adv. Mater. 25 (2013) 2326–2331.

[46] L. Dong, et al., Simultaneous production of high-performance flexible textile electrodes and fiber electrodes for wearable energy storage, Adv. Mater. 28 (2016) 1675–1681.

[47] S. Huang, et al., Electrodeposition of polypyrrole on carbon nanotube-coated cotton fabrics for all-solid flexible supercapacitor electrodes, RSC Adv. 6 (2016) 13359–13364.

[48] K. Jost, et al., Knitted and screen printed carbon-fiber supercapacitors for applications in wearable electronics, Energy Environ. Sci. 6 (2013) 2698–2705.

[49] S. Shi, et al., Flexible asymmetric supercapacitors based on ultrathin two-dimensional nanosheets with outstanding electrochemical performance and aesthetic property, Sci. Rep. 3 (2013).

[50] Y. Lin, Y. Gao, Z. Fan, Printable fabrication of nanocoral-structured electrodes for high-performance flexible and planar supercapacitor with artistic design, Adv. Mater. 29 (2017) 1701736.

[51] IEEE. Powering IoT Devices: Technologies and Opportunities—IEEE Internet of Things. Available at: https://iot.ieee.org/newsletter/november-2015/powering-iot-devices-technologies-and-opportunities.html, 2015.

[52] Y.-M. Choi, M.G. Lee, Y. Jeon, Wearable biomechanical energy harvesting technologies, Energies 10 (2017) 1483.

[53] Sekretaryova, A.N., Facilitating Electron Transfer in Bioelectrocatalytic Systems. PhD Theses. Linköping: Linköping University Electronic Press, 2016.

[54] J.A. Cracknell, K.A. Vincent, F.A. Armstrong, Enzymes as working or inspirational electrocatalysts for fuel cells and electrolysis, Chem. Rev. 108 (2008) 2439–2461.

[55] D. Leech, P. Kavanagh, W. Schuhmann, Enzymatic fuel cells: recent progress, Electrochim. Acta 84 (2012) 223–234.

[56] C.J. Harvey, R.F. LeBouf, A.B. Stefaniak, Formulation and stability of a novel artificial human sweat under conditions of storage and use, Toxicol. in Vitro 24 (2010) 1790–1796.

[57] W. Jia, G. Valdés-Ramírez, A.J. Bandodkar, J.R. Windmiller, J. Wang, Epidermal biofuel cells: energy harvesting from human perspiration, Angew. Chem. Int. Ed. 52 (2013) 7233–7236.

[58] W. Jia, et al., Wearable textile biofuel cells for powering electronics, J. Mater. Chem. A 2 (2014) 18184–18189.

[59] A.J. Bandodkar, et al., Soft, stretchable, high power density electronic skin-based biofuel cells for scavenging energy from human sweat, Energy Environ. Sci. 10 (2017) 1581–1589.

[60] D. Pankratov, E. González-Arribas, Z. Blum, S. Shleev, Tear based bioelectronics, Electroanalysis 28 (2016) 1250–1266.

[61] M. Falk, et al., Biofuel cell as a power source for electronic contact lenses, Biosens. Bioelectron. 37 (2012) 38–45.

[62] M. Falk, V. Andoralov, M. Silow, M.D. Toscano, S. Shleev, Miniature biofuel cell as a potential power source for glucose-sensing contact lenses, Anal. Chem. 85 (2013) 6342–6348.

[63] M. Falk, D. Pankratov, L. Lindh, T. Arnebrant, S. Shleev, Miniature direct electron transfer based enzymatic fuel cell operating in human sweat and saliva, Fuel Cells 14 (2014) 1050–1056.

[64] P. Bollella, et al., A glucose/oxygen enzymatic fuel cell based on gold nanoparticles modified graphene screen-printed electrode. Proof-of-concept in human saliva, Sensors Actuators B Chem. 256 (2018) 921–930.

[65] A.T. Yahiro, S.M. Lee, D.O. Kimble, Bioelectrochemistry: I. Enzyme utilizing bio-fuel cell studies, Biochim. Biophys. Acta 88 (1964) 375–383.

[66] E. Katz, I. Willner, A.B. Kotlyar, A non-compartmentalized glucose|O2 biofuel cell by bioengineered electrode surfaces, J. Electroanal. Chem. 479 (1999) 64–68.

[67] E. Katz, A.F. Bückmann, I. Willner, Self-powered enzyme-based biosensors, J. Am. Chem. Soc. 123 (2001) 10752–10753.

[68] G. Valdés-Ramírez, et al., Microneedle-based self-powered glucose sensor, Electrochem. Commun. 47 (2014) 58–62.

[69] I. Jeerapan, J.R. Sempionatto, A. Pavinatto, J.-M. You, J. Wang, Stretchable biofuel cells as wearable textile-based self-powered sensors, J. Mater. Chem. A 4 (2016) 18342–18353.

[70] A.N. Sekretaryova, et al., Cholesterol self-powered biosensor, Anal. Chem. 86 (2014) 9540–9547.

[71] A. Koushanpour, M. Gamella, E. Katz, A biofuel cell based on biocatalytic reactions of lactate on both anode and cathode electrodes—extracting electrical power from human sweat, Electroanalysis 29 (2017) 1602–1611.

[72] M. Zhou, J. Wang, Biofuel cells for self-powered electrochemical biosensing and logic biosensing: a review, Electroanalysis 24 (2012) 197–209.

[73] M. Zhou, S. Dong, Bioelectrochemical interface engineering: toward the fabrication of electrochemical biosensors, biofuel cells, and self-powered logic biosensors, Acc. Chem. Res. 44 (2011) 1232–1243.

[74] K. Sode, T. Yamazaki, I. Lee, T. Hanashi, W. Tsugawa, BioCapacitor: a novel principle for biosensors, Biosens. Bioelectron. 76 (2016) 20–28.

[75] T. Miyake, et al., Enzymatic biofuel cells designed for direct power generation from biofluids in living organisms, Energy Environ. Sci. 4 (2011) 5008–5012.

[76] T. Miyake, S. Yoshino, T. Yamada, K. Hata, M. Nishizawa, Self-regulating enzyme−nanotube ensemble films and their application as flexible electrodes for biofuel cells, J. Am. Chem. Soc. 133 (2011) 5129–5134.

[77] W. Zeng, et al., Fiber-based wearable electronics: a review of materials, fabrication, devices, and applications, Adv. Mater. 26 (2014) 5310–5336.

[78] J.-H. Lee, et al., All-in-one energy harvesting and storage devices, J. Mater. Chem. A 4 (2016) 7983–7999.

[79] V. Leonov, R.J.M. Vullers, Wearable electronics self-powered by using human body heat: the state of the art and the perspective, J. Renew. Sustain. Energy 1 (2009) 062701.

[80] C. Dagdeviren, Z. Li, Z.L. Wang, Energy harvesting from the animal/human body for self-powered electronics, Annu. Rev. Biomed. Eng. 19 (2017) 85–108.

[81] A.R.M. Siddique, S. Mahmud, B.V. Heyst, A review of the state of the science on wearable thermoelectric power generators (TEGs) and their existing challenges, Renew. Sust. Energ. Rev. 73 (2017) 730–744.

[82] T. Torfs, V. Leonov, C.V. Hoof, B. Gyselinckx, Body-heat powered autonomous pulse oximeter, in: *2006 5th IEEE Conference on Sensors*, 2006, pp. 427–430, https://doi.org/10.1109/ICSENS.2007.355497.

[83] V. Leonov, T. Torfs, P. Fiorini, C.V. Hoof, Thermoelectric converters of human warmth for self-powered wireless sensor nodes, IEEE Sensors J. 7 (2007) 650–657.

[84] T. Torfs, et al., Wearable autonomous wireless electro-encephalography system fully powered by human body heat, in: *2008 IEEE Sensors*, 2008, pp. 1269–1272. https://doi.org/10.1109/ICSENS.2008.4716675.

[85] Z. Lou, L. Li, L. Wang, G. Shen, Recent progress of self-powered sensing systems for wearable electronics, Small 13 (2017) 1701791.

[86] A. Lay-Ekuakille, G. Vendramin, A. Trotta, G. Mazzotta, Thermoelectric generator design based on power from body heat for biomedical autonomous devices, in: *2009 IEEE International Workshop on Medical Measurements and Applications*, 2009, pp. 1–4. https://doi.org/10.1109/MEMEA.2009.5167942.

[87] M. Lossec, B. Multon, H.B. Ahmed, C. Goupil, Thermoelectric generator placed on the human body: system modeling and energy conversion improvements, Eur. Phys. J. Appl. Phys. 52 (2010).

[88] J.H. We, S.J. Kim, B.J. Cho, Hybrid composite of screen-printed inorganic thermoelectric film and organic conducting polymer for flexible thermoelectric power generator, Energy 73 (2014) 506–512.

[89] L. Francioso, et al., PDMS/Kapton interface plasma treatment effects on the polymeric package for a wearable thermoelectric generator, ACS Appl. Mater. Interfaces 5 (2013) 6586–6590.

[90] K. Suemori, S. Hoshino, T. Kamata, Flexible and lightweight thermoelectric generators composed of carbon nanotube–polystyrene composites printed on film substrate, Appl. Phys. Lett. 103 (2013) 153902.

[91] F. Suarez, et al., Flexible thermoelectric generator using bulk legs and liquid metal interconnects for wearable electronics, Appl. Energy 202 (2017) 736–745.

[92] Z. Lu, H. Zhang, C. Mao, C.M. Li, Silk fabric-based wearable thermoelectric generator for energy harvesting from the human body, Appl. Energy 164 (2016) 57–63.

[93] M. Hyland, H. Hunter, J. Liu, E. Veety, D. Vashaee, Wearable thermoelectric generators for human body heat harvesting, Appl. Energy 182 (2016) 518–524.

[94] S. Jin Kim, J. Hyung We, B. Jin Cho, A wearable thermoelectric generator fabricated on a glass fabric, Energy Environ. Sci. 7 (2014) 1959–1965.

[95] Y.J. Kim, et al., Realization of high-performance screen-printed flexible thermoelectric generator by improving contact characteristics, Adv. Mater. Interfaces 4 (2017) 1700870.

[96] A. Ben Amar, A.B. Kouki, H. Cao, Power approaches for implantable medical devices, Sensors 15 (2015) 28889–28914.

[97] W.-S. Jung, et al., Powerful curved piezoelectric generator for wearable applications, Nano Energy 13 (2015) 174–181.

[98] X. Lu, H. Qu, M. Skorobogatiy, Piezoelectric micro- and nanostructured fibers fabricated from thermoplastic nanocomposites using a fiber drawing technique: comparative study and potential applications, ACS Nano 11 (2017) 2103–2114.

[99] G. Zhu, A.C. Wang, Y. Liu, Y. Zhou, Z.L. Wang, Functional electrical stimulation by nanogenerator with 58 V output voltage, Nano Lett. 12 (2012) 3086–3090.

[100] Z.L. Wang, J. Song, Piezoelectric nanogenerators based on zinc oxide nanowire arrays, Science 312 (2006) 242–246.

[101] W. Zeng, et al., Highly durable all-fiber nanogenerator for mechanical energy harvesting, Energy Environ. Sci. 6 (2013) 2631–2638.

[102] R. Yang, Y. Qin, L. Dai, Z.L. Wang, Power generation with laterally packaged piezoelectric fine wires, Nat. Nanotechnol. 4 (2009) 34.

[103] A. Proto, M. Penhaker, S. Conforto, M. Schmid, Nanogenerators for human body energy harvesting, Trends Biotechnol. 35 (2017) 610–624.

[104] J. Zhong, et al., Fiber-based generator for wearable electronics and mobile medication, ACS Nano 8 (2014) 6273–6280.

[105] F.-R. Fan, Z.-Q. Tian, Z. Lin Wang, Flexible triboelectric generator, Nano Energy 1 (2012) 328–334.

[106] R.I. Haque, P.-A. Farine, D. Briand, Fully casted soft power generating triboelectric shoe insole, J. Phys. Conf. Ser. 773 (2016) 012097.

[107] L. Dhakar, P. Pitchappa, F.E.H. Tay, C. Lee, An intelligent skin based self-powered finger motion sensor integrated with triboelectric nanogenerator, Nano Energy 19 (2016) 532–540.

[108] S. Jung, J. Lee, T. Hyeon, M. Lee, D.-H. Kim, Fabric-based integrated energy devices for wearable activity monitors, Adv. Mater. 26 (2014) 6329–6334.

[109] K. Ylli, et al., Energy harvesting from human motion: exploiting swing and shock excitations, Smart Mater. Struct. 24 (2015) 025029.

[110] S. Wu, et al., An electromagnetic wearable 3-DoF resonance human body motion energy harvester using ferrofluid as a lubricant, Appl. Energy 197 (2017) 364–374.

[111] M. Geisler, et al., Human-motion energy harvester for autonomous body area sensors, Smart Mater. Struct. 26 (2017) 035028.

[112] R.R. Mather, J.I.B. Wilson, Fabrication of photovoltaic textiles, Coatings 7 (2017) 63.

[113] T.M. Clarke, J.R. Durrant, Charge photogeneration in organic solar cells, Chem. Rev. 110 (2010) 6736–6767.

[114] N. Zhang, et al., A wearable all-solid photovoltaic textile, Adv. Mater. 28 (2016) 263–269.

[115] S. Pan, J. Ren, X. Fang, H. Peng, Integration: an effective strategy to develop multifunctional energy storage devices, Adv. Energy Mater. 6 (2016) 1501867.

[116] Y. Sun, X. Yan, Recent advances in dual-functional devices integrating solar cells and supercapacitors, Sol. RRL 1 (2017) 1700002.

[117] P. Dong, et al., A flexible solar cell/supercapacitor integrated energy device, Nano Energy 42 (2017) 181–186.

[118] A. Scalia, et al., A flexible and portable powerpack by solid-state supercapacitor and dye-sensitized solar cell integration, J. Power Sources 359 (2017) 311–321.

[119] Z. Chai, et al., Tailorable and wearable textile devices for solar energy harvesting and simultaneous storage, ACS Nano 10 (2016) 9201–9207.

[120] Z. Liu, et al., Novel integration of perovskite solar cell and supercapacitor based on carbon electrode for hybridizing energy conversion and storage, ACS Appl. Mater. Interfaces 9 (2017) 22361–22368.

[121] C. Li, et al., Wearable energy-smart ribbons for synchronous energy harvest and storage, Nat. Commun. 7 (2016).

[122] A.P.S. Hasanzadeh, P.S. Vaez-Zadeh, A review of contactless electrical power transfer: applications, challenges and future trends, Automatika 56 (2015) 367–378.

[123] D. Kim, A. Abu-Siada, A. Sutinjo, State-of-the-art literature review of WPT: current limitations and solutions on IPT, Electr. Power Syst. Res. 154 (2018) 493–502.

[124] H. Zhang, F. Lu, H. Hofmann, C. Mi, An LC compensated electric field repeater for long distance capacitive power transfer, in: *2016 IEEE Energy Conversion Congress and Exposition (ECCE)*, 2016, pp. 1–5. https://doi.org/10.1109/ECCE.2016.7854858.

[125] N. Tesla, Apparatus for Transmitting Electrical Energy, US patent no. 1119732, 1907

[126] A. Kurs, et al., Wireless power transfer via strongly coupled magnetic resonances, Science 317 (2007) 83–86.

[127] J. Kim, et al., Miniaturized flexible electronic systems with wireless power and near-field communication capabilities, Adv. Funct. Mater. 25 (2015) 4761–4767.

[128] G. Iddan, G. Meron, A. Glukhovsky, P. Swain, Wireless capsule endoscopy, Nature 405 (2000) 417.

[129] J.S. Ho, et al., Wireless power transfer to deep-tissue microimplants, Proc. Natl. Acad. Sci. 111 (2014) 7974–7979.

[130] T. Le, K. Mayaram, T. Fiez, Efficient far-field radio frequency energy harvesting for passively powered sensor networks, IEEE J. Solid State Circuits 43 (2008) 1287–1302.

[131] S.I. Park, et al., Ultraminiaturized photovoltaic and radio frequency powered optoelectronic systems for wireless optogenetics, J. Neural Eng. 12 (2015) 056002.

[132] H. Jabbar, Y.S. Song, T.T. Jeong, RF energy harvesting system and circuits for charging of mobile devices, IEEE Trans. Consum. Electron. 56 (2010) 247–253.

[133] X. Huang, et al., Epidermal radio frequency electronics for wireless power transfer, Microsyst. Nanoeng. 2 (2016) 16052.

[134] P. Simon, Y. Gogotsi, Materials for electrochemical capacitors, Nat. Mater. 7 (2008) 845.

[135] X. Xue, S. Wang, W. Guo, Y. Zhang, Z.L. Wang, Hybridizing energy conversion and storage in a mechanical-to-electrochemical process for self-charging power cell, Nano Lett. 12 (2012) 5048–5054.

[136] Y. Zi, et al., Effective energy storage from a triboelectric nanogenerator, Nat. Commun. 7 (2016).

[137] M. Rasmussen, S. Abdellaoui, S.D. Minteer, Enzymatic biofuel cells: 30 years of critical advancements, Biosens. Bioelectron. 76 (2016) 91–102.

[138] P. Scodeller, et al., Layer-by-layer self-assembled osmium polymer-mediated laccase oxygen cathodes for biofuel cells: the role of hydrogen peroxide, J. Am. Chem. Soc. 132 (2010) 11132–11140.

[139] F. Mao, N. Mano, A. Heller, Long tethers binding redox centers to polymer backbones enhance electron transport in enzyme "wiring" hydrogels, J. Am. Chem. Soc. 125 (2003) 4951–4957.

[140] E. González-Arribas, et al., Transparent, mediator- and membrane-free enzymatic fuel cell based on nanostructured chemically modified indium tin oxide electrodes, Biosens. Bioelectron. 97 (2017) 46–52.

[141] J. Vivekananthan, R.A. Rincón, V. Kuznetsov, S. Pöller, W. Schuhmann, Biofuel-cell cathodes based on bilirubin oxidase immobilized through organic linkers on 3D hierarchically structured carbon electrodes, ChemElectroChem 1 (2014) 1901–1908.

[142] M. Shao, et al., Mutual enhancement of the current density and the coulombic efficiency for a bioanode by entrapping bi-enzymes with Os-complex modified electrodeposition paints, Biosens. Bioelectron. 40 (2013) 308–314.

[143] F.C. Macazo, S.D. Minteer, Enzyme cascades in biofuel cells, Curr. Opin. Electrochem. 5 (2017) 114–120.

[144] I. Mazurenko, A. de Poulpiquet, E. Lojou, Recent developments in high surface area bioelectrodes for enzymatic fuel cells, Curr. Opin. Electrochem. 5 (2017) 74–84.

[145] J.N. Renner, S.D. Minteer, The use of engineered protein materials in electrochemical devices, Exp. Biol. Med. 241 (2016) 980–985.

[146] C. Hou, A. Liu, An integrated device of enzymatic biofuel cells and supercapacitor for both efficient electric energy conversion and storage, Electrochim. Acta 245 (2017) 303–308.

[147] M. Zhou, M.S.H. Al-Furjan, J. Zou, W. Liu, A review on heat and mechanical energy harvesting from human—principles, prototypes and perspectives, Renew. Sust. Energ. Rev. 82 (2018) 3582–3609.

[148] C. Dagdeviren, et al., Recent progress in flexible and stretchable piezoelectric devices for mechanical energy harvesting, sensing and actuation, Extreme Mech. Lett. 9 (2016) 269–281.

[149] R. Hinchet, W. Seung, S.-W. Kim, Recent progress on flexible triboelectric nanogenerators for selfpowered electronics, ChemSusChem 8 (2015) 2327–2344.

[150] C. Xu, X. Wang, Z.L. Wang, Nanowire structured hybrid cell for concurrently scavenging solar and mechanical energies, J. Am. Chem. Soc. 131 (2009) 5866–5872.

[151] J. Bae, et al., Single-fiber-based hybridization of energy converters and storage units using graphene as electrodes, Adv. Mater. 23 (2011) 3446–3449.

[152] S. Lee, et al., Flexible hybrid cell for simultaneously harvesting thermal and mechanical energies, Nano Energy 2 (2013) 817–825.

[153] N. Wang, L. Han, H. He, N.-H. Park, K. Koumoto, A novel high-performance photovoltaic–thermoelectric hybrid device, Energy Environ. Sci. 4 (2011) 3676–3679.

[154] T. Park, et al., Photothermally activated pyroelectric polymer films for harvesting of solar heat with a hybrid energy cell structure, ACS Nano 9 (2015) 11830–11839.

[155] J.-H. Lee, et al., Thermally induced strain-coupled highly stretchable and sensitive pyroelectric nanogenerators, Adv. Energy Mater. 5 (2015) 1500704.

[156] Z. Wang, et al., Light-induced pyroelectric effect as an effective approach for ultrafast ultraviolet nanosensing, Nat. Commun. 6 (2015) 8401.

Further reading

[157] C. Liu, Z.G. Neale, G. Cao, Understanding electrochemical potentials of cathode materials in rechargeable batteries, Mater. Today 19 (2016) 109–123.

CHAPTER 5

E-skin and wearable systems for health care

William Navaraj, Clara Smith, Ravinder Dahiya

School of Engineering, University of Glasgow, Glasgow, United Kingdom

Chapter outline

5.1 Introduction

Seamless integration of biological systems with electronics has huge implications for basic research from reverse engineering the brain to applications such as bidirectional interfaces with prosthesis. This will enable instant processing and analysis of biological signals in the form of electrical signals, as well as for real-time bioelectronic actuation. Thanks to the advancements in bioelectronics technology, in a not too distant future, it may become possible to restore vision or reverse the effects of spinal cord injury. The bioelectronic interfaces could be in various integrable forms namely wearables, implantables, or ingestibles. Skin, the largest external organ, is an excellent site for bioelectronic interfaces. Artificial electronic skin (e-skin) with various components such as sensors, actuators, communication, signal processing, energy harvesting and storage capabilities, and conformable and flexible-form factor could form a topical or implantable second skin that integrates with natural skin. With integration into prostheses and health-care devices such as catheters, the e-skin could address several existing problems in health care as well as lead to the realization of many

Wearable Bioelectronics. https://doi.org/10.1016/B978-0-08-102407-2.00006-0

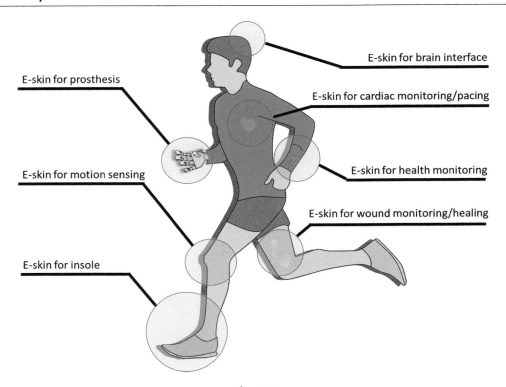

Fig. 5.1
Typical applications of electronic skin [1–9].

concepts previously considered science fiction. This chapter presents some of the key features of the e-skin and along with potential applications, particularly related to health care. The chapter is organized as follows: Section 5.2 presents various components of flexible e-skin including various sensors, active devices, interconnects/electrode, communication structures, etc. Section 5.3 presents various applications of e-skin, mainly related to health care. This section is divided into topical (over the skin), implantable (under the skin), and inanimato (for inanimate objects such as prostheses and surgical tools) applications. Fig. 5.1 summarizes the typical applications of e-skin systems namely, (i) topical e-skin (e-skin for health monitoring, insole), (ii) implantable e-skin (e-skin for brain or heart interface), and (iii) inanimato-e-skin (e-skin for prosthesis). Finally, a summary of the chapter is presented in the final section.

5.2 Components of e-skin systems

E-skin requires heterogeneous integration between sensors, active devices, interconnects, communication interfaces, energy management circuits, data storage, processing components, energy harvesting components, etc. (Fig. 5.2). Some of the common requirements of these components are biocompatibility, conformability to skin topography, flexibility, and,

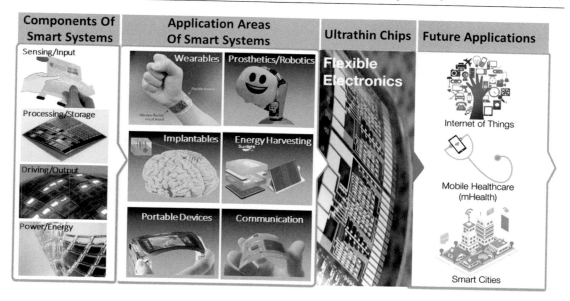

Fig. 5.2

Applications enabled by inorganic micro-/nanostructures-based high-performance flexible electronics through underpinning research in areas such as sensing, computing, data storage, and energy. *Adapted from Ref. S. Gupta, et al., Ultra-thin chip technologies for high performance flexible electronics, NPJ Flex. Electr. 2(8) (2018) 1-8. NPJ:CC by 4.0. Refs. Q. Cao, et al., Medium-scale carbon nanotube thin-film integrated circuits on flexible plastic substrates, Nature 454 (7203) (2008) 495; T. Sekitani, et al., Stretchable active-matrix organic light-emitting diode display using printable elastic conductors, Nat. Mater. 8 (6) (2009) 494; T. Saxena, R.V. Bellamkonda, Implantable electronics: a sensor web for neurons, Nat. Mater. 14 (12) (2015) 1190; J. Lee, et al., Stretchable GaAs photovoltaics with designs that enable high areal coverage, Adv. Mater. 23 (8) (2011) 986–991; W. Gao, et al., Fully integrated wearable sensor arrays for multiplexed in situ perspiration analysis, Nature 529 (7587) (2016) 509.*

where needed, stretchability to various degree, sustainability to various strains due to body motion, minimal discomfort, reasonable adhesion, reasonable shelf life and service life, lightweight. In some cases, there may be some special-requirements such as bio-resorbability, permeability to water vapor, specific molecules or biofluids.

The two important aspects to be considered for realizing most common electronic systems are shown in Fig. 5.3A and B, namely the system development cycle and the key components; the same applies for the development of a flexible e-skin. The cycle starts with system specifications followed by the design of the system architecture which typically involves considerations of various functional modules, computing requirements, energy/power requirements, speed, form factor, design, and compatibility. Then, various device architectures must be decided, considering the system specifications and the performance needed. The various interrelated components given in Fig. 5.3B, namely, the materials, microstructure,

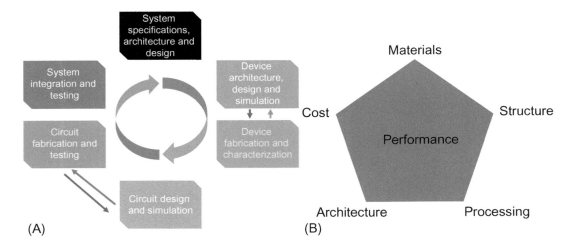

Fig. 5.3

(A) Flexible electronics system development cycle and (B) components to be considered for flexible electronics system.

processing, architecture, and cost, play an important role in deciding the device performance. For example, the architecture and material used detemine the processing requirements which, in turn, affect the microstructure of the material and eventually the associated cost. Advanced flexible electronic system development requires modeling/simulation studies on device, circuit, and system levels. The device-level workflow (involving simulation, fabrication, and characterization) may require iterations before finalizing a device component. For example, empirical parameters, such as fixed oxide charges, interface trap density of gate dielectric and mobility of channel material, are required to be fed as input to MOSFET models in order to obtain accurate device simulation characteristics. The overall flow goes through cycles of device, circuit, and system for further advancements and price-performance enhancement. In the following section, some of the key components of e-skin are discussed namely, active switching devices, sensors, and interconnects.

5.2.1 Substrates

Table 5.1 compares typical substrates/packaging materials considered for e-skin development. Optimal substrates are chosen based on the processing and deployment considerations. Polymer substrates offer substantially reduced processing temperature window. Degradation temperature (T_d) (shown in Table 5.1), gives an estimate of the maximum fabrication temperature. For most materials T_d relates to glass transition temperature (T_g), above which inelastic deformation takes place and the substrate no longer retains its original dimension. This affects subsequent fabrication steps such as photolithography [15]. The mechanical properties of polymer substrates offer a varying degree of flexibility and stretchability as

Table 5.1: Typical flexible substrates for e-skin development.

Substrate material	T_d (°C)	Young's modulus Pa	ε	CTE (ppm/K)	Density g/cm³	Color/ transparency	WVTR g/m²day	OTR cm³/m²day	σ_t Wm⁻¹K⁻¹	WA %	Other relevant properties	Ref.
Poly-(dimethyl-siloxane) PDMS	150	0.3–3 M	2.3–2.8	300	0.97	Transp.	72.8–100.1	3740–4895	0.15–0.17		Non-irritating to skin, no adverse effect on rabbits and mice, only mild inflammatory reaction when implanted.	[10–14]
Poly-(ethylene tereph-thalate) PET	120	2800–3100 M	2.8–3.2	70	1.38	90% Transp.	21	6	0.15–0.24	0.3		[10, 15, 16]
Poly-(ethylene napthalate) PEN	160	2500 M	3.2	44	1.35	87% Transp.	6.9	2	0.15	0.4	1 μm thin foil of PEN was used to realize imperceptible skin electronics	[10, 15–17]
Poly-(ether-sulfone) PES	190	2400–2800 M	3.5	97–101	1.37	89% Transp.	73	235	0.18		Good dimensional stability, poor solvent resistance	[10, 15, 16]
Poly-(ether-ether-ketone) PEEK	240	3600 M	3.2–4.5	161	1.26–1.4	—			0.25			[10, 15]
Poly-carbonate (PC)	150	2400 M	3.0			92% Transp.	60	300	0.19	0.2		[16]
Poly-imide PI (Kapton® HN)	>300	2500 M	3.4–3.5	20	1.42	30%–60% Orange	64	22	0.12	1.3		[10, 15, 16, 18]
Colorless poly-imide CPI (Neopulim)	303	NA	2.9	58	1.23	90% Transp.	93	NA		2.1		[16]

Continued

Table 5.1: Typical flexible substrates for e-skin development—cont'd

Substrate material	T_d (°C)	Young's modulus Pa	ε	CTE (ppm/K)	Density g/cm³	Color/transparency	WVTR g/m²day	OTR cm³/m²day	σ_t Wm⁻¹K⁻¹	WA %	Other relevant properties	Ref.
Liquid crystal polymer (LCP)	>350		2.9	3–17	1.4	Opaque			0.3	0.02	High interfacial adhesion, extremely low degree of moisture absorption, small volume, light weight, cost-effective	[18]
Ecoflex 00-30		0.027–0.029 M	2.8	NA	1.07	Translucent	NA	NA	NA	NA	Biodegradable polymer based on potato starch, corn and polylactic acid	[19–21]

T_d, degradation temperature; ε, dielectric constant; WVTR, water vapor transmission rate; OTR, oxygen transmission rate; CTE, coefficient of thermal expansion; σ_t, thermal conductivity; WA, water absorption; NA, not available.

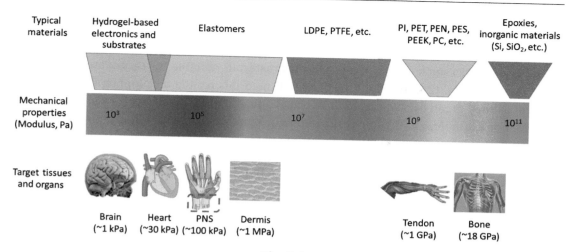

Fig. 5.4

Comparison of modulus of various flexible electronics materials compared to that of various biological tissues/organs. Modulus matching can guide the choice of materials. *Adapted from C.J. Bettinger, Recent advances in materials and flexible electronics for peripheral nerve interfaces, Bioelectr. Med. 4(1) (2018) 6.*

given by the Young's modulus of typical materials in the Table 5.1. This is an important consideration to achieve conformability to the skin and for implantable to conform to tissue/organ topography and to sustain various strains due to body motion. Study of tissue-device interactions suggests that matching the mechanical properties of the biotic-abiotic interface can contribute to the improvement of the reliability and performance of biointegration [22, 23]. One approach followed is the modulus matching (illustrated in Fig. 5.4). Another aspect is permeability to water or oxygen which may be advantageous or disadvantageous depending on the applications. For example, in the case of implantable devices, the packages made of polyimide (PI), polydimethylsiloxane (PDMS), and parylene-C do not effectively prevent moisture infiltration through the discrete boundary of lamination [18]. This may lead to device failure or toxic elements from the device to be leaked and incorporated within the human body. Materials such as liquid crystal polymers (LCPs) are advantageous because of high interfacial adhesion, biocompatibility, extremely low degree of moisture absorption, lightweight, and cost-effectiveness. Transparency may also be required for some application such as on-skin display and pulse oximetry, etc. In this regard, some of the given materials in Table 5.1 may be suitable. While not ideal for packing moisture-sensitive components, elastomers like PDMS, Ecoflex are advantageous for distribution of sensors due to their biocompatibility, chemical inertness, and conformability to uneven surfaces. For example, PDMS implementations with a high degree of stretchability (up to 452% [24] and 280% [25]) have been demonstrated. Ecoflex is advantageous owing to its biodegradability [19]. Nonconventional substrates [26], such as textiles [27], papers [28, 29], electrospun fibers [30] have also been used for realizing flexible skin electronics.

5.2.2 Active switching devices

One of the primary features of e-skin, which makes it smart and functional, is the active switching devices such as transistors. Various materials suitable for e-skin are discussed in reviews in Refs. [26, 31, 32]. The choice of materials for the development of e-skin is critical as they greatly influence both the mechanical and electrical performance of the device. For example, the organic semiconductor materials and amorphous silicon have been widely used to obtain flexible electronic devices due to their inherent mechanical flexibility and relatively low material and processing costs. Thin film transistors (TFTs) can be realized from organic materials for application in e-skin [33]. Such materials will typically include an aromatic or otherwise conjugated π-electron system. The π-electron system facilitates the delocalization of orbital wave functions to which electron-donating or withdrawing groups can be attached to realize n- or p-type organic semiconductors. Some of the typical materials include small molecules such as rubrene, pentacene, tetracene, tetracyanoquinodimethane (TCNQ), diindenoperylene, perylenediimides, and polymers such as polythiophenes (especially poly(3-hexylthiophene) (P3HT)), poly(p-phenylene vinylene) (PPV), polyfluorene, polydiacetylene, and poly(2,5-thienylene vinylene) [26, 34].

However, organic materials typically have low charge-carrier mobility ($0.0001–10\,cm^2/V\,s$ in contrast to $100–3000\,cm^2/V\,s$ of inorganic semiconductors) [35–38], which limits their application in areas requiring high-performance flexible electronics. A range of alternative solutions is, therefore, being explored for high-performance flexible electronics. For example, very high charge-carrier mobility materials such as graphene or silicon nanowires (NWs) are being explored as channel materials for field effect transistors (FETs) [39–42]. In the case of graphene, the zero bandgap and difficulties with its synthesis and transfer over large flexible areas pose a huge challenge [39].

E-skin would require fast communication and computation. For example, wireless communication in mobile health (mHealth) or Internet-of-things (IoTs) will require switching in frequency bands up to ultrahigh frequencies (0.3–3 GHz) [43]. The faster communication, higher bandwidth, and efficient distributed computation implemented with very high switching speeds required for IoT or smart cities will make the high-performance requirements inevitable to achieve smart connected objects with flexible nodes. In this regard, micro/nanostructures, such as ultrathin chips (UTCs), thin membranes, ribbons, NWs, etc. from single-crystal silicon and compound semiconductors can offer better solutions as they exhibit high charge-carrier mobility and the technology for devices based on these materials is mature [31, 38, 40, 42, 44–48]. Fig. 5.5 shows multiple forms of Si and other inorganic micro/nanostructures (IMNSs) for high-performance flexible electronics. Bulk silicon is normally rigid and brittle; but, in thin form factors, it starts to become flexible [e.g., ultrathin silicon wafer

(Fig. 5.5) or chips (Fig. 5.5)]. Thin silicon was initially explored as a means to realize photovoltaic arrays for space applications [49]. The technology readiness available to obtain devices down to nanoscale dimensions and the possibility to exponentially scale the device densities with ultra-large-scale integration (ULSI) up to billions of devices per mm^2, makes silicon-based microelectronics a good candidate for addressing immediate high-performance needs in flexible electronics in the form of UTCs [31]. Furthermore, recent advances, such as the printing of silicon and compound semiconductor micro/nanostructures on flexible substrates make them an attractive alternative for high-performance large-area flexible electronics [50–53]. To realize electronics by printing, silicon-based membranes/ribbons and wires as active components (e.g., FETs) are among the best potential candidates (FETs structures schematically illustrated in Fig. 5.5A). Other approaches such as thick chip array on foil (Fig. 5.5B) and polycrystalline inorganic materials (Fig. 5.5C) such as poly-silicon or metal oxides [15] on flexible substrates are also potential candidates depending on the application of interest. The above implies that IMNS-based bendable high-performance electronics could lead to a wide range of applications.

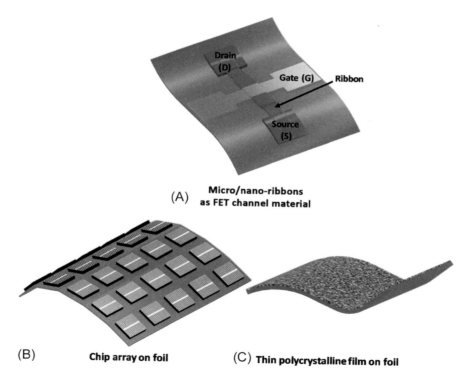

(A) Micro/nano-ribbons as FET channel material

(B) Chip array on foil

(C) Thin polycrystalline film on foil

Fig. 5.5
Illustration of (A–C) multiple forms of inorganic semiconductors for flexible electronics.

5.2.3 Sensors

A range of sensors is required to realize the smart functionalities of the e-skin. This includes mechanical (e.g., tactile, pressure, strain, acoustic), magnetic, thermal, optical [such as ultraviolet (UV) dose measurement explained in Section 5.3.1.2], and chemical sensors. Two typical examples of sensor categories are given below.

5.2.3.1 Tactile sensors

Flexible touch screens are one of the components required for interactive topical e-skin. By measuring the change in resistance, capacitance, optical, mechanical, charge, or magnetic properties of the material being touched, the act of touch can be detected [54]. Based on this, there are various types of touch-screen strategies namely resistive, capacitive (self and mutual), acoustic, and optical [55]. Resistive touch screens majorly work in single-finger touch mode and need complex designs/architectures for implementing multi-touch—at a significantly high cost. Air gaps that must be maintained in resistive touch screens could lead to false inputs in flexible layers and hence cannot be used for bending applications. Capacitive touch screens allow multitouch operations but at the expense of increased per-cycle readout time. Other touch-screen technologies such as acoustic touch screens and infrared touch screens suffer from ambient light interference and are sensitive to liquids and contaminants.

CNTs, organic polymers, graphene, and silicon are typical materials that have been used for making tactile e-skin elements [7, 8, 32, 56–61]. A wide spectrum of touch sensors that are currently available is listed in Table 5.2. Despite a large number of sensor types, the touch sensing has not been widely implemented in prosthetic and robotics. This is partly because of challenges associated with the distributed nature of tactile sensing and the associated computational requirements, the requirement for bendability, the varying spatiotemporal resolutions at different parts of the body, and the need to detect multiple contact parameters [55, 69]. A solution which addresses all these issues does not exist as of yet and likely to emerge from research projects such as neuPRINTSKIN that are specifically targeting these challenges [70]. The IMNSs-based flexible electronics technology could help address these challenges. For example, UTC technology could find application as the flexible IC element of e-skin electronics (a flexible and transparent e-skin for sensing/input as illustrated in Fig. 5.2) [8, 26, 71, 72], especially to mimic tactile sensing in fingertips. In order to achieve biomimetic tactile sensing, about $250\,MRs/cm^2$ (plus additional thermoceptors- and nociceptors-equivalent) are required in the fingertip of a prosthetic limb [73], which could be achieved by high-density tactile sensors such as flexible piezoelectric oxide semiconductor field effect transistor (POSFET) that can conform to the fingertips [74] (Fig. 5.6). For areas where a lower density of tactile sensors is required, an IMNS-based macroelectronics strategy is useful [76]. Some of the prior implementations of materials used for tactile sensing are summarized in Table 5.2 [58].

Table 5.2: Prior art of demonstrations of electronic skin.

Technology	Sensor density (cm^{-2})						
	Temp.	Pressure	Strain	Dynamic forces	Humidity	Mechanics	Ref.
Human fingertips	4	70	48	163	Intra-sensory interaction	Stretchable, durable, self-healing, biodegradable, neural architecture	[62] [63]
Human palm	4	8	16	34	Intra-sensory interaction	-do-	[62] [63]
Carbon nanotubes (CNT)	–	25	–	–	–	Stretchable	[57]
Self-healing sensor	–	1	–	–	–	Self-healing	[64]
Biodegradable polymer	–	13	–	–	–	Biodegradable	[65]
Stretchable silicon	11	44	44	–	1	Stretchable, nanoribbons	[7]
Piezotronic	–	8464	–	–	–	Flexible	[66]
All-graphene	25	25	–	–	25	Stretchable	[67]
CNT active matrix	–	8.9	–	–	–	Flexible	[68]
Organic active matrix	7.3	7.3	–	–	–	Flexible	[56]
Organic digital	–	1	–	–	–	Flexible	[33]
POSFET	–	–	–	100	–	Rigid	[59]
Coplanar graphene	–	1	–	1	0	Flexible, transparent, energy autonomous	[8]

Adapted from Ref. [58].

IMNSs in the form of FETs can contribute to both dynamic and static sensor arrays. The POSFET is an example of a dynamic sensor that can mimic FA-I and FA-II with its implementation as a silicon-based FET is used [59] as a subelement. In the case of POSFETs, a piezoelectric material is used over the top of a MOSFET gate as shown in Fig. 5.7A. Akin to FA mechanoreceptors in human skin, the POSFETs are capable of sensing and (partially) processing the tactile signal at the same site. There are several advantages in the marriage of sensing material and the electronics such as event-driven signaling, better integration, better signal-to-noise ratio, faster response, wider bandwidth, better force sensitivity, and no interconnect is required between the transducer and electronic devices [59, 79]. Further, such transistors could directly form a component of an amplifier or a higher-order circuit [80]. So far, POSFETs have been fabricated using bulk silicon. Using CMOS fabrication strategy, POSFET technology could be used for high-density taxels. The wafers or chips could also be thinned as schematically illustrated in Fig. 5.5 to make them flexible. Alternatively, the printing of NWs could be used to realize a POSFET. Such devices are expected to have higher sensitivity due to the higher surface-to-volume ratio of NWs compared to the silicon chips-based POSFETs.

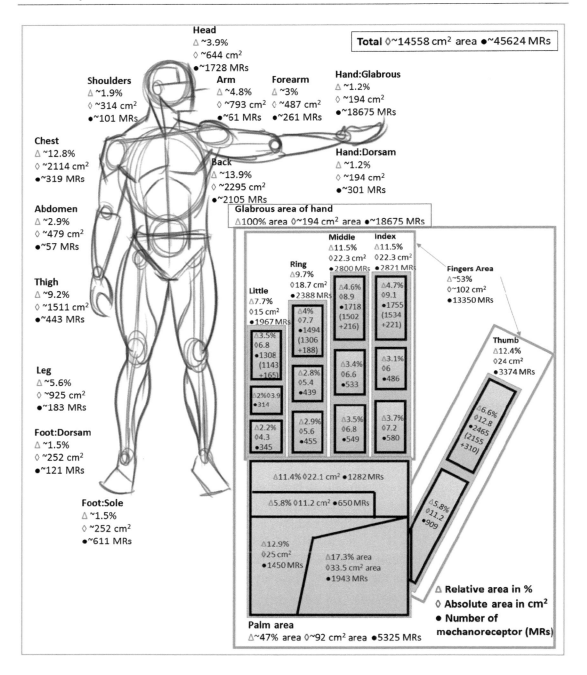

Fig. 5.6
The estimated distribution of mechanoreceptors in various parts of human skin [75].
Frontiers: CC by 4.0.

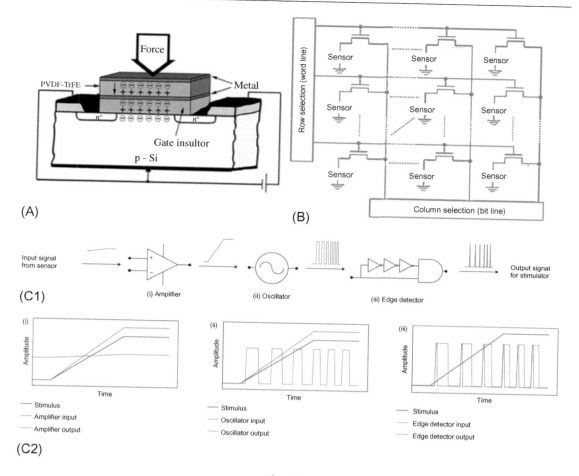

Fig. 5.7

Sensor integration strategies with inorganic micro/nanostructures FETs (A) POSFET [59], (B) row column addressing of transducers (e.g., Refs. [77, 78]) (C) signal to spike or AP convertor for biomimetic tactile signal transducer: (C1-i to C1-iii) shows the components for the spike converter, namely (C-i) amplifier (C-ii) oscillator (C-iii) edge detector (C2-i to C2-iii) shows the input-output of each stage corresponding to (C1-i to C1-iii). *Reprinted with permission from Springer Nature, Copyright, 2016 A. Chortoss, J. Liu, Z. Bao, Pursuing prosthetic electronic skin, Nat. Mater. 15 (9) (2016) 937–950.*

Fig. 5.7B shows the second strategy where inorganic nanostructures are used as active-matrix addressing elements of the sensor array. The row selectors activate the gates while the column selectors are useful to read individual sensor elements. The use of high-performance inorganic flexible FETs is promising here as the high mobility leads to low ON resistance, which favors a low signal-to-noise-ratio (SNR) and efficient readout. The high on-to-off ratio contributes toward lower leakage and hence results in lower power consumption and cross talk.

Fig. 5.7C shows the third strategy which involves a biomimetic signal-to-spike rate conversion where an IMNS-based approach could offer a high-performance and highly efficient solution.

The spike rate conversion is achieved by three components, namely: amplifier, oscillator, and edge detector (C-i to C-iii connected in series). The amplifier is an optional component for this conversion. The transducer could be a part of the oscillator (e.g., a ring oscillator based on silicon NWs) and finally connected to an inorganic nanostructured material-based inverter. Inorganic nanostructures are promising for printable highly efficient spike rate coders. Alternate innovative strategies are also possible such as the one involving ν-NWFET [75].

To summarize, UTC technology finds application in realizing e-skin elements for highly sensitive and high-resolution areas such as the finger-tip of a robotic hand. A micro/nanostructures-based printing approach finds application for macro-e-skin for the rest of the robot's surface. Both, static and dynamic sensors are realizable with IMNSs which are key in achieving human-like tactile sensing in robots. In the next section the application of e-skin with reference to bidirectional prostheses are discussed.

5.2.3.2 Field effect transistor-based sensors

FET-based sensors that are used for sensing ions and biochemicals are ideal for use in e-skin because of their compactness, ease of large-scale repeatable fabrication capability, tunability, and ability to interface with smart electronics such as a neural network. There are various configurations of such sensors and two of these that closely align with e-skin are (1) ion-sensitive field effect transistor (ISFET) and (2) chemiresistor. Nanostructures such as NWs (Fig. 5.8 and Table 5.3) are ideal for realizing such field-effect sensors because of the high surface-to-volume ratio, which leads to very high sensitivity.

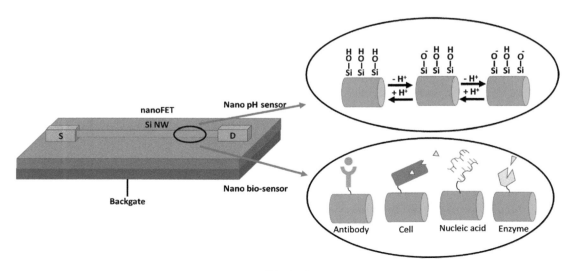

Fig. 5.8
Schematic illustration of NW-FET-based pH sensor and biosensor (BioFET).

Table 5.3: SiNW biosensors (Prior art).

Analytical performance of SiNW biosensors					
Device specification	Fabrication	Mechanism	Application	Detection limit	References
p-Type SiNW; diameter: 20 nm	Bottom-up	Biotin-avidin binding	Streptavidin	10 pM	[1]
n-Type SiNW, p-type SiNW; diameter: 20 nm	Bottom-up	Antibody-antigen interaction	PSA, CEA, Mucin-1	PSA: 2 fM, CEA: 0.55 fM. Mucin-1: 0.49 fM	[25]
p-Type SiNW; diameter: 20 nm	Bottom-up	PNA-DNA hybridization	DNA	10 fM	[9]
p-Type SiNW; diameter: 20 nm	Bottom-up	Antibody-virus interaction	Influenza A virus	Single virus	[32]
n-Type SiNW, p-type SiNW; thickness: 40 nm, width: 50–150 nm	Top-down	Biotin-avidin binding	Streptavidin	10 fM	[19, 50]
n-Type SiNW, p-type SiNW; thickness: 40 nm. width: 50–150 nm	Top-down	Antibody-antigen interaction	PSA, CA 15.3	PSA: 2.5 ng mL^{-1}, CA 15.3: 30 U mL^{-1}	[55]
n-Type SiNW, p-type SiNW; width: 20 nm, length: 30 nm	Top-down	DNA-DNA hybridization	DNA	10 pM	[81]
n-Type SiNW, p-type SiNW; width: 50 nm, length: 20 nm	Top-down	DNA–DNA hybridization	DNA	25 pM	[31, 82]
n-Type SiNW; thickness: ≤40 nm	Top-down	Antibody-antigen interaction	PSA	30 aM	[26]
p-Type SiNW; diameter: 30–60 nm	Bottom-up	Protein-protein interaction	TnI	7 nM	[11]
n-Type SiNW; width: 50 nm, thickness: 60 nm, length: 100 nm	Top-down	PNA-DNA hybridization	DNA	10 fM	[15, 83]
n-Type SiNW; width: 50 nm, thickness: 60 nm, length: 100 nm	Top-down	Antibody-antigen interaction	cTnT	1 fg mL^{-1}	[27]
n-Type SiNW; width: 50 nm, thickness: 60 nm, length: 100 nm	Top-down	PNA-DNA hybridization	RT-PCR product of DEN-2	10 fM	[18]
n-Type SiNW; width: 50 nm, thickness: 60 nm, length: 100 nm	Top-down	PNA-RNA hybridization	microRNA	1 fM	[22]
n-Type SiNW; width: 50 nm, thickness: 60 nm, length: 100 nm	Top-down	Protein-DNA interaction	ERα	10 fM	[14]
n-Type SiNW; width: 50 nm, thickness: 60 nm, length: 100 nm	Top-down	Antibody-antigen interaction	cTnT, CK-MM, CK-MB	1 pg mL^{-1}	[12]

Reprinted from Ref. G.-J. Zhang, Y. Ning, Silicon nanowire biosensor and its applications in disease diagnostics: a review, Anal. Chim. Acta 749 (2012) 1–15.

5.2.4 Interconnects

Interconnects are critical to power and allow communication between various components of the e-skin. In e-skin, there is an additional requirement that the interconnects should be stretchable as some of the body parts it conforms to (e.g., elbow) experience significant stretching. Several strategies have been devised and reported in the literature for flexible and stretchable electronics. As an example, a stretchable system concept using the popular strategy of connecting rigid islands with wavy stretchable interconnects is shown in Fig. 5.9. The rigid islands in this scheme can be considered as the components of e-skin. It is recommended that these islands should have a flexible form factor, which along with the stretchability of the substrate and interconnects should allow better conformability with soft and curved surfaces.

A similar strategy of interconnects (also involves a stretchable wireless antenna.) has been used to realize a stretchable wireless system for sweat pH monitoring which is presented in Section 5.3.1.1 (Fig. 5.10). A detailed review of printable stretchable interconnects is presented in Ref. [85].

5.2.5 Actuators

Various kinds of actuators are also useful as a component in e-skin. For example, topical e-skin with an array of tactile actuators finds application for sensory substitution in prosthesis and for deaf-blind communication. In such cases, the tactile feedback is provided through various forms of stimulation such as skin stretch, vibration, force or painless

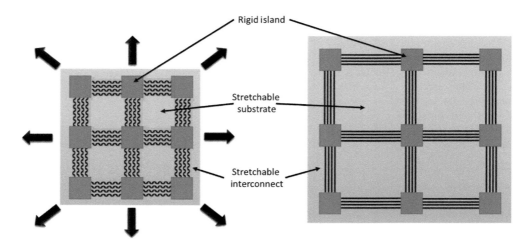

Fig. 5.9
Illustration of the stretchable system concept using rigid islands and stretchable interconnects/substrate.

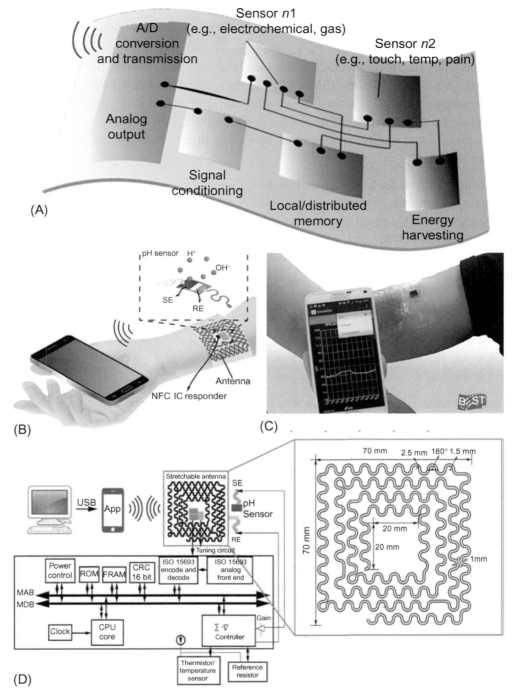

Fig. 5.10

(A) E-skin concept with multiple functionalities integrated over ultrathin flexible substrates, Copyright (2019) [84]. (B) Schematic illustration of a topical pH sensing e-skin patch with mobile readout. (C) Realized e-skin patch. (D) System-level block diagram for wireless pH data transmission with the inset (antenna design). *Reprinted from Ref. W. Dang, et al., Stretchable wireless system for sweat pH monitoring, Biosens. Bioelectron. 107 (2018) 192–202, Copyright (2018), with permission from Elsevier.*

electric shock [86, 87] substitutes the hearing and vision modalities [88]. These include electromagnetic, electrocutaneous, electrostatic, piezoelectric, pneumatic, rheological fluids, and shape-memory alloy (SMA), etc. Early research and development in this area were mainly to provide a sensory substitution for the blind using Braille devices. Recently, application of tactile displays has expanded to fields such as robotics, haptics, teleoperation, virtual reality, video games, as well as in prosthesis for the restoration of feeling to amputees.

Alternate applications for actuators include transdermal drug delivery through a closed-loop theranostic system which continuously monitors the physiological status of the body and delivers appropriate therapeutic agents when needed. For example, such devices as smart-patches with microneedles can be programed to deliver a precise volume of the drug (via actuating micropumps) in a controlled manner [89]. Such devices will blur the line between topical and implantable devices.

5.3 Applications of e-skin

Our skin is essential in allowing us to interact with the natural world and the objects around us. Electronically mimicking the skin's function and/or augmenting the skin with additional smart capabilities would have profound implications for health care.

Electronic devices and integrated circuits are conventionally fabricated on rigid and flat substrates, such as silicon (Si) wafers as current micro/nanofabrication technology allow realizing devices on planar substrates only. The resulting planar electronics has revolutionized our lives through fast communication and computing, but the lack of bendability in these devices presents challenges for using them in emerging applications such as wearable and implantable electronics, and robotic skin. These applications require high-performance electronics to conform to curved surfaces [8, 32, 44, 55, 59, 72, 73, 90–93]. For this reason, there is a huge interest in obtaining electronics on flexible and nonconventional substrates such as soft plastics and even paper [15, 28]. Flexible electronics is changing the way we make and use electronics. For example, the convergence of flexible electronics and biology has immense potential for many exciting future applications, some of these are implants, actuators, tools for surgical procedures, electrodes, sensors, and neural interfaces. The key enablers for realizing such exciting applications are electronics that can be integrated intimately and conformably to the soft, curvilinear surfaces of biological tissues. Many existing applications such as wearable/ implantable systems that require bendability to conform to the curved surface of tissues and organs [94] are driving the progress in the field, which in turn enable the development of numerous futuristic applications, such as mHealth, wearable systems, smart cities, and IoTs. For example, the convergence of flexible electronics and biology has immense potential for many exciting future applications some of which are given in Table 5.4 and

Table 5.4: Biomedical applications of flexible electronics [2, 95–102].

Surgical procedures	Implants	Actuators
Video endoscopes Smart catheters Swallowable smart pill	Subretinal implants Smart pace makers Electrical recording of heart signals Other systems for blind vision	ICD defibrillator Electroceuticals Flexible Haptics e-Skin for robots Wound healing
Flexible electrodes	**Sensors**	**Neural interface and prosthetics**
Electrocardiography (ECG) Electromyography (EMG) Electroencephalography (EEG) Electrocorticography or intra-cranial EEG (iEEG) Intra/extracellular recording using electrodes Nanowire FETs based cellular recording	Blast sensor patch in sports/military helmets to detect trauma injury Ultraviolet (UV) sensor patch to sense the UV dose exposure throughout the day Pulse oximetry sensor patch Fruit freshness sensor Sensing H_2S gas from fruits Oxygen sensor patch Magnetic resonance imaging (MRI) coils Ocular pressure sensors Smart contact lens Wound monitoring Wireless implantable pressure sensor Other diagnostic and health-monitoring sensor patches	Tactile functional prosthetics Neuroprosthetics Brain machine interface for exciting and sensing neurons Neuromorphic implantable biomedical system Optogenetics

categorized as tools for surgical procedures, implants, actuators, electrodes, sensors, and neural interfaces. Smartphones with roll up displays and health-care patches attached to the skin to deliver drugs or monitor vital signs, etc. are some other areas which will benefit from electronics on flexible substrates [5, 15, 44]. The various medical devices (and associated e-skin systems) could be divided into four categories: (i) diagnostic, (ii) therapeutic, (iii) health monitoring and preventive care, and (iv) assistive or rehabilitative devices [103]. Several initiatives from governments and industry have contributed to the progress in this important futuristic area and it is now estimated that the market for flexible electronics will reach $300 billion by 2028 [104–106].

5.3.1 Topical e-skin systems

Topical e-skin is an ultrathin and lightweight structure comprising mainly electronic and/ or sensing components on flexible/bendable substrates that can conform over the skin (illustrated in Fig. 5.10). Topical e-skin systems are mainly useful for diagnosis, preventive care, and health-monitoring applications.

5.3.1.1 Diagnostic/monitoring patch

Recent technological advances in the field of biomedical electronics are enabling a shift in the health-care paradigm toward individual-centric management of health through platforms such as mHealth [107]. Noninvasive methods for continuous monitoring of key physiological parameters—such as heart rate and rhythm, blood pressure, temperature, and respiration rate—as well as analytes such as glucose, urea, pyruvate, in various body fluids are of interest [31, 103, 108, 109]. By conforming to the body surface, the bendable electronics can improve the reliability of noninvasive data collection as well as offers ease of use, even under low-resource settings, without the need for highly trained medical staff. As a result, there has been increased interest recently in monitoring health conditions through body fluids such as sweat, tears, and urine [108, 110].

As given in Table 5.5 [5], there is a correlation among various analytes such as glucose, urea, and ascorbate in the blood, tears, and sweat. Several diseases (including chronic diseases), could be monitored or diagnosed based on the concentration of these analytes in sweat or tears, thereby eliminating the need for acquiring blood samples, at least for initial diagnosis. Sweat is particularly attractive as it is strongly correlated to the blood [113] which mainly consists of water and electrolytes including sodium, chloride, potassium, urea, lactate, amino acids, bicarbonate, and calcium [114]. Various diseases such as diabetes, hypocalcemia, hypochloremia, etc. can be diagnosed by measuring some of these analytes in the sweat.

A typical illustration of a topical pH sensing e-skin patch with mobile readout is shown in Fig. 5.10B and the realized e-skin patch in Fig. 5.10C corresponding to the system-level block diagram Fig. 5.10C [5].

Table 5.5: Analytes in blood, tears, and sweat with their diagnostic significance [5, 110–112].

Analytes	Blood (mM)	Tear (mM)	Sweat (mM)	Diagnostic-application
Glucose	3.3–6.5	0.013–0.051	0.33–0.65	Hyper/hypo glycaemia/diabetes
Lactate	3.6–7.5	1.1–2.1	13.4–26.7	Ischemia, sepsis, liver disease, cancer
Urea	6.2 ± 0.9	3.0–6.0	22.2 ± 8.0	Uraemia indicating renal dysfunction
Creatinine	0.077–0.127	0.014–0.051	0.014–0.051	Renal dysfunction
Na^+	140.5 ± 2.2	120–165	66.3 ± 46.0	Hyper/hyponatremia
K^+	4.8 ± 0.8	20–42	9.0 ± 4.8	Indicator of ocular disease
Ca^{2+}	2.0–2.6	0.4–1.1	4–60	Hyper/hypo calcemia
Mg^{2+}	0.7–1.1	0.5–0.9	0.6	Acidosis and muscle contraction
Cl^-	98.9 ± 6.7	118–135	59.4 ± 30.4	Hyper/hypo chloremia
Pyruvate	0.1–0.2	0.05–0.35	0.003–1	Disorders of energy metabolism
Ascorbate	0.04–0.06	0.22–1.31	0.43	Diabetes

5.3.1.2 Preventive care: Wearable UV dosimeter

The topical e-skin system also finds application for preventive care. An example application is a wearable dosimeter for measuring UV exposure or other harmful radiation monitoring. Exposure to UV has several health benefits such as increased vitamin D levels, improvement in skin ailment (psoriasis, eczema, dermatitis, etc.) and enhanced mood (higher levels of a beta-endorphin molecule activating feel-good processes in the brain) [115]. Furthermore, deliberate tanning is a common practice worldwide. However, overexposure to UV radiation can be damaging, particularly to the skin and eyes. The acute effects of UV damage to the skin can be recognized as sunburn, but in the long-term skin damage can lead to the acceleration of skin aging and skin cancers such as squamous cell carcinoma, basal cell carcinoma, and malignant melanoma [115–117]. Monitoring the level of exposure of the body to UV light is therefore important. A flexible UV photodetector (PD) system based on zinc oxide (ZnO) NWs was developed for wearable UV dosimetry [40, 101, 102] shown in Fig. 5.11. The PDs exhibited $>10^3\%$ photocurrent-to-dark current ratios, high sensitivity, fast response times (<1 s), excellent stability under several UV/dark irradiation cycles, and extreme bending conditions. Their robust response justifies their suitability for high-performance wearable UV dosimetry application.

5.3.1.3 Plantar pressure monitoring insole

Topical e-skin has good potential in applications for biomechanical profiling. One example of a medical condition where such information is valuable is diabetic neuropathy. Diabetes

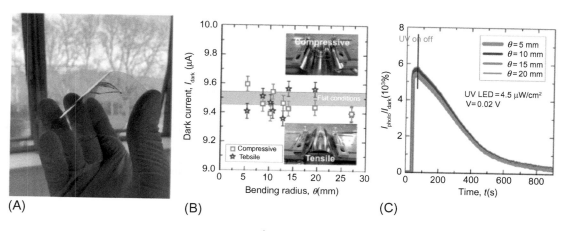

Fig. 5.11
Characteristics of UV Photodetectors under Bending Conditions for application in wearable dosimetry. (A) Photograph of the WB UV PD based on Si/ZnO NWs fabricated on a flexible PI substrate. (B) Dynamic bending characterization of flexible WB UV PDs, comprising compressive (top inset) and tensile bending (bottom inset) of the device and at different bending radii (θ). (C) I_{photo}/I_{dark} of WB UV PDs vs θ (under tensile conditions), CC by 4.0 [40].

mellitus is the sixth leading cause of death worldwide according to the World Health Organization (WHO). Diabetic peripheral neuropathy is the most common complication of diabetes and is considered the greatest source of morbidity and mortality in diabetic patients [118]. Symmetrical loss of sensorimotor function of the lower limbs, in a stocking-like distribution, is the most common pattern of neuropathy in diabetes [119]. A consequence of an insensate foot is the inability to detect pressure points when walking. Altered gait combined with biomechanical changes to soft tissue leads to an increased risk of ulcer formation. Diabetes is associated with poor wound healing meaning that, once present, ulcers are slow to heal and often chronic in nature. Therefore, ulceration often precedes infection and, ultimately, amputation [120].

Changes in foot loading characteristics are responsible for the aforementioned soft tissue changes. Therefore, objective evaluation of plantar pressure distribution is a useful tool for predicting the risk of ulceration in the diabetic foot [121]; elevated pressures are considered a major risk factor for ulceration [120]. Previous examples of platforms for monitoring or assessing plantar pressure patterns have been described in the literature. Generally, these platforms can be divided into insoles or plates although discrete sensors that can be positioned on the sole of the foot are also available [122]. Not only do such systems allow assessment of plantar pressures but they also provide a means of quantitatively assessing the effectiveness of interventions for load redistribution.

e-Skin that is the result of flexible and stretchable electronics, fabricated on soft materials, could be utilized in this context for biomechanical profiling. Furthermore, the increased conformability and improved skin contact would result in better fitting insoles compared to traditional insoles. Poor-fitting insoles ironically have the potential to cause skin injury due to the patient's inability to detect points of friction. Early detection of change in foot loading patterns could facilitate earlier intervention, in the form of physiotherapy, to attempt to reverse abnormal loading patterns. Furthermore, an e-skin insole designed to provide the patient with meaningful real-time sensory feedback would empower the patient to engage more effectively with physiotherapy and gait remedying exercises. It could also provide health-care practitioners with a means for long-term monitoring and provide useful quantitative data in-between appointments.

Sensory information could be relayed to the patient through sensory substitution, for example, as visual information displayed to the user on a screen, or by coupling the insole with a device that interfaces with the nervous system. The problem with the latter solution in the context of diabetes is that the presence of further neuropathies may prevent successful interface.

As described above, one of the crucial problems of an insensate foot is the inability to detect pressure points or pain. This means that diabetic patients often lose the involuntary reflex that protects the foot in response to a painful stimulus. For example, a painful stimulus, such as stepping on a pin, will normally stimulate sensory neurons which transmit a signal to the dorsal column in the spinal cord. Here, the signal is relayed by an interneuron to a motor neuron. The motor neuron carries the signal to the relevant muscles which then contract and lift the foot off the ground. An e-skin insole for sensory substitution coupled with functional electrical stimulation (FES) to stimulate muscle contraction could restore this important protective reflex.

The value of in-shoe plantar pressure monitoring in the context of diabetes is well recognized. Within diabetic foot medicine, there is a current strive toward identifying patients at risk of ulceration based on their biomechanical profile [120]. Flexible, conformable electronics that can provide real-time quantitative feedback on foot loading characteristic have great potential to serve as a useful tool for reducing the incidence of diabetic foot ulceration, or even amputation.

A simpler version of insole was used to control upper limb prosthesis (see Fig. 5.12) based on toe-gesture [123]. It is suitable for people with upper limb amputation without much residual limb area where myoelectric output is not accessible (e.g., shoulder disarticulation). Other than a prosthesis, the insole could be used to control other appliances, such as an input device to a personal computer.

5.3.1.4 Bio-electric recording

Other applications of epidermal e-skin systems include electrode systems for bioelectric recording such as s-electromyogram (EMG), electroencephalogram (EEG), and electrocardiogram (ECG) [124]. Here, conformable contact enables high fidelity efficient measurement with high signal-to-noise ratios of recorded signals [125]. The case of ECG and EMG are discussed here some of which are also applicable for EEG and iEEG (Intracranial EEG) or ECoG (electro-corticography). E-skin-based photoplethysmography sensors and on-screen displays have also been demonstrated by researchers [1].

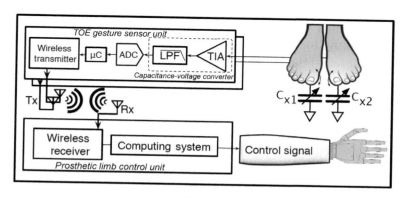

Fig. 5.12
Block diagram illustrating system for control of an upper-limb prosthesis using toe gestures applied on pressure sensors underneath the big toe in a insole. *Reprinted with permission from IEEE, Copyright (2015) W.T. Navaraj, et al. Upper limb prosthetic control using toe gesture sensors, IEEE Sensors, Korea, 2015.*

Electrocardiogram

Recording biological signals provide a preferential doorway to a wider understanding of the physiological phenomena within the human body, either under normal or pathological conditions. For instance, the rhythmical activity of the heart could be analyzed by measuring the difference of electric potential between two locations on the surface of the body also known as electrocardiogram (ECG). By suitably, recording and processing of the signal through associated software subsystems it is possible to infer the energy consumption while exercising as well as to detect several abnormalities such as bradycardia, tachycardia, and other arrhythmias. Both recording hardware and associated software subsystems have to withstand rigorous testing and several iterations to match established recording standard practice, whereas the collected data usually undergo several post-processing stages until the studied phenomena can be displayed in a clean and satisfactory manner. Such standards for the conditioning, acquisition, and processing of biological signals have been consolidated throughout the history of medical practice. Conformal contact with high signal-to-noise ratio via e-skin enables reliable readout and processing of these biological signals to carry out appropriate actions. For example, real-time monitoring of heart arrhythmia is essential to counter the phenomenon through pacemakers and other stimuli thereby saving life in a timely manner.

Electromyography

"Myography" refers to the medical technique of recording of muscular activities. Studying the activation of the skeletal muscles by means of recording the electrical potentials produced during muscular contractions, is of primary interest to practitioners in rehabilitation medicine and engineering in the form of electromyography (EMG) as well as study of muscle fatigue [125a]. The technique is performed by means of an array of electrodes placed either on the skin surface or directly inserted in the muscular tissue of interest, compensating for the adverse effects of skin impedance, the former called as surface EMG (s-EMG) and the latter, intramuscular EMG (IM-EMG). EMG has become widely accepted among clinicians and physiotherapists for its useful features in the study and assessment of neuromuscular diseases and disorders of motor control. Furthermore, EMG offers insight on the force contribution of individual and groups of muscles (e.g., study of interosseous muscles of the hand, the flexor and extensor pollicis longus of the thumb [125a, 125b]). EMG is very useful in combination with biomechanical models that explain the function of portions of the musculoskeletal system. In essence, the possibility to develop systems and devices that can interface bioelectric activities to external devices holds an incredible clinical promise, especially when related to the emerging field of neural prosthetics that to this day strive to restore muscular activity and function in disabled patients with limited limb mobility. This is achievable by interfacing EMG activity to external devices and actuators.

e-Skin's potential for high signal-to-noise ratio, less discomfort/irritation is suitable for s-EMG compared to conventional wet electrode patches-based system (Fig. 5.13). Recently, inflammation-free, highly gas-permeable, ultrathin, lightweight, and stretchable electrodes based on nanomesh were demonstrated [126]. The electrode's impedance was found to be comparable with that of gel electrodes with stability >30,000 bending cycles. A 1-week skin patch test revealed that nanomesh electrodes have far less risk of inflammation. The nanomesh electrodes were used to carryout EMG recordings with minimal discomfort to the user.

5.3.2 Implantable e-skin

Implantable e-skin systems are intended to interface directly with various tissue types for diagnostic, therapeutic, and other health-care monitoring applications. Examples include flexible systems for the neural interface, electrocorticography, intramuscular electromyography, pacemaker devices, etc.

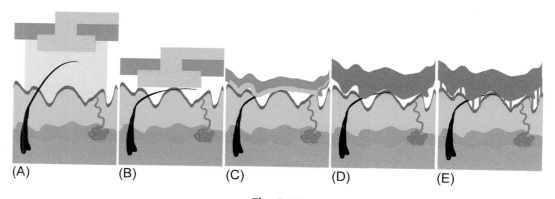

Fig. 5.13
Schematic illustration of different types of electrodes: (A) Rigid electrodes with conductive gel that can penetrate into the wrinkles in the stratum corneum of the skin. (B) Dry rigid electrodes (e.g., Myo band from Thalmic Lab, needs compression band to form intact contact with skin). (C) Flexible and stretchable electrodes on thin polymer substrates can conform to the uneven surface of the skin creating better interface compared to dry and rigid electrodes. (D) Gel-like polymer electrodes can form a better interface with skin similar to wet gel-based electrodes. (E) Micro/ nanostructured ultrasoft polymer conductive electrodes with repetitive dry adherence and removal capability.

5.3.2.1 Neurotechnology

Neurotechnology refers to the field of medical electronics that deals with electronic interaction and interface with the human nervous system. It involves a set of tools, methodologies, and approaches to monitor, access, restore, augment, and/or stimulate the nervous system [127]. Neurotechnology works on the basis that the brain uses electrical signals to send and receive messages and process information. E-skin based neural interface can be used to monitor electrical signals, block undesired signals, and carry out FES. For example, electrical stimuli may be used to restore function to inanimate muscle in cases of paralysis. E-skin based bidirectional neural interface may also help to restore functionality in the next-generation of prosthetic devices, as explained in the next section.

The bendability, stretchability, and conformability of e-skin to curved, soft surfaces improve biocompatibility for neural interface (Fig. 5.14). This will enable advanced research related to applications such as traumatic brain injury and monitoring the brain's response to trauma; induced learning in brain cells; novel pharmacological treatments; the understanding of neural signal propagation, processing, and coding; interpretation of thoughts and intentions for the control of prosthetic devices.

5.3.2.2 Neural implants

Much research has been dedicated to the use of implantable electrodes as a means of accessing neural information for control of prosthetic limbs or assistive devices [128]. These devices are

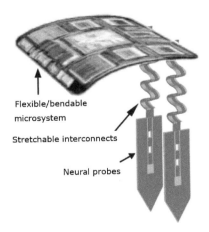

Flexible/bendable
microsystem

Stretchable interconnects

Neural probes

Fig. 5.14
An example of a flexible/bendable version of neural recording microsystem with stretchable interconnects between probes and the chip to reduce the comfortability related issues in using implants. *Copyright (2015), Reprinted with permission R. Dahiya, Epidermal electronics: flexible electronics for biomedical applications, in: S. Carrara and K. Iniewski (Eds.), Handbook of Bioelectronics: Directly Interfacing Electronics and Biological Systems, Cambridge University Press, 2015.*

either implanted within the brain, to interface with the central nervous system, or within peripheral nerves. Neural circuitry within the brain is less well understood than in the periphery and damage to surrounding brain tissue can have profound side effects. Peripheral nerve interfaces are less invasive with a far smaller side effect profile. In any case, the factors complicating the bio-integration of electrodes are the same whether the target tissue is brain or peripheral nerve.

The fact that cells are able to detect the mechanical properties of their physical environment is well recognized. Furthermore, mechanical cues are known to direct cell differentiation. Therefore, it is important to attempt to minimize any discrepancy between the mechanical properties of electrode implants and their surrounding tissue as a means of diminishing disruption to the cellular environment, and, consequently, improving biocompatibility and device stability.

Rigid materials like silicon and tungsten were traditionally used for electrode implants [4] but poor compliance with the micro-movement of surrounding soft brain tissue in the central nervous system, or sheer stresses in the periphery would trigger a foreign body response. These rigid electrodes cause cell damage, inflammation, and eventually scar tissue formation. Scar tissue encapsulates the device and impedes signal strength. In addition to this, activation of a foreign body response would result in migration of surrounding neurons or axons away from the implant [129]. In other words, the inflammatory response ultimately leads to device failure [4].

Brain tissue is one of the softest of human tissue types with Young's modulus somewhere in the range of 0.5–1.0 Pa [130, 131]. Ultrasoft microelectrodes fabricated from elastomers and conducting polymers have been reported with Young's modulus lower than 1 MPa [4]. Recently, electrodes consisting of conducting hydrogels, with modulus in the KPa range, have been fabricated [132]. These softer, more flexible electrodes have demonstrated improved biocompatibility and device longevity when compared to the more rigid, traditional equivalents [4, 132].

Advances in fabrication technologies, such as photolithography and electron beam lithography, permit increased fabrication resolution. This allows more electrodes to be accommodated on a single probe without increasing the dimensions of the probe [133]. Thus, the selectivity of the electrodes increases allowing differentiation of acquired information and more meaningful signal interpretation.

These technologies are similarly employed in the fabrication of ultrathin, ultraflexible e-skin with dense array patterns. In terms of neural interface, e-skin can be employed in the periphery as a multielectrode array that can be wrapped around the nerve with good compliance and, as such, minimal risk of nerve damage.

An extensive body of research now supports efforts to reduce implant rigidity as a means of achieving seamless bio-integration. The result would be soft, ultrathin, flexible electrodes able to record action potentials (APs) and modulate populations of neurons whilst remaining chronically stable.

5.3.2.3 Intramuscular EMG skin

Myoelectric prostheses have traditionally relied on s-EMG to provide control signals [134, 135] because of the ease-of-use, noninvasiveness, and convenience. However, s-EMG have some shortcomings in terms of maintaining a firm electrical contact with the skin, poor differentiability between different muscles owing to cross talk, inability to reliably record deep muscles. IM-EMG while not explored widely as S-EMG can compensate all the above shortcomings with the difference being an invasive process where conventionally specialized percutaneous electrodes shaped as needles are used to reliably record signals from deep muscles [135]. Fig. 5.15 shows the comparison between the s-EMG and IM-EMG signal. Implanted e-skin mesh as IM-EMG interface with wireless readout can offer a solution to the problem of the requirement of percutaneous electrodes. The main features of the comparison between both the techniques are displayed in Table 5.6.

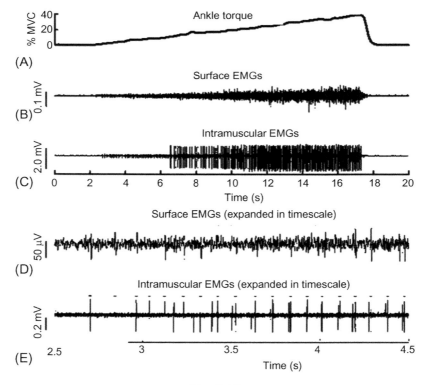

Fig. 5.15

Electromyograms and motor unit APs recordings. (A) shows a plantar flexion torque during a single isometric contraction. (B) and (C) show sEMG and intramuscular EMG recordings from the gastrocnemius muscle respectively, whereas (D) and (E) show the expanded time scale of the previous recordings. *Copyright, 2011, Elsevier M.C. Garcia, T. Vieira, Surface electromyography: why, when and how to use it, Rev. Andal. Med. Deporte 4 (1) (2011) 17–28.*

Table 5.6: Comparison of the main features of sEMG and IM EMG.

	Surface EMG	Intramuscular EMG
Advantages	Workhorse of modern EMG especially related to rehabilitation medicine Noninvasive Allows for effective pattern recognition in gesture control applications such as prosthetic devices	Can accurately discriminate between muscles No risk of muscle cross talk during contraction Useful to analyze deep muscular activity
Disadvantages	Sensible to electrode displacement during motions Highly affected by changes in skin impedance of the subject Highly sensible to muscle cross talk	Highly invasive Clinically unfeasible due to constant contact with the muscle required Prolonged contact may result in tissue inflammation

Similar to iEMG, a conformal e-skin on the heart can be used for cardiac diagnostics, monitoring, and therapeutics. An e-skin having real-time sensing, processing, and actuation will be a boon and a lifesaver for heart patients without inhibiting their physical mobility.

5.3.2.4 Treatment of neuropathic pain

The use of transcutaneous electrical nerve stimulation (TENS) for the non-pharmacological treatment of various types of painful conditions, including chronic neuropathic pain, is well established. A traditional TENS machine is a hand-held, battery-operated device, with lead wires that connect to bulky electrode pads. E-skin could be exploited as a more practical, more discrete, alternative to traditional TENS machines. The fact that e-skin can function as a wireless wearable device appears more attractive and convenient for on-the-go use.

Furthermore, this could pose a relatively simple and noninvasive means of restoring sensory feedback to amputees. The use of TENS in aiding perceptual embodiment of prosthetic limbs has been described [136, 137]. E-skin would represent a superior alternative to the relatively arbitrary, non-discriminate, electrode pads previously tested. The much denser electrode array patterns afforded by E-skin could allow for selective stimulation of specific nerve afferents and perception of a greater variety of sensory stimuli. Improved electrode contact would also facilitate a reduction in the strength of stimulating current required reducing the risk of pain.

5.3.3 Inanimato e-skin

E-skin enables additional functionalities to already existing inanimate tools/objects used for health care such as prosthesis, surgical catheters, and other tools.

5.3.3.1 Prosthetic skin

Prosthetics is one of the important research areas where robotic technology is oriented to rehabilitate the disabled and physically challenged, thereby improving the quality of lives of millions. Current robotic prostheses can mimic the mechanical functionality of human hands and legs.

A 2013 survey of amputees indicated that the two most critical elements for a widespread acceptance of prosthetics are (1) the ability to feel with their prosthesis and (2) enhanced, intuitive motor control [138]. Without sensory feedback, the prosthetic will be just like any other tool and won't become a "part of the body" of the amputee for intuitive use. Research shows that subjects tend to apply much more force than necessary when carrying out tasks involving their fingers and hands when the hands are temporarily anesthetized [139]. Research also suggests that those who lose their sense of touch constantly suffer bruises, burns, and broken bones due to the lack of sensory feedback [139]. It is estimated that up to 80% of amputees are affected by phantom limb pain. Stimulating residual sensory pathways helps in alleviating phantom limb pain [140]. The above indicates that the sense of touch plays an important role in understanding and interacting with various objects, environment, and the associated motor behavior.

Humans and other biological organisms use tactile feedback to interact with the environment [71]. Inspired by nature, numerous research groups are harnessing the technological advances to develop artificial e-skin with features mimicking the human skin [8, 26, 32, 141–144]. These works find application in prosthetics, to potentially bestow lost sensory feelings to amputees [145] and in robotics, to provide the touch sensory capability allowing them to interact physically and safely with real-world objects [72]. Both these applications are discussed below and are followed by a discussion on schemes and specification of e-skin. Thus far, the major focus of artificial skin research has been on the development of various types of sensors (e.g., contact pressure, temperature, etc.) and their integration on large and flexible or conformable substrates [26, 54]. In order to design an efficient tactile sensitive neuro-prosthetic system, it is vital to understand how tactile sensing works in biological systems [71].

In humans, the skin area can be divided into glabrous and non-glabrous areas and each of them has different types of sensory receptors.

The glabrous (hairless) areas of the human skin comprise of four main types of mechanoreceptors, namely Meissner corpuscles, Pacinian corpuscles, Merkel cells, and Ruffini corpuscles, also schematically illustrated in Fig. 5.16. Meissner corpuscles (FA-I) and Pacinian corpuscles (FA-II) come under Fast adapting (FA) mechanoreceptors (i.e., they fire bursts of APs during the onset and offset of various tactile stimuli but remain silent during steady state). They are also known as rapid adapting (RA) mechanoreceptors. Merkel cells (SA-I) and Ruffini corpuscles (SA-II) are slow adapting (SA) mechanoreceptors.

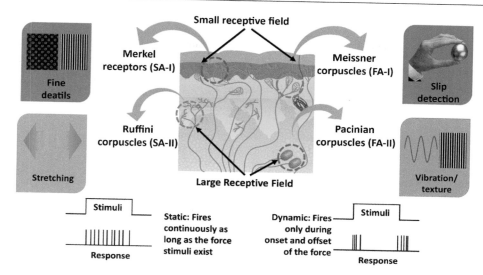

Fig. 5.16

Mechanoreceptors in glabrous area of human skin.

Both static and dynamic sensors are needed to mimic biological tactile sensors. Merkel cells and Meissner corpuscles are closer to the surface of the glabrous skin with a smaller receptive field (<3 mm) whereas, Ruffini and Pacinian corpuscles are deeper in the skin and have a larger receptive field. Table 5.7 summarizes the various receptors in the glabrous area of human skin and their functionalities. SA-I are useful for sensing fine details and for discrimination of object shape and textures. FA-II can also help in discriminating object textures with aid from the sliding motion of the fingers against the object's surface. Fingerprints have been found to play a key role in the tactile perception of fine textures (spatial scale <200 μm) [146].

Another important factor to consider is the density and the number of mechanoreceptors in the human skin. This is needed to find how sensors have to be distributed, readout and hierarchy planned for a full-body robotic skin in par with a human. Also, the density and the sensor count will set what technology should be used for realizing e-skin at different parts of the robot [72].

Fig. 5.6 shows that an estimated 45k mechanoreceptors are distributed across ~1.5 m² area of human skin, based on reports in the literature [62, 139, 156, 157]. Out of 45k receptors, an estimated ~21k sensors are in each upper limb area—mainly concentrated on the glabrous skin of the upper limb (~18k sensors). This is an estimate of only mechanoreceptors, and the number of sensors will be much higher if we consider that tactile sensing also involves thermo-receptors and nociceptors [139] responsible for sensing temperature and pain. With the recent shift in the focus of tactile skin research in robotics from hands to whole-body tactile feedback, a need has arisen for new techniques to manage the tactile data. Currently, limited solutions

Table 5.7: Mechanoreceptors in human skin and their functions.

Sense receptor	Function	Reference
Mechano-ceptors slow adapting SA-I or Merkel corpuscle	Innocuous mechanical stimuli (static forces, very sensitive, high resolution, sensing fine details, useful for discrimination of object shape and texture, receptive field size ~2–3 mm)	[139, 147–150]
Mechano-ceptors slow adapting SA-II or Ruffini corpuscle	Innocuous mechanical stimuli (static forces, skin textures, proprioception, receptive field size ~10–15 mm)	[147, 148]
Mechano-ceptors fast adapting FA-I or Meissner corpuscle	Innocuous mechanical stimuli (dynamic forces and vibrations, low-frequency (5–50 Hz), object manipulation, texture discrimination, slip detection, controlling hand grip, receptive field small)	[139, 147, 148, 151]
Mechano-ceptors fast adapting FA-II or Pacinian corpuscle or Vater-Pacinian corpuscles or Lamellar corpuscles	Innocuous mechanical stimuli (dynamic forces and vibrations, measure high-frequency vibrations (up to 400 Hz), slip detection, fine texture when figure moves, receptive field very large)	[146–149, 151]
Noci-ceptors	Polymodal (noxious cold, noxious heat or more than one noxious stimulus modality)	
Warm thermo-ceptors	Innocuous thermal stimuli	[152]
Cold thermo-ceptors	Innocuous thermal stimuli	[152, 153]
Combination of mechanoceptors and proprioceptive sensors (muscle spindles and fibrous capsules, partly from SA-II)	Hardness, joint positions in space	[154]
Combination of mechanoceptors (SA-I, FA-I, FA-II, SA-II) and thermoceptors	Wetness	[155]

are available to deal with large data generated in tactile skin. In the case of the prosthesis, it is important not only to collect the tactile data for critical feedback but also to decode the user's intentions in real time [145]. For this, neuron-like inferences early on from the tactile data, thus reducing the data along the sensory pathway could help. A significant downstream reduction in the number of neurons transmitting stimuli is observed in early sensory pathways in humans [158–160]. Research suggests that within the biological tactile sensory system, distributed computing takes place [71]. The distributed local processing of tactile data allowing it to be partially processed close to the sensing elements and sending the smaller amounts of summary data to higher-perceptual level as in biological skin is advantageous [55, 160]. The tactile related neural spikes are found to have locally encoded information of the force's magnitude, direction, and the local curvature [147, 161]. In this regard, the hardware-implemented neuromorphic tactile data processing along with neural networks like algorithms within the e-skin could be helpful and may have many advantages. The key challenges in realizing e-skin are: (1) distributed multi-sensors, (2) processing of large data distributed over a large area, and (3) encoded data transfer to a higher level.

IMNSs-based flexible electronics could be used for realizing neural mimicking e-skin. A sample implementation scenario and further futuristic directions are presented in Ref. [75] involving the concept of neural nanowire FET (ν-NWFET).

For bidirectional prostheses interface technologies beyond tactile sensing are required where IMNS could be used, as explained in this section.

The key blocks of the e-skin system for closed-loop neuro-prosthetics (illustrated in Fig. 5.17) are:

(1) distributed flexible tactile data sensing system.
(2) distributed data acquisition and processing system.
(3) interface between the residual limb and the prosthetics.
(4) control of prosthesis.

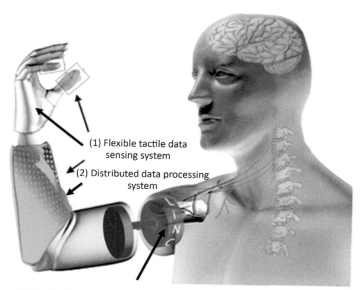

(1) Flexible tactile data
     sensing system

(2) Distributed data processing
     system

(3) Interface between residual limb and the prosthetics
(4) Control output of motorized prosthesis

Fig. 5.17
Schematic representation of electronic skin system for closed-loop bidirectional prosthesis.
Copyright (2015), reprinted with permission R. Dahiya, Epidermal electronics: flexible electronics for biomedical applications, in: S. Carrara and K. Iniewski (Eds.), Handbook of Bioelectronics: Directly Interfacing Electronics and Biological Systems, Cambridge University Press, 2015.

IMNS-based FETs could find application in various forms at each stage for the above application. Fig. 5.18 depicts how IMNS as e-skin elements could be used for various components of closed-loop bidirectional neural prosthesis.

In block 1, a large-area printed IMNS-based flexible FET array is envisaged to be used as an addressable readout interface to address the tactile sensors of the e-skin. Further, the IMNS itself could form as a part of a static or dynamic sensor [59, 78, 162] as explained in the previous section.

In block 2, a biomimetic tactile data processing strategy has been proposed based on a ν-NWFET device as a building block [75]. This is in order to mimic the local data processing in the early sensory pathways of the tactile sensing nervous system.

In block 3, there are two key components; (1) reading the neural signals and interpreting them reliably to decode the prosthesis user's intention, and (2) writing to the neurons to give feedback to the user. Nanowire FETs find application in reading from the neurons [163, 164], thanks to the higher sensitivity offered by the surface-to-volume ratio as well as for decoding the neural signals such as spike sorting. Currently, there is no stable, long-lasting, reliable solution for writing to the neurons. A promising solution is an optogenetic neural interface which uses genetically modified microbial opsins, or light-sensitive ion channels that are specific to nerves, for control of neural signaling [138]. The nerves can be excited or inhibited by specific wavelengths of light. Signal control at the biochemical level can be achieved with optogenetics interface without physical contact between the nerve and the electrode. Toward optogenetic neural interface, ultrathin silicon membrane-based JLFETs or equally UTCs could be used as μLED drivers.

Fig. 5.18 shows a typical application where IMNSs as e-skin elements find application in various components of closed-loop bidirectional neural prosthesis. It comprises of:

(1) IMNS-based e-skin with row/column readout and biomimetic data processing
(2) e-Skin for bidirectional neural interface with the capability of

(a) reading the neural signals and interpreting them reliably to decode the prosthesis user's intention.
(b) writing to the neurons to give feedback to the user.

Nanowire FETs find application in reading from the neurons [163, 164], thanks to the higher sensitivity offered by the surface-to-volume ratio, as well as for decoding the neural signals such as spike sorting. UTCs can also be used for this application. There is already progress in this direction as presented in a conference publication [165], where flexible UTCs for the neural interface was realized based on the technology developed during this doctoral thesis. Currently, there is no stable, long lasting, and a reliable solution for writing to the neurons. Conventionally, direct neural stimulation through longitudinal intrafascicular electrodes and more recently transverse intrafascicular multichannel electrodes, have been used to interface

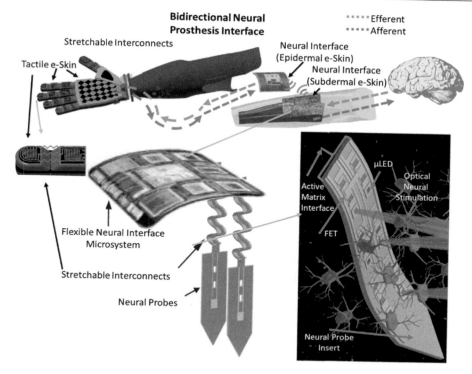

Fig. 5.18

IMNS as electronic skin elements for various components of closed-loop bidirectional neural prosthesis.

with peripheral nerves for sensory feedback [138, 145, 166, 167]. Current direct neural stimulation has disadvantages in terms of causing structural changes within the nerve and the foreign body response to the electrode may induce encapsulation by scar tissue. This is observed in a recent human study with thin-film longitudinal intrafascicular electrodes where the sensory detection completely ceased after 10 days of electrical stimulation [168]. A promising solution is an optogenetic neural interface which uses genetically modified microbial opsins or light-sensitive ion channels that are specific to nerves, for control of neural signaling [138]. The nerves can be excited or inhibited by specific wavelengths of light. Signal control at the biochemical level can be achieved with the optogenetics interface without physical contact between the nerve and the electrode. Toward optogenetic neural interface, ultrathin silicon ribbon-based JLFETs or UTCs presented on this thesis could be used as μLED drivers schematically illustrated in Fig. 5.18.

Optogenetic neural stimulation currently seems to be an interesting pathway to achieve this [138] where signal control at the biochemical level can be achieved with the optogenetics interface without physical contact between the nerve and the electrode. Optogenetics requires compact light sources that can deliver light with an excellent spatial, temporal, and spectral resolution to deep brain structures [6]. Optogenetics pulses of light with spatiotemporal precision are needed to stimulate the neurons. Typically, optogenetic stimulation is carried out by an external light source with fiber-optics to deliver the light to the targeted location. Typical driving requirements in such application are precise temporal requirement, that is, rise time and fall time (10%–90% and vice versa) of current pulses $<100\,\mu s$ and in some specific applications $<1\,\mu s$ with current level up to 1.5 A. Such an arrangement is cumbersome and involves tether.

Tether-free implantable miniaturized optogenetic systems are preferred in such cases and IMNSs-based drivers could provide the required temporal and spatial resolution. Further, with IMNSs it will be possible to achieve multi-wavelength and multiarray microLEDs (μLEDs) targeting various optogenetic channels (corresponding to various opsins), such as channelrhodopsin [169], halorhodopsin [170], archaerhodopsin [171], and bacteriorhodopsin [47]. Toward an optogenetic neural interface, IMNS compound semiconductor structures, and FET technology could lead to high-density active arrays or matrix probes where IMNS-based FETs are proposed to be used as μLED drivers.

Also, UTCs finds application as a gateway or interfacing chip between the neural interface (implantable) e-skin and external wireless transceiver (topical) e-skin (Fig. 5.18) as well as for controlling the prosthesis in an efficient way. The high-performance of the UTCs serve to drive RF circuits and act as wireless powering circuits for the interface between the epidermal neural interface e-skin and the implantable neural interface e-skin.

Other applications include a smart tactile communication system for deaf-blind people [172]. Such smart assistive systems will not only enable bidirectional communication between people to people (disabled as well as normal) [172] but also between people to futuristic assistive robots [173].

5.3.3.2 Surgical tools and robotic surgery

Tactile e-skin wrapped around the surgical tools such as catheters (Fig. 5.19) will enable remote measurement/feeling of tactile sensations [72]. The use of surgical robots and image guidance in minimally invasive surgery (MIS) has experienced gradual exponential growth since the 1990s [174]. Current trends demonstrate the technology is now being investigated more widely for its potential across most surgical specialties and even represents the gold standard for a few specific interventions [175].

Robotics in surgery currently serves a primarily assistive purpose. Medical interventions are informed by a combination of patient-specific data and applied general medical knowledge; currently, only human reasoning and judgment can accurately interpret and rationalize such information. Robots can facilitate decision-making and improve the accuracy of actions by increasing the quantity and quality of information available to the operator.

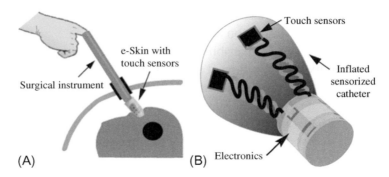

Fig. 5.19

(A) The concept of surgical instrument wrapped with e-skin, allowing surgeons to feel the tissues and organs inside the body. (B) The scheme of inflatable balloon catheter with sensors and electronics on the balloon to allow soft mechanical contact in angioplasty, septostomy, and other standard procedures. *Copyright (2015), reprinted with permission R. Dahiya, Epidermal electronics: flexible electronics for biomedical applications, in: S. Carrara and K. Iniewski (Eds.), Handbook of Bioelectronics: Directly Interfacing Electronics and Biological Systems, Cambridge University Press, 2015.*

They are intended to augment the surgeon's skills to achieve greater accuracy and precision in complex procedures [176]. Their use is not restricted to the operating theatre where the robot resides; remote access enables the surgeon to perform tele-surgery without being physically present at the side of the patient [177]. Such technology has tremendous potential to transform the standard of surgical care, and surgical training, particularly in developing countries.

Despite interest from surgeons and health care organizations, astronomical costs, and lack of haptic feedback are cited as the two major factors preventing the widespread adoption of robotic assistive technology for routine use in surgery [175, 178].

Haptics describes force and tactile feedback. Such feedback is essential for precise tissue handling. The improved visual feedback associated with robotic techniques has thus far provided some compensation for diminished haptic feedback, but fine manipulation of tissue will continue to be compromised unless this shortfall is addressed [175].

Whereas promising progress has been demonstrated in restoring force feedback, relatively little research has been reported for tactile haptic feedback [179]. Tactile sensors measure properties such as pressure, vibration, stiffness, texture, and shape [178]. As such, tactile haptic feedback is essential for the detection of local mechanical properties of tissues, such as compliance and surface texture. If realized, haptic feedback combined with robotic precision would allow the potential of MIS to be exploited in full [175, 179].

Restoring haptic feedback to the surgeon through electronics requires both haptic sensors on the patient side of the instrument, to acquire information from the tissues, and an interface at the operational side to relay this information to the surgeon.

Advances in flexible electronics, material science, and fabrication technologies combine to present a viable cost-effective solution to current constraints. E-skin allows for greater array density, increasing the sensory capability of miniaturized devices. The flexible nature of the e-skin means that it could be wrapped around the tip of surgical instruments to contact with the patient's body and acquire useful information about tissue properties. This information could then be relayed to the surgeon, providing a meaningful substitute to manual palpation. An inflatable balloon catheter, with heterogeneously integrated high-performance semiconductor devices, sensors, actuators, and other components forming an e-skin is presented in [180] schematically illustrated in Fig. 5.19B. Such tools facilitate the elimination of blockages in the stenotic blood vessel in peripheral or coronary angioplasty and in the diagnosis of biological tissues and intraluminal surfaces through direct, soft mechanical contact in septostomy and other standard procedures [180, 181].

The fabrication of biocompatible, biodegradable e-skin that is cheap to produce and easily disposable could solve the problem of sterilization that currently complicates the use of electronic components in surgery. The realization of reliable haptic feedback in the field of surgical robotics would expand human capabilities to improve precision in surgical procedures and advance provision of health care in developing countries and areas where trained health care personnel are scarce. Flexible electronics enable promising progress toward this direction.

While there are interesting futuristic applications, it is to be noted that there are major challenges and hurdles for IMNS-based technologies which have to be addressed and overcome. These include packaging, modeling, and dealing with thermal and stress-strain effects. A major reason behind the success of CMOS technology has been the availability of accurate models to predict the device response. This led to abstract models for use in CAD tools. However, this is challenging in the case of IMNS-based flexible electronics as stress and various device architecture-related effects must be considered in the model. Another important challenge where more and more research innovations and breakthroughs are required is in the scalability of the fabrication process. In conclusion, despite many challenges, the IMNS-based technology holds great promise for advances in many areas where high-performance flexible and conformable electronics are needed.

5.4 Summary

Natural skin has vast and highly discriminate sensory capabilities. This, combined with its large surface area, and direct communication with both the human nervous system and the external world, makes it an ideal site for interfacing electronics with the human body. Such was the inspiration for the development of topical e-skin systems.

Attempts to mimic the function of natural skin have triggered the demand for flexible, conformable electronics that can seamlessly integrate with biological systems.

Natural skin also provides a good example of an effective interface design, whereby, a system of electrical sensors directly contacts and stimulates underlying tissue. This concept has inspired implantable and inanimate-e-skin applications where, for example, the e-skin is wrapped around a nerve, and covers a prosthetic device respectively.

Elements impacting upon the e-skin system design, are highlighted: materials, compatibility, architecture, energy/power requirements, and cost are all factors to consider. Each of these elements is interrelated and have an impact on one another. Therefore, to achieve significant progress in the field as a whole, further research is required into each. Further advances in fabrication technologies are also required if the full potential of e-skin systems is to be realized.

This chapter has provided examples of applications within each of the categories of e-skin described above. It indicates the huge potential of such applications within health-care diagnostics, disease monitoring, assistive technologies, and rehabilitation. E-skin in these contexts could provide individuals with data to inform their lifestyle practices or indicate the need for treatment. It could also aid in an earlier and less invasive diagnosis. There is a great demand for soft, flexible electronics within the field of surgical robotics in order to restore haptic feedback to the operating surgeon, and facilitate progress in the subfields of MIS and tele-surgery. E-skin represents a viable solution to this particular challenge.

Implantable e-skin represents a potentially life-changing intervention for patients suffering from spinal injuries or disability. With further research, it offers a solution to help overcome the limits of the human body to repair itself after such catastrophic injuries.

Similarly, inanimato e-skin offers a potential means of restoring sensory feedback to users of prosthetic devices. UTCs and the POSFET are described as examples representing recent progress within this field. The need for a bidirectional interface in this setting was discussed.

Here, the development of hardware-implemented neuromorphic tactile data processing with neural network-like algorithms within e-skin would be advantageous in combating the challenges facing readout and processing of neural signals in this context.

References

[1] T. Yokota, et al., Ultraflexible organic photonic skin, Sci. Adv. (2016) 2(4).
[2] G.-T. Hwang, et al., In vivo silicon-based flexible radio frequency integrated circuits monolithically encapsulated with biocompatible liquid crystal polymers, ACS Nano 7 (5) (2013) 4545–4553.
[3] R.C. Webb, et al., Ultrathin conformal devices for precise and continuous thermal characterization of human skin, Nat. Mater. 12 (10) (2013) 938–944.
[4] Z.J. Du, et al., Ultrasoft microwire neural electrodes improve chronic tissue integration, Acta Biomater. 53 (2017) 46–58.
[5] W. Dang, et al., Stretchable wireless system for sweat pH monitoring, Biosens. Bioelectron. 107 (2018) 192–202.

[6] L.E. Osborn, et al., Prosthesis with neuromorphic multilayered e-dermis perceives touch and pain, Sci. Robot. 3 (19) (2018).

[7] J. Kim, et al., Stretchable silicon nanoribbon electronics for skin prosthesis, Nat. Commun. 5 (2014).

[8] C.G. Núñez, et al., Energy autonomous flexible and transparent tactile skin, Adv. Funct. Mater. 1606287 (2017).

[9] E. Hosseini, L. Manjakkal, R. Dahiya, Bio-organic glycine based flexible piezoelectric stress sensor for wound monitoring, in: IEEE Sensors, New Delhi, 2018.

[10] J. Mark, Polymer Data Handbook, Oxford University Press, New York, 1999.

[11] M.C. Bélanger, Y. Marois, Hemocompatibility, biocompatibility, inflammatory and in vivo studies of primary reference materials low-density polyethylene and polydimethylsiloxane: a review, J. Biomed. Mater. Res. 58 (5) (2001) 467–477.

[12] B.A. Grzybowski, S.T. Brittain, G.M. Whitesides, Thermally actuated interferometric sensors based on the thermal expansion of transparent elastomeric media, Rev. Sci. Instrum. 70 (4) (1999) 2031–2037.

[13] T.N. Tran, et al., Bioelastomers based on cocoa shell waste with antioxidant ability, Adv. Sustain. Syst. 1 (7) (2017) 1700002.

[14] D. Sun, Characterization of Medical Grade Poly-Dimethylsiloxane as Encapsulation Materials for Implantable Microelectromechanical Systems, Case Western Reserve University, 2014.

[15] A. Nathan, et al., Flexible electronics: the next ubiquitous platform, Proc. IEEE 100 (Special Centennial Issue) (2012) 1486–1517.

[16] J.-G. Liu, et al., Colorless and transparent high–temperature-resistant polymer optical films–current status and potential applications in optoelectronic fabrications, in: Optoelectronics-Materials and Devices, InTech, 2015.

[17] M. Kaltenbrunner, et al., An ultra-lightweight design for imperceptible plastic electronics, Nature 499 (7459) (2013) 458.

[18] C.J. Lee, et al., Neural signal recording using microelectrode arrays fabricated on liquid crystal polymer material, Mater. Sci. Eng. C 24 (1-2) (2004) 265–268.

[19] M. Irimia-Vladu, et al., Environmentally sustainable organic field effect transistors, Org. Electron. 11 (12) (2010) 1974–1990.

[20] P. Boonvisut, M.C. Çavuşoğlu, Estimation of soft tissue mechanical parameters from robotic manipulation data, IEEE/ASME Trans. Mechatr. 18 (5) (2013) 1602–1611.

[21] Ecoflex Series, Super-Soft, Addition Cure Silicone Rubbers, Smooth-On, 2015, p. 6.

[22] C.J. Bettinger, Recent advances in materials and flexible electronics for peripheral nerve interfaces, Bioelectr. Med. 4 (1) (2018) 6.

[23] I.R. Minev, et al., Electronic dura mater for long-term multimodal neural interfaces, Science 347 (6218) (2015) 159–163.

[24] J. Lee, et al., Stretchable semiconductor technologies with high areal coverages and strain-limiting behavior: demonstration in high-efficiency dual-junction GaInP/GaAs photovoltaics, Small 8 (12) (2012) 1851–1856.

[25] T. Yamada, et al., A stretchable carbon nanotube strain sensor for human-motion detection, Nat. Nanotechnol. 6 (2011) 296.

[26] M.L. Hammock, et al., 25th anniversary article: The evolution of electronic skin (e-skin): a brief history, design considerations, and recent progress, Adv. Mater. 25 (42) (2013) 5997–6038.

[27] K. Cherenack, L. van Pieterson, Smart textiles: challenges and opportunities, J. Appl. Phys. 112 (9) (2012) 091301.

[28] D. Tobjörk, R. Österbacka, Paper electronics, Adv. Mater. 23 (17) (2011) 1935–1961.

[29] J.M. Nassar, et al., Paper skin multisensory platform for simultaneous environmental monitoring, Adv. Mater. Technol. 1 (1) (2016) 1600004.

[30] M. Park, et al., Highly stretchable electric circuits from a composite material of silver nanoparticles and elastomeric fibres, Nat. Nanotechnol. 7 (12) (2012) 803.

[31] S. Gupta, et al., Ultra-thin chip technologies for high performance flexible electronics, NPJ Flex. Electr. 2 (8) (2018) 1–8.

[32] N. Yogeswaran, et al., New materials and advances in making electronic skin for interactive robots, Adv. Robot. 29 (21) (2015) 1359–1373.

[33] B.C.-K. Tee, et al., A skin-inspired organic digital mechanoreceptor, Science 350 (6258) (2015) 313–316.

[34] Z. Bao, J. Locklin, Organic Field-Effect Transistors, CRC Press, 2007.

[35] X. Liu, et al., Large-scale integration of semiconductor nanowires for high-performance flexible electronics, ACS Nano 6 (3) (2012) 1888–1900.

[36] J. Lewis, Material challenge for flexible organic devices, Mater. Today 9 (4) (2006) 38–45.

[37] H. Zhou, et al., Fast flexible electronics with strained silicon nanomembranes, Sci. Rep. 3 (2013).

[38] Y. Sun, J.A. Rogers, Inorganic semiconductors for flexible electronics, Adv. Mater. 19 (15) (2007) 1897–1916.

[39] E.O. Polat, et al., Synthesis of large area graphene for high performance in flexible optoelectronic devices, Sci. Rep. 5 (2015).

[40] C. García Núñez, et al., Heterogeneous integration of contact-printed semiconductor nanowires for high-performance devices on large areas, Microsyst. Nanoeng. 4 (1) (2018) 22.

[41] D. Shakthivel, C. García Núñez, R. Dahiya, Inorganic Semiconducting Nanowires for Flexible Electronics, 2016.

[42] C.G. Nunez, et al., Integration Techniques for Micro/Nanostructures Based Large-area Electronics, in Elements of Flexible and Large Area Electronics, Cambridge University Press, 2018.

[43] D. Bandyopadhyay, J. Sen, Internet of things: applications and challenges in technology and standardization, Wirel. Pers. Commun. 58 (1) (2011) 49–69.

[44] D.-H. Kim, et al., Epidermal electronics, Science 333 (6044) (2011) 838–843.

[45] K.J. Yu, et al., Inorganic semiconducting materials for flexible and stretchable electronics, NPJ Flex. Electr. 1 (1) (2017) 4.

[46] W.T. Navaraj, et al., Wafer scale transfer of ultrathin silicon chips on flexible substrates for high performance bendable systems, Adv. Electr. Mater. (2018) 1700277.

[47] W.T. Navaraj, et al., Simulation study of junctionless silicon nanoribbon FETs for high-performance printable electronics, in: IEEE European Conference on Circuit Theory and Design (ECCTD), IEEE, Catania, 2017.

[48] S. Khan, et al., Flexible FETs using ultrathin Si microwires embedded in solution processed dielectric and metal layers, J. Micromech. Microeng. 25 (12) (2015) 125019.

[49] R. Crabb, F. Treble, Thin silicon solar cells for large flexible arrays, Nature 213 (5082) (1967) 1223.

[50] S. Khan, L. Lorenzelli, R. Dahiya, Technologies for printing sensors and electronics over large flexible substrates: a review, IEEE Sensors J. 15 (6) (2015) 3164–3185.

[51] D. Shakthivel, et al., Transfer printing Si nanowires for flexible large area electronics, in: Innovations in Large Area Electronics (InnoLAE) Conference, Cambridge, UK, 2016.

[52] R. Dahiya, G. Gottardi, N. Laidani, PDMS residues-free micro/macrostructures on flexible substrates, Microelectron. Eng. 136 (2015) 57–62.

[53] R.S. Dahiya, et al., Fabrication of single crystal silicon micro-/nanostructures and transferring them to flexible substrates, Microelectron. Eng. 98 (2012) 502–507.

[54] R. Dahiya, M. Valle, Robotic Tactile Sensing—Technologies and System, Springer, Dordrecht, 2013, p. 245.

[55] R. Dahiya, et al., Developing electronic skin with the sense of touch, Inform. Display 31 (4) (2015) 5.

[56] T. Someya, et al., Conformable, flexible, large-area networks of pressure and thermal sensors with organic transistor active matrixes, Proc. Natl. Acad. Sci. U. S. A. 102 (35) (2005) 12321–12325.

[57] D.J. Lipomi, et al., Skin-like pressure and strain sensors based on transparent elastic films of carbon nanotubes, Nat. Nanotechnol. 6 (12) (2011) 788–792.

[58] A. Chortos, J. Liu, Z. Bao, Pursuing prosthetic electronic skin, Nat. Mater. 15 (9) (2016) 937–950.

[59] R. Dahiya, et al., POSFET tactile sensing arrays using CMOS technology, Sensors Actuators A 202 (2013) 226–232.

[60] N. Yogeswaran, et al., Piezoelectric graphene field effect transistor pressure sensors for tactile sensing, Appl. Phys. Lett. 113 (1) (2018) 014102-1–014102-4.

[61] S. Khan, et al., Flexible tactile sensors using screen printed P(VDF-TrFE) and MWCNT/PDMS composites, IEEE Sensors J. 15 (6) (2014) 3146–3155.

[62] R.S. Johansson, Å.B. Vallbo, Tactile sensibility in the human hand: relative and absolute densities of four types of mechanoreceptive units in glabrous skin, J. Physiol. 286 (1) (1979) 283–300.

[63] D. Filingeri, et al., Thermal and tactile interactions in the perception of local skin wetness at rest and during exercise in thermo-neutral and warm environments, Neuroscience 258 (2014) 121–130.

[64] B.C. Tee, et al., An electrically and mechanically self-healing composite with pressure- and flexion-sensitive properties for electronic skin applications, Nat. Nanotechnol. 7 (12) (2012) 825–832.

[65] C.M. Boutry, et al., A sensitive and biodegradable pressure sensor array for cardiovascular monitoring, Adv. Mater. 27 (43) (2015) 6954–6961.

[66] W. Wu, X. Wen, Z.L. Wang, Taxel-addressable matrix of vertical-nanowire piezotronic transistors for active and adaptive tactile imaging, Science 340 (6135) (2013) 952–957.

[67] D.H. Ho, et al., Stretchable and multimodal all graphene electronic skin, Adv. Mater. (2016).

[68] C. Yeom, et al., Large-area compliant tactile sensors using printed carbon nanotube active-matrix backplanes, Adv. Mater. 27 (9) (2015) 1561–1566.

[69] L.W. Wei, A Neuromorphic Approach to Tactile Perception, 2016.

[70] NeuPrintSkin, Available from: https://gow.epsrc.ukri.org/NGBOViewGrant.aspx?GrantRef=EP/R029644/1. (cited 13 December 2018).

[71] R. Dahiya, et al., Tactile sensing—from humans to humanoids, IEEE Trans. Robot. 26 (1) (2010) 1–20.

[72] R. Dahiya, et al., Directions toward effective utilization of tactile skin: a review, IEEE Sensors J. 13 (11) (2013) 4121–4138.

[73] R. Dahiya, et al., Towards tactile sensing system on chip for robotic applications, IEEE Sensors J. 11 (12) (2011) 3216–3226.

[74] S. Gupta, et al., Towards bendable piezoelectric oxide semiconductor field effect transistor based touch sensor, in: IEEE ISCAS, IEEE, 2016.

[75] W.T. Navaraj, et al., Nanowire FET based neural element for robotic tactile sensing skin, Front. Neurosci. 11 (2017) 501.

[76] G. Cannata, et al., Modular skin for humanoid robot systems, in: Int. Conf. on Cognitive Systems, 2010.

[77] T. Someya, et al., A large-area, flexible pressure sensor matrix with organic field-effect transistors for artificial skin applications, Proc. Natl. Acad. Sci. U. S. A. 101 (27) (2004) 9966–9970.

[78] K. Takei, et al., Nanowire active-matrix circuitry for low-voltage macroscale artificial skin, Nat. Mater. 9 (10) (2010) 821–826.

[79] S. Caviglia, et al., Spike-based readout of POSFET tactile sensors, IEEE Trans. Circuits Syst. I: Regul. Pap. 64 (6) (2016) 1421–1431.

[80] S. Gupta, et al., Device modelling for bendable piezoelectric FET-based touch sensing system, IEEE Trans. Circuits Syst. I: Regul. Pap. 63 (12) (2016) 2200–2208.

[81] T. Saxena, R.V. Bellamkonda, Implantable electronics: a sensor web for neurons, Nat. Mater. 14 (12) (2015) 1190.

[82] Q. Cao, et al., Medium-scale carbon nanotube thin-film integrated circuits on flexible plastic substrates, Nature 454 (7203) (2008) 495.

[83] J. Lee, et al., Stretchable GaAs photovoltaics with designs that enable high areal coverage, Adv. Mater. 23 (8) (2011) 986–991.

[84] R. Dahiya, E-skin: from humanoids to humans, Proc. IEEE (2019).

[85] W. Dang, et al., Printable stretchable interconnects, Flex. Print. Electr. 2 (1) (2017) 1–17.

[86] M.A. Srinivasan, C. Basdogan, Haptics in virtual environments: taxonomy, research status, and challenges, Comput. Graph. 21 (4) (1997) 393–404.

[87] M. Sreelakshmi, T.D. Subash, Haptic technology: a comprehensive review on its applications and future prospects, Mater. Today: Proc. 4 (2) (2017) 4182–4187.

[88] M. Srinivasan, et al., Human and machine haptics, RLE Progr. Rep. 147 (1999).

[89] C.O. Mahony, et al., Embedded sensors for micro transdermal interface platforms (microTIPs), in: 2016 Symposium on Design, Test, Integration and Packaging of MEMS/MOEMS (DTIP), 2016.

[90] T. Sekitani, T. Someya, Stretchable, large-area organic electronics, Adv. Mater. 22 (2010) 2228–2246.

[91] J.A. Rogers, T. Someya, Y. Huang, Materials and mechanics for stretchable electronics, Science 327 (5973) (2010) 1603–1607.

[92] S. Khan, L. Lorenzelli, R. Dahiya, Flexible MISFET devices from transfer printed Si microwires and spray coating, IEEE J. Electr. Dev. Soc. 4 (4) (2016) 189–196.

[93] J.N. Burghartz, Ultra-Thin Chip Technology and Applications, Springer, 2011.

[94] L. Martiradonna, Implantable devices: a solid base, Nat. Mater. 14 (10) (2015) 962.

[95] J.N. Burghartz, et al., HDR CMOS imagers and their applications, in: 8th International Conference on Solid-State and Integrated Circuit Technology, ICSICT 2006, 2006.

[96] J.N. Burghartz, et al., CMOS imager technologies for biomedical applications, in: IEEE International Solid-State Circuits Conference, 2008. ISSCC 2008. Digest of Technical Papers, 2008.

[97] G. Kunkel, et al., Ultra-flexible and ultra-thin embedded medical devices on large area panels, in: 3rd Electronic System-Integration Technology Conference (ESTC), 2010, 2010.

[98] E. Zrenner, et al., Can subretinal microphotodiodes successfully replace degenerated photoreceptors? Vis. Res. 39 (15) (1999) 2555–2567.

[99] T. Cohen-Karni, et al., Flexible electrical recording from cells using nanowire transistor arrays, Proc. Natl. Acad. Sci. 106 (18) (2009) 7309–7313.

[100] B.P. Timko, et al., Electrical recording from hearts with flexible nanowire device arrays, Nano Lett. 9 (2) (2009) 914–918.

[101] C.G. Núñez, et al., ZnO nanowires-based flexible UV photodetector system for wearable dosimetry, IEEE Sensors J. 18 (19) (2018) 7881–7888.

[102] C.G. Nunez, et al., ZnO nanowires based flexible UV photodetectors for wearable dosimetry, in: 2017 IEEE Sensors, 2017.

[103] R. Dahiya, Epidermal electronics: flexible electronics for biomedical applications, in: S. Carrara, K. Iniewski (Eds.), Handbook of Bioelectronics: Directly Interfacing Electronics and Biological Systems, Cambridge University Press, 2015.

[104] S. Madhusudan, et al., Inkjet printing—process and its applications, Adv. Mater. 22 (6) (2010) 673–685.

[105] I.C. Cheng, S. Wagner, Overview of flexible electronics technology, in: Flexible Electronics, Springer, 2009, pp. 1–28.

[106] R. Das, P. Harrop, Printed, Organic & Flexible Electronics Forecasts, Players & Opportunities 2013–2023, IDTechEx, Cambridge, 2013.

[107] D. Quesada-González, A. Merkoçi, Mobile phone-based biosensing: an emerging "diagnostic and communication" technology, Biosens. Bioelectron. 92 (2017) 549–562.

[108] W. Gao, et al., Fully integrated wearable sensor arrays for multiplexed in situ perspiration analysis, Nature 529 (7587) (2016) 509.

[109] Y. Liu, M. Pharr, G.A. Salvatore, Lab-on-skin: a review of flexible and stretchable electronics for wearable health monitoring, ACS Nano 11 (10) (2017) 9614–9635.

[110] N.M. Farandos, et al., Contact lens sensors in ocular diagnostics, Adv. Healthc. Mater. 4 (6) (2015) 792–810.

[111] S. Tinku, et al., Smart contact lens using passive structures, in: IEEE Sensors Conference, 2014.

[112] S. Corrie, et al., Blood, sweat, and tears: developing clinically relevant protein biosensors for integrated body fluid analysis, Analyst 140 (13) (2015) 4350–4364.

[113] D.A. Sakharov, et al., Relationship between lactate concentrations in active muscle sweat and whole blood, Bull. Exp. Biol. Med. 150 (1) (2010) 83–85.

[114] M.J. Patterson, S.D.R. Galloway, M.A. Nimmo, Variations in regional sweat composition in normal human males, Exp. Physiol. 85 (6) (2000) 869–875.

[115] R.K. Sivamani, L.A. Crane, R.P. Dellavalle, The benefits and risks of ultraviolet tanning and its alternatives: the role of prudent sun exposure, Dermatol. Clin. 27 (2) (2009) 149–154.

[116] B.K. Armstrong, A. Kricker, The epidemiology of UV induced skin cancer, J. Photochem. Photobiol. B Biol. 63 (1-3) (2001) 8–18.

[117] F. De Gruijl, Skin cancer and solar UV radiation, Eur. J. Cancer 35 (14) (1999) 2003–2009.

[118]   H.M. Al-Angari, et al., Novel dynamic peak and distribution plantar pressure measures on diabetic patients during walking, Gait Posture 51 (2017) 261–267.

[119]   M.J. Fowler, Microvascular and macrovascular complications of diabetes, Clin. Diabetes 26 (2008) 77.

[120]   K. Deschamps, et al., Classification of forefoot plantar pressure distribution in persons with diabetes: a novel perspective for the mechanical management of diabetic foot? PLoS ONE 8 (11) (2013) e79924.

[121]   Y.C. Lu, Q.C. Mei, Y.D. Gu, Plantar loading reflects ulceration risks of diabetic foot with toe deformation, Biomed. Res. Int. 2015 (2015) 6.

[122]   L. Claverie, A. Ille, P. Moretto, Discrete sensors distribution for accurate plantar pressure analyses, Med. Eng. Phys. 38 (12) (2016) 1489–1494.

[123]   W.T. Navaraj, et al., Upper limb prosthetic control using toe gesture sensors, in: IEEE Sensors, Korea, 2015.

[124]   A. Vilouras, et al., At-home computer-aided myoelectric training system for wrist prosthesis, in: EuroHaptics: International Conference on Human Haptic Sensing and Touch Enabled Computer Applications, Springer, 2016.

[125]   H. Han, et al., Trends in epidermal stretchable electronics for noninvasive long-term healthcare applications, Int. J. Autom. Smart Technol. 7 (2) (2017) 37–52.

[125a] C.J. De Luca, The use of surface electromyography in biomechanics, J. Appl. Biomech. 13 (2) (1997) 135–163.

[125b] Y. Li, X. Zhang, Y. Gong, Y. Cheng, X. Gao, X. Chen, Motor function evaluation of hemiplegic upper-extremities using data fusion from wearable inertial and surface EMG sensors, Sensors 17 (3) (2017) 582.

[126]   A. Miyamoto, et al., Inflammation-free, gas-permeable, lightweight, stretchable on-skin electronics with nanomeshes, Nat. Nanotechnol. 12 (2017) 907.

[127]   V.N. Nukala, W.E. Halal, Emerging neurotechnologies: trends, relevance and prospects, Synesis: J. Sci. Technol. Ethics Policy 1 (1) (2010).

[128]   A.E. Schultz, T.A. Kuiken, Neural interfaces for control of upper limb prostheses: the state of the art and future possibilities, PM&R 3 (1) (2011) 55–67.

[129]   H.C. Lee, et al., Histological evaluation of flexible neural implants; flexibility limit for reducing the tissue response? J. Neural Eng. 14 (3) (2017).

[130]   A. Gefen, S.S. Margulies, Are in vivo and in situ brain tissues mechanically similar? J. Biomech. 37 (9) (2004) 1339–1352.

[131]   N.D. Leipzig, M.S. Shoichet, The effect of substrate stiffness on adult neural stem cell behavior, Biomaterials 30 (36) (2009) 6867–6878.

[132]   J. Goding, et al., Interpenetrating conducting hydrogel materials for neural interfacing electrodes, Adv. Healthc. Mater. 6 (9) (2017).

[133]   L. Luan, et al., Ultraflexible nanoelectronic probes form reliable, glial scar–free neural integration, Sci. Adv. 3 (2) (2017).

[134]   F. Tenore, et al., Towards the control of individual fingers of a prosthetic hand using surface EMG signals, in: 2007 29th Annual International Conference of the IEEE Engineering in Medicine and Biology Society, 2007.

[135]   L.H. Smith, L.J. Hargrove, Comparison of surface and intramuscular EMG pattern recognition for simultaneous wrist/hand motion classification, in: Conference proceedings: Annual International Conference of the IEEE Engineering in Medicine and Biology Society. IEEE Engineering in Medicine and Biology Society. Conference, NIH Public Access, 2013.

[136]   M.R. Mulvey, et al., The use of transcutaneous electrical nerve stimulation (TENS) to aid perceptual embodiment of prosthetic limbs, Med. Hypotheses 72 (2) (2009) 140–142.

[137]   M.R. Mulvey, et al., Perceptual embodiment of prosthetic limbs by transcutaneous electrical nerve stimulation, Neuromodul.: Technol. Neural Interface 15 (1) (2012) 42–47.

[138]   B.T. Nghiem, et al., Providing a sense of touch to prosthetic hands, Plast. Reconstr. Surg. 135 (6) (2015) 1652–1663.

[139]   E.B. Goldstein, J. Brockmole, Sensation and Perception, Cengage Learning, 2016.

[140] H. Flor, et al., Effect of sensory discrimination training on cortical reorganisation and phantom limb pain, Lancet 357 (9270) (2001) 1763–1764.

[141] B.C.K. Tee, et al., An electrically and mechanically self-healing composite with pressure- and flexion-sensitive properties for electronic skin applications, Nat. Nanotechnol. 7 (12) (2012) 825–832.

[142] S. Bauer, Flexible electronics: sophisticated skin, Nat. Mater. 12 (10) (2013) 871–872.

[143] C. Wang, et al., User-interactive electronic skin for instantaneous pressure visualization, Nat. Mater. 12 (10) (2013) 899–904.

[144] J.J. Boland, Flexible electronics: within touch of artificial skin, Nat. Mater. 9 (10) (2010) 790–792.

[145] S. Raspopovic, et al., Restoring natural sensory feedback in real-time bidirectional hand prostheses, Sci. Transl. Med. 6 (222) (2014) 222ra19.

[146] J. Scheibert, et al., The role of fingerprints in the coding of tactile information probed with a biomimetic sensor, Science 323 (5920) (2009) 1503–1506.

[147] R.S. Johansson, J.R. Flanagan, Coding and use of tactile signals from the fingertips in object manipulation tasks, Nat. Rev. Neurosci. 10 (5) (2009) 345–359.

[148] V.E. Abraira, D.D. Ginty, The sensory neurons of touch, Neuron 79 (4) (2013) 618–639.

[149] A.I. Weber, et al., Spatial and temporal codes mediate the tactile perception of natural textures, Proc. Natl. Acad. Sci. 110 (42) (2013) 17107–17112.

[150] P. Jenmalm, et al., Influence of object shape on responses of human tactile afferents under conditions characteristic of manipulation, Eur. J. Neurosci. 18 (1) (2003) 164–176.

[151] R. Johansson, G. Westling, Signals in tactile afferents from the fingers eliciting adaptive motor responses during precision grip, Exp. Brain Res. 66 (1) (1987) 141–154.

[152] H. Hensel, Thermoreceptors, Annu. Rev. Physiol. 36 (1) (1974) 233–249.

[153] M. Campero, H. Bostock, Unmyelinated afferents in human skin and their responsiveness to low temperature, Neurosci. Lett. 470 (3) (2010) 188–192.

[154] W.M.B. Tiest, Tactual perception of material properties, Vis. Res. 50 (24) (2010) 2775–2782.

[155] R. Ackerley, et al., Wetness perception across body sites, Neurosci. Lett. 522 (1) (2012) 73–77.

[156] F. Mancini, et al., Whole-body mapping of spatial acuity for pain and touch, Ann. Neurol. 75 (6) (2014) 917–924.

[157] M. Boniol, et al., Proportion of skin surface area of children and young adults from 2 to 18 years old, J. Investig. Dermatol. 128 (2) (2008) 461–464.

[158] L.B. Buck, Information coding in the vertebrate olfactory system, Annu. Rev. Neurosci. 19 (1) (1996) 517–544.

[159] V.J. Barranca, et al., Sparsity and compressed coding in sensory systems, PLoS Comput. Biol. 10 (8) (2014) e1003793.

[160] H.B. Barlow, The ferrier lecture, 1980: critical limiting factors in the design of the eye and visual cortex, Proc. R. Soc. Lond. B Biol. Sci. 212 (1186) (1981) 1–34.

[161] R.S. Johansson, I. Birznieks, First spikes in ensembles of human tactile afferents code complex spatial fingertip events, Nat. Neurosci. 7 (2) (2004) 170–177.

[162] R. Dahiya, et al., CMOS implementation of POSFET tactile sensing arrays with on chip readout, in: Proc. Int. Conf. Sensor Technologies and Applications (SENSORCOMM), 2010.

[163] Q. Qing, et al., Nanowire transistor arrays for mapping neural circuits in acute brain slices, Proc. Natl. Acad. Sci. 107 (5) (2010) 1882–1887.

[164] J. Judy, DARPA RE-NET Government Oversight Program Review, Defense Advanced Research Projects Agency, Arlington, VA, 2013.

[165] J. Sales, et al., Multi-modal 64x peripheral nerve active probe & micro-stimulator with on-chip dual-coil power/data transmission and 2nd-order Opamp-less $\Delta\Sigma$ ADC, in: Submitted to International Solid-State Circuits Conference, San Francisco, 2019.

[166] G.S. Dhillon, K.W. Horch, Direct neural sensory feedback and control of a prosthetic arm, IEEE Trans. Neural Syst. Rehabil. Eng. 13 (4) (2005) 468–472.

[167] G.S. Dhillon, et al., Residual function in peripheral nerve stumps of amputees: implications for neural control of artificial limbs, J. Hand Surg. 29 (4) (2004) 605–615.

[168] P.M. Rossini, et al., Double nerve intraneural interface implant on a human amputee for robotic hand control, Clin. Neurophysiol. 121 (5) (2010) 777–783.

[169] T. Tchumatchenko, et al., Delivery of continuously-varying stimuli using channelrhodopsin-2, Front. Neural Circuits 7 (2013).

[170] S. Zhao, et al., Improved expression of halorhodopsin for light-induced silencing of neuronal activity, Brain Cell Biol. 36 (1-4) (2008) 141–154.

[171] I.B. Witten, et al., Cholinergic interneurons control local circuit activity and cocaine conditioning, Science 330 (6011) (2010) 1677–1681.

[172] O. Ozioko, et al., Smart Finger Braille: a tactile sensing and actuation based communication glove for deafblind people, in: IEEE ISIE, IEEE, 2017.

[173] O. Ozioko, et al., Tactile communication system for the interaction between deafblind and robots, in: IEEE International Conference on Robot and Human Interactive Communication, Nanjing, China, 2018.

[174] A. Hughes-Hallett, et al., Quantitative analysis of technological innovation in minimally invasive surgery, Br. J. Surg. 102 (2) (2015) e151–e157.

[175] A. Wedmid, E. Llukani, D.I. Lee, Future perspectives in robotic surgery, BJU Int. 108 (6 Pt 2) (2011) 1028–1036.

[176] M. Siddaiah-Subramanya, K.W. Tiang, M. Nyandowe, A new era of minimally invasive surgery: progress and development of major technical innovations in general surgery over the last decade, Surg. J. 3 (4) (2017) e163–e166.

[177] J. Marescaux, et al., Transatlantic robot-assisted telesurgery, Nature 413 (6854) (2001) 379–380.

[178] N. Enayati, E.D. Momi, G. Ferrigno, Haptics in robot-assisted surgery: challenges and benefits, IEEE Rev. Biomed. Eng. 9 (2016) 49–65.

[179] A.M. Okamura, Haptic feedback in robot-assisted minimally invasive surgery, Curr. Opin. Urol. 19 (1) (2009) 102–107.

[180] D.-H. Kim, et al., Materials for multifunctional balloon catheters with capabilities in cardiac electrophysiological mapping and ablation therapy, Nat. Mater. 10 (4) (2011) 316.

[181] R.L. Mueller, T.A. Sanborn, The history of interventional cardiology: cardiac catheterization, angioplasty, and related interventions, Am. Heart J. 129 (1) (1995) 146–172.

Further reading

[182] T. Sekitani, et al., Stretchable active-matrix organic light-emitting diode display using printable elastic conductors, Nat. Mater. 8 (6) (2009) 494.

[183] G.-J. Zhang, Y. Ning, Silicon nanowire biosensor and its applications in disease diagnostics: a review, Anal. Chim. Acta 749 (2012) 1–15.

[184] M.C. Garcia, T. Vieira, Surface electromyography: why, when and how to use it, Rev. Andal. Med. Deporte 4 (1) (2011) 17–28.

CHAPTER 6

Wearable device for thermotherapies

Minyoung Suh[a], Sergio Curto[b], Punit Prakash[c], Gerard van Rhoon[b]
[a]Textile and Apparel, Technology and Management, North Carolina State University, Raleigh, NC, United States [b]Radiation Oncology, Erasmus MC Cancer Institute, Rotterdam, The Netherlands [c]Electrical and Computer Engineering, Kansas State University, Manhattan, KS, United States

Chapter Outline

6.1 Introduction

There has been a sustained interest in the development and adoption of technologies to track physiological and activity parameters related to health conditions. Wearable electronic technologies, such as smart watches and fitness trackers, are now in widespread use as

Wearable Bioelectronics. https://doi.org/10.1016/B978-0-08-102407-2.00007-2

wellness monitoring devices [1]. A few wearables have also recently been approved as medical devices, establishing their utility for providing clinical-grade feedback related to specific indications [2]. Physiological quantities of interest for continuous monitoring in daily living include heart rate, respiratory rate, oxygen saturation, and blood pressures.

Textile-based technologies lend themselves well to applications where there is a need for monitoring of physiological parameters. Textile-based sensors are comfortable, likely to be unobtrusive, and offer the potential to conform to a wide range of body sizes and shapes. These may be stand-alone sensors made from fabric, or integrated within clothing [3]. Therapeutic devices and systems deliver controlled doses of external energy to a region of the body to induce desired therapeutic effects. Similar to diagnostic sensors and technologies, the use of textile-based devices for therapeutic technologies has potential to improve comfort and conformity. Examples of therapeutic technologies include functional electrical stimulation technologies and thermal therapy devices and systems. Electrical stimulation technologies deliver pulsed electric currents at frequencies in the range of 1 to 1000 Hz for neuromuscular stimulation and are often employed on a demand-based setting. For example, Crema et al. [4] recently developed a garment incorporating an electrode array to deliver electrical stimulation to hand muscles, with application to hand-grasp training and assistance.

In contrast to electrical stimulation applications, thermal therapy devices are typically employed in a medical setting to deliver electromagnetic or acoustic energy to a region of the body for controlled modification of the local tissue temperature. Depending on the intensity and duration of heating, biological effects include modifications of local blood flow, and associated changes in local oxygenation and pH, and thermally induced damage and cell death. Applications include the use of moderate heating in sports medicine [5] and hyperthermia adjuvant to chemotherapy or radiation therapy for cancer treatment [6, 6a]. For these applications, the treatment is often delivered in a clinical setting for careful delivery of energy to achieve the desired biological and clinical effects, while minimizing damage to nontarget tissues. Even though these treatments are often administered within the clinical environment, wearable applicators, and technologies stand to offer substantial benefits to user, including, conformity of the device to individual patient anatomy and comfort, as well as ease of use for the operators.

As illustrated in Fig. 6.1, conventional devices and systems for delivering hyperthermia employ a power source that supplies electromagnetic energy to an applicator which incorporates antennas for coupling the energy to the body. The systems often employ a water bolus to cool the surface of the skin in contact with the applicator, while permitting heating of deeper tissue. Although some of these technologies are in clinical use, the applicators are often rigid and bulky, have limited means to conform to the patient's body, and may be restricted to use within specialized medical facilities. Since these treatments are often

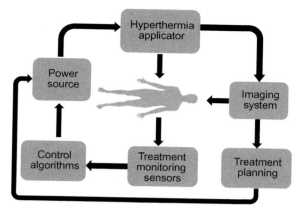

Fig. 6.1
System structure for thermal therapy.

performed for long duration up to 90 min, and repeatedly, there is a substantial motivation to make them more comfortable, customize energy delivery for individual patients, and potentially contribute to improved patient adherence to the treatment regimen. On the other hand, rigid applicators ensure that the applicator geometry remains consistent across treatment; variations in energy delivery across treatments are thus limited to discrepancies in how the applicator interfaces with the patient, as well as spatial and temporal heterogeneity in tissue biophysical properties [7].

This chapter focuses on the technological considerations for the design of wearable devices for delivering thermal therapies. Antennas are transducers that convert electromagnetic energy transferred within guided structures, to waves propagating. Conventional antennas are fabricated from metals with high electrical conductivity (e.g., copper) and have a high efficiency. When constructed, these antennas are rigid and retain their geometry, and thus can be expected to deliver a consistent electromagnetic radiation pattern. As detailed in other chapters, there has been substantial progress in integrating conductive materials within textiles and fabrics to fabricate antennas suitable for a variety of applications, including on-body communication and wireless sensing. Using similar approaches, textile-based antennas have strong potential to serve as conformal applicators for delivering thermal therapy. However, the conformity poses as an added challenge in that the antenna's radiation characteristics may change as its geometry relative to the patient's body changes while self-heating due to low efficiency may change the antenna characteristics.

This chapter discusses the design, fabrication, and application of textile-based technologies for therapeutic applications, with an emphasis on thermal therapies. Section 6.2 introduces diverse occasions in which continuous thermal treatments are involved. Sections 6.3 and 6.4

cover the fundamental materials and techniques for incorporating antennas within wearable devices. Being a key element in the system, the design of wearable antennas is followed in Section 6.5. Section 6.6 discusses requirements of the system specific to thermal therapy applications, and introduces considerations to implement wearable thermal therapy technologies.

6.2 Thermal applications

In wearable devices, heat is generated by electrical resistance, chemical reaction, or microwaves and transferred by conduction, convection, or conversion [8], respectively. Conductive material of high resistance is desirable to produce more resistive heat, but there is a risk of thermal damage to the system because resistive heat keeps being accumulated on the conductor due to limited thermal conduction. Polymer substrates would melt down and this harms other components within the system. Convectional devices such as hot packs with heating liquid are efficient heaters but cause considerable discomfort to the wearers due to its weight and bulk as well as stiffness. An alternative approach has been to radiate electromagnetic energy to a specific target tissue. Unlike resistive heat, radiative heat does not warm the conductor itself up, and can be emitted to a distant target spot. However, there could be a concern related to potential negative influence of electromagnetic field on human health.

6.2.1 Thermal monitoring

Human body thermography is a good resource of diverse pathological indicators. It can tell about the risk for patients to develop certain pathological conditions, for instance, in breast cancer investigation, or for monitoring vascular, dermatological, and rheumatic disorders [9]. Another possible use of thermography is to optimize thermal comfort within clothing environment. The change of heat carried by a person can be monitored in real time and this makes it possible to adjust the temperature in microenvironment before thermal overload or shortage is detected by the person and unpleasant physiological reactions take place.

The most common technique for thermal monitoring is based on infrared, which is currently not feasible for wearable applications [9]. In contrast, thermal contact sensors can take a wearable form, such as thermocouples and thermistors. By the thermoelectric effect, a thermocouple produces a voltage depending on temperature difference between two conductors and this voltage can be interpreted to measure temperature. Recent wearable thermocouples are small in size enough to be embedded into textiles without adding weight and bulk. On the other hand, a wearable thermistor consists of a length of fine wire embedded on polymer substrates [10], and this component has a known relationship between electrical resistance and temperature, which is used to provide an indication of temperature.

Smartness of e-textiles is defined by its capability to sense and actuate [11]. Based on the data collected by thermal sensors, smart devices can make different types of decisions helpful for the wearer; for example, whether to warm up or cool down, or if she needs in-depth medical examinations for breast cancer. Accurate and reliable thermal sensing is vital in this process and actively investigated by researchers in diverse fields.

6.2.2 Thermal comfort

Relying on conduction or convection heating mostly, technologies to generate on-demand heat have been administered in arctic clothes or outdoor winter clothing for a long time. As a consequence, considerable commercial products have been introduced to market [12]. Some recent investigations to fabricate textile heating elements were achieved by weaving [13] and printing [14, 15]. Emphasizing the use in large-scale film heaters, these attempts aimed more at overcoming mechanical limitations of heating elements, such as breathability, flexibility, and endurance to mechanical deformations, and providing better physical comfort to the wearer. Invisible appearance and short response time are other concerns highlighted in those applications [14, 15].

6.2.3 Pain management

Thermal treatment can be applied for medicine-free pain management. Some nerve endings, such as thermoreceptors or proprioceptors, are known to initiate nerve signals that block nociception within the spinal cord [8] and the activation of these receptors reduces muscle tone, relaxes painful muscles, and enhances tissue blood flow. Thermotherapy relies on this physiological mechanism that skin temperature change can inhibit the transmission of nociceptive signals to the brain.

A wearable device takes huge advantages in topical heat treatment that it has broad and close contact interface with the skin, and is considered to be the most effective to treat against persistent pain [16]. Thermotherapy patches are placed on articular regions, such as lower back and knees, and conductive or conventional heat is applied directly to the skin. Therapeutic effect includes improving blood circulation, preventing inflammation, and therefore, alleviating pain. Applied frequently to joint injuries, those wearable devices also have to be soft and stretch enough to prevent physical discomfort [17–19]. Conformal geometry of the device is critical for this application as well.

6.2.4 Cancer therapy

Thermal therapy can be applied for further therapeutic effects such as cancer diagnosis and treatment. Breast cancer thermography was introduced in 1956 as a screening tool and was initially well accepted by medical communities. However, controversial studies were published about the sensitivity of thermography in the 1970s, and the interest in this diagnostic approach rapidly diminished. Later in 1982, FDA approved thermography as a breast cancer risk assessment tool [20], and there have been continuous research on cancer thermography until today for the early detection of breast cancer as well as discrimination of tumor density and size, and response to chemotherapy [21].

Unlike other screening techniques such as mammography or clinical breast exams, thermography is a noninvasive procedure that does not involve compression of the breast tissue or exposure to radiation. Using high-resolution temperature measurements of breast tissue, thermography can provide functional information on thermal and vascular conditions of the breast tissue. These functional changes are considered as physiological changes in tissues, which precede pathological changes. Giansanti et al. [21] study supports thermography's potential role in the early detection of breast abnormalities that may lead to cancer. Especially, a wearable device takes advantages for the long-term monitoring of the thermal activity and is able to check the presence of thermal abnormal patterns in breast tissues. Design and fabrication of a wearable device for breast cancer thermography can be found from Wang et al. [22].

A similar thermal approach can be taken toward hyperthermia treatments. Hyperthermia is a type of treatment that exposes cancer tissues to external heat to increase its temperature to ~42°C. The temperature between 40°C and 44°C is known to be impactful, not to the normal cells, but to cancer cells. Hyperthermia is administered in combination with conventional therapies such as chemotherapy and radiotherapy. It helps drugs penetrate better into cancer cells in chemotherapy and makes them more sensitive to ionized radiation in radiotherapy. A significantly reduced size of tumor cells were reported when hyperthermia was combined with radiation therapy [23]. Conformal hyperthermia applicators for large area of the torso was also proven to be effective for chest wall recurrence of breast cancer [24].

Wearable devices provide unique technological capabilities that are not possible with conventional electronics. The most beneficial nature of wearable devices is that it keeps in close contact with the skin for a long time. This allows treatments for chronic diseases as well as real-time monitoring of physiological parameters. Wearable devices are designed to be unobtrusive and comfortable, and could be customized for individual patients. Consequently, it can potentially contribute to improved patient adherence to the treatment regimen.

6.3 Material

Electronic textiles are fabricated by embedding a conductor into a textile structure. As it takes bigger portion of conductive component, it loses the typical textile properties such as flexibility or drapability and it becomes more electrically conductive. Property characterization of nonconductive material is another critical factor to consider in conductive textiles. As the demand of wireless connectivity grows, textile dielectric properties become important.

6.3.1 Conductors

Traditionally, metal powder or thin wires have been applied as a conductor in electro-textiles. Being equivalently resistive at the level of $1.6 \times 10^{-8} \Omega\,m$ [25], silver and copper are the most common metals in conductive textiles. Silver has the advantage of healthfulness, while copper offers great affordability. Stainless steel is significantly more resistive ($7.4 \times 10^{-7} \Omega\,m$) than copper and silver [25], but is favored by textile industry since it does not become discolored or rusty easily. The nonconductive materials usually consist of polyester or polyamide.

Conventional conductive yarns are either pure metal yarns or composites of metals and nonconductive fibers which help improving mechanical properties [11]. Fine metal wires, whose typical diameters range from 1 to 80 μm [26], are popularly used to form a conductive yarn because they are most similar to typical textile fibers in physical shapes and fineness while providing a high conductivity. Those metal wires wrap around the yarn along its axis [13] or become a core as a bundle [27]. A finer spun yarn results in better flexibility and drapability, but the conductor contents and processability becomes critical to produce those types of yarns.

Conductive textiles can be obtained from nonmetallic materials as well, such as carbon. For example, graphite, an allotrope of carbon, is a good nonmetal electrical conductor. Derived from graphene, carbon nanotubes (CNTs) have received much attention in research and development over the past decade for its superior electrical conductivity, high mechanical strength, and fair flexibility. Electrical resistivity of CNTs is known to be as low as $1.0 \times 10^{-8} \Omega\,m$. Recent advance in CNT processing techniques enables the production of CNT for 3D printable inks [28, 29] as well as in sheet structures [30] for more fabric-oriented applications.

6.3.2 Dielectrics

Due to the intensive spotlight on material innovations in mechanically excellent conductors, nonconductive portions of conductive textiles did not receive much attention from academia and industry. For a long time, in wearable electronics, fabrics were merely understood as a physical carrier of technological components to make them wearable. However, nonconductive material also plays a key role in conductive textiles; in term of not only its mechanical property but also its electrical property. Especially, electrical property of nonconductive textiles becomes increasingly important as the wearable device market and demand of wireless connectivity between various wearable devices grow.

Being electrically resistive, most polymeric materials are dielectrics. Dielectric materials interact with microwave energy due to the dipolar polarization phenomenon. Polarization takes place when polar molecules try to align themselves with the external electromagnetic

Table 6.1: Dielectric materials [33–35].

	ε'	ε''	Condition
Vacuum	1.0	0	
Air	~1.0	~0	
Polypropylene	2.2	1.4×10^{-4}	25°C, 1 kHz
Polyethylene	2.3	3.0×10^{-4}	25°C, 1 kHz
Rubber	3.0	5.0×10^{-3}	
Polyester	3.2	5.0×10^{-3}	25°C, 1 kHz
Nylon 6	3.7	1.6×10^{-2}	25°C, 1 kHz
Nylon 66	4.0	1.4×10^{-3}	25°C, 60 Hz
Silicon	11.7	5.0×10^{-3}	25°C, 1 kHz
Distilled water	77.0	1.6×10^{-1}	20°C, 3 GHz

field [31]. Different types of polarization are dominant depending on the frequency of electromagnetic field, such as electronic, atomic, dipolar, and ionic polarizations [32]. The overall polarization ability is characterized by permittivity (ε'), and electric energy loss due to the polarization is defined as dielectric loss (ε'').

Dielectric permittivity and loss of polymeric materials are summarized in Table 6.1. Polymeric materials are characterized by their fairly low dielectric loss. Polymeric materials have advantages to be easily processed into mechanically robust but flexible structures, but they generally suffer from a low dielectric constant [36]. According to their dielectric nature, polymeric material is classified into three different groups [37]. The first group is represented by polyethylene, polypropylene, and polyester, which are difficult to polarize due to their nonpolar molecular structure. Multimolecular substances such as rubbers and polybutadiene belong to the second group, which yields polarization at high frequencies, but weak polarization at low frequencies. The last group is characterized as being polar at low frequency and includes polyamide and polyvinylchloride.

The majority of dielectrics exist in the world as spatially disordered mixtures of two or more components, and textiles are not an exception. Textiles are not a simple homogeneous polymeric system, but a heterogeneous three-phase system, which consists of fiber, air, and moisture. Hence, in order to understand the dielectric properties of fabrics, it is useful to consider the fabric as a composite of materials of fiber, moisture, and air [38].

6.4 Fabrication methods and challenges

Photolithography has been a traditional technique in electronic industry to create delicate metal patterns on nonconductive surface. This is still a valid technique when flexible polymer films are considered [15], but cannot be applied to textiles substrates. Aiming at seamless embedment of metallic components into textile structures, there have been a few different approaches (Fig. 6.2) tried in previous attempts for wearable devices.

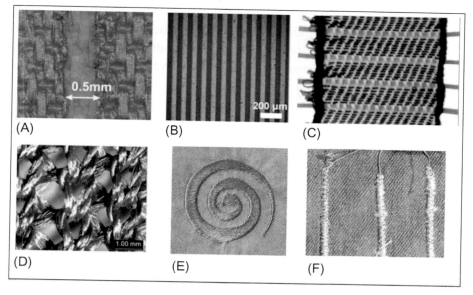

Fig. 6.2

E-textile examples of different fabrication techniques. (A) Printed structure [39]; (B) etched structure [15]; (C) woven structure [40]; (D) knitted structure [41]; (E) embroidered structure [42]; and (F) couched structure [43]. *(B) Copyright© 2017 American Chemical Society. (E) Reprinted with permission from Ohio State News. (F) Reprinted with permission from IBM System Journal.*

6.4.1 Conductive printing

Conductive printing might have been the most common techniques across disciplines. Conductive inks are prepared with metal nanoparticles in water-based solutions [25]. The inks are deposited directly over the fabric surface by diverse means (Fig. 6.2A), such as screen printing [14, 39], inkjet printing [10, 44], or 3D printing [28, 45]. Thermal sintering needs to be followed after printing for solvent evaporation and structure densification [25, 46].

Printability, which describes the efficiency of conductive printing, is largely determined by whether conductive ink penetrates a substrate or remains on the surface. According to Karaguzel et al. [46], conductive printing is optimized when it takes place mostly on the surface, not being dispersed into the internal structure of the textiles. It is highly related to how micropores are distributed over the surface. Having more flat and smooth surfaces similar to films and papers, high-density fabrics woven with fine synthetic filament yarns, such as nylon taffeta, have an advantage in that they have few printability issues. Coarse fabrics woven or knitted relatively loosely with uneven spun yarns of natural fibers, such as linen canvas, might be less favorable in terms of printability.

A heavier thickness of the conductive ink layer would decrease the electrical resistance, but excessive release of ink may result in serious defects in printing resolution. Thick ink layer could be easily peeled and damaged in durability. Corrosion and oxidation are also pointed out to be overcome in terms of durability. Since most conductive inks and pastes are based on silver filler having high brittleness, reliable conductivity is difficult to achieve [47]. Repeated bending load destroys conductive connections in the ink layer [39] and causes stability issues in long-term conductivity [47].

6.4.2 Laminating and etching

Similar to traditional textile finishing processes such as dyeing and coating, lamination is a technique to deposit a thin layer of conductive materials on the exterior surface of textiles regardless of its pattern. Diverse methods have been applied to achieve this such as dipping [48], spinning [19], plasma treatment [49], and chemical vapor deposition [50]. Thin and uniform distribution of conductive materials over the large surface is the core technology.

The laminated textiles go through further processes to acquire the desired conductive patterns for functional elements in specific electronics (Fig. 6.2B). For simple geometries relatively low in resolution such as a circular and rectangular shapes, laser cutting could be used to trim the conductive surface. However, more complicated techniques are required for microfabrication. Similar to photolithography, the desired conductive pattern of high resolution is engraved on the conductive surface through photoresist masking and chemical etching [10, 15].

6.4.3 Weaving

One of the simplest ways to embed conductive yarns into a fabric is to weave them as a warp or a weft [13, 27, 40, 51]. Empirically, plain weave has been preferred because its construction represents the most elementary and simple textile structure [27]. Plain weave has warp yarns most frequently interlaced with the weft yarns in under-one-over-one order (Fig. 6.2C). Since no lateral yarn movement is possible, a very sturdy fabric structure can be created [52].

Conductive yarns can be inserted along either warp (longitudinal) or weft (transverse) directions within woven fabrics. However, it is possible to let electrical current flow through a designated path by selective connections and disconnections at the contact points between conductive warps and wefts. Welded interconnection points are known to make huge improvement in the overall conductivity of woven fabrics [13, 51]. Final resistance of the copper-woven fabric with unwelded intersection points (2.31 Ω/m) is 10 times higher than that of welded points [51].

6.4.4 Knitting

Knitted structure consists of interconnected loops which usually results in a very stretchy fabric. This method requires more flexible conductive yarns than any other structures because the yarn is highly curved to form a loop. Formed with loops of a long continuous yarn entangled each other (Fig. 6.2D), knitted structure yields high resistance across the fabric, although the yarn itself is highly conductive [53]. It is because electrical contacts are not sturdy or robust between loops. Due to high resistivity, the use of knitted e-textile is often limited to certain applications that do not require high conductivity, such as electromagnetic interference (EMI) shielding [54, 55] or sensing [53].

Electrical resistance of knit fabrics has been investigated theoretically by considering a geometrical structure of knitted yarns as a resistive network [41, 56]. In a resistive network model, linear resistance is defined by the yarn resistance, while contact resistance is decided by both yarn resistance and contacting environment. Contact resistance is known to be much higher than linear resistance [41], and therefore contributes much to the overall increase of fabric resistance. Within single jersey, which is the simplest knit structure, the electrical resistance of fabrics changed in a same manner to conventional conductors; as the length becomes doubled, the resistance is doubled as well [56].

6.4.5 Embroidery

Referred as e-broidery [43], electronic embroidery is a technique to create linear or planar patterns of conductive threads with various stitches. Embroidery was previously understood only for decorative purposes, but now has been creating a lot of potentials for smart textiles. Unlike weaving and knitting methods, embroidery arranges a conductive thread in any shape and direction crossing over seams and boundaries (Fig. 6.2E).

One of the important technical issues associated with e-broidery is whether a conductive thread is mechanically flexible and soft enough to be machine stitched [52]. Metal-composite wires inherently lack in cohesion and deformability, and twists above certain levels have to be applied to combine metal wires and form a thread. Because of that, metal yarns are easy to get untwisted unless there is enough yarn tension preventing the thread from unraveling. Unstable structure of conductive threads causes problems to create unnecessary loops or knots and get stuck in the sewing machine. Limited shape recovery is another challenge of conductive thread to overcome to be machine-stitched. Current machine-stitchable conductive threads can be used only as a bobbin thread in conventional 301 stitch machine, but not as a needle thread [57].

Due to the limited mechanical properties of conductive threads, e-broidery often takes a couched structure where two totally unrelated threads are involved; one for covering and the other for being covered [40, 43]. A covering thread does not have to be conductive but has to go through with mechanically challenging processes. Remaining intact without any twists, loops, and tangles, covered threads are okay to be rigid with high conductivity. The covering thread does nothing but hosts the conductive thread (Fig. 6.2F).

Those fabrication techniques can be either extrinsic or intrinsic [52]. Extrinsic embedment refers to a superficial attachment of conductive elements to conventional textile surfaces such as printing or laminating, while conductive materials go through with traditional textile processing such as weaving and knitting, for intrinsic embedment. In general, intrinsic methods yield more mechanically robust but flexible e-textiles, and extrinsic e-textiles are more electrically conductive and easy to fabricate. According to Zysset et al. [40], mechanical strain of e-textiles was improved much when the embedment took place earlier in fabrication stages; 25% at fiber, 15% at fabric, and 6% at postfabric levels. Depending on the end application requirements, researchers and developers are choosing different fabrication techniques for their wearable device.

6.5 Antenna (electrode)

The antenna is a key element of a wearable device for thermotherapy. A specific antenna design is essential to enhance energy coupling and achieve preferential temperature increments in a specific target.

A challenge for many external devices for thermotherapy is that energy needs to be coupled into deep tissues without overheating the skin and superficial tissues [58]. Overheating of superficial tissues is a potential source of pain and can develop subcutaneous burns and damage the skin as well. Water bolus are used to control the skin temperature, and to adapt the antenna surface of the wearable device to the irregular skin surface (see Section 6.6.1). Due to the heterogeneous dielectric properties of the different tissues in human body, there is a complex electrical load to an antenna when it is located in its near field region. This complex load may result in the antenna detuning from the system frequency and interfere with the optimum energy deposition [59]. An antenna that remains sufficiently matched to the source frequency during variably loaded conditions can improve the overall system stability [60].

The electromagnetic field can penetrate deeper if the system operates at low frequency; however, the frequency of system operation is inversely proportional to the antenna size. This limits the antenna location at curved sites of the body, while a large antenna size is not desirable for wearable devices. Consequently, a compromise between operation frequency and physical dimension of the antenna needs to be considered. Small elements will provide high spatial resolution of power control and are capable of conforming to body contour. As is well known and generally accepted [61, 62], the penetration depth decreases with smaller aperture size. On the other hand, the large wavelength associated with low frequency makes it difficult to deliver energy into specific targets in small regions, and consequently large volumes become heated [59]. To avoid enhanced energy deposition on superficial tissues and interfaces, the antenna should generate tangentially aligned electric fields. Antennas that do not require a balanced-to-unbalanced (balun) transition are preferred to reduce volume and simplify the fed system [63].

Various antenna designs have been considered for superficial thermotherapy. Energy transfers from the antenna to the tissue by circular or linear field polarization using E- or H-field coupling.

Antennas using E-field coupling are most common and include waveguides [64], microstrip [24, 65], patch [63, 66], spiral [67], dipoles [68, 69], and others. While waveguide applicators offer an excellent heating pattern, their dimensions and weight limit their usability as a wearable device. Benefits of a patch antenna are its compactness, lightweight, impedance matching, and ability to generate tangential electric fields. They have been extensively characterized in the previous research and are in clinical use for the treatment of tumors in head and neck area [70, 71]. Antennas using H-field coupling are less commonly used, and a current sheet antenna is the most well-known. A few different types of antennas are discussed in the following sections.

6.5.1 Contact flexible microstrip applicators

Contact flexible microstrip applicators (CFMAs) are based on microstrip technology and are developed to operate at 27, 40, 70, and 434 MHz [65]. Fig. 6.3A shows CFMA of different sizes. Due to the high flexibility of the applicators, it is possible to adjust them to follow the body contour. A water bolus is incorporated to the system with the purpose of improving the

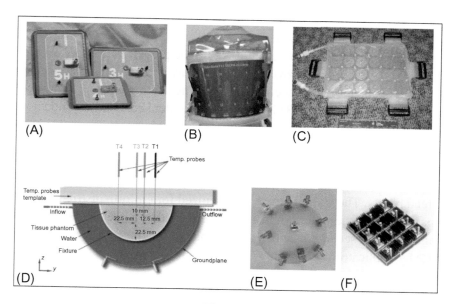

Fig. 6.3

Examples of wearable applicators. (A) Contact flexible microstrip applicator [72]; (B) conformal microwave array [24]; (C) spiral antenna [73]; (D) phased antenna array [74]; (E) conformal microwave antenna; (F) current sheet applicator. *(A) Copyright© 2018 Informa UK Limited. (B) From P. Stauffer, P. Maccarini, K. Arunachalam, O. Craciunescu, C. Diederich, T. Juang, F. Rossetto, J. Schlorff, A. Milligan, J. Hsu, P. Sneed, Z. Vujaskovic, Conformal microwave array (CMA) applicators for hyperthermia of diffuse chest wall recurrence, Int. J. Hyperth. 26 (7) (2010) 686–698. http://dx.doi.org/10.3109/02656736.2010.501511. (C) From G. Rhoon, External electromagnetic methods and devices, in: E. Moros (Ed.), Physics of Thermal Therapy: Fundamentals and Clinical Applications, CRC Press, Boca Raton, FL, 2013. (D) Copyright© 2018 Informa UK Limited. (E) Photo courtesy of Prof. Erdem Topsakal, Virginia Commonwealth University.*

matching and cooling the skin. The applicators generate a tangentially aligned electric field component to treat deep tissues and avoid overheating of subcutaneous fat layers. The CFMA generate effective heating in field sizes of 64–400 cm². Two coplanar active electrodes are separated from a shield electrode by a layer of substrate. At the 434 MHz operating band, the two active electrodes are excited as a plane dipole-like microstrip antenna by a slot of approximately 5 mm. A short circuit is located about $1/4\lambda_{substrate}$ away from the exciting slot [72]. Bending is possible around the axis perpendicular to the exiting slot (e.g., on the axis of the main E-field) [73]. The CFMA single element antennas have been evolved into the CFMA-12, which consists of 12 capacitor-type mini antennas placed in a 3×4 array [75]. Each mini antenna operates in same way as a single antenna in CFMA. The full arrangement of applicators allows spatial control of energy distribution by modulating amplitude for each element.

6.5.2 Conformal microwave array

The conformal microwave array (CMA) was designed to conform to body contours while it facilitates the treatment of superficial disease in large areas, such as diffuse chest wall recurrence [24], as shown in Fig. 6.3B. The CMA has been specifically designed to be wearable and allows patients to move around within the predetermined distance from the device. It consists of a flexible microwave antenna array with an integrated water bolus for skin surface cooling and electromagnetic coupling. The heating element is fabricated from a flexible printed circuit board (PCB) in an array of the dual concentric conductor (DCC) with multifed $\lambda/4$ square slot aperture elements and it operates at 433 and 915 MHz [76]. Buried in coplanar waveguides, feed lines were implemented to improve matching and power efficiency. Four tuning stubs match the 50 Ω coplanar waveguide transmission lines to the feed impedance of the DCC slot and provide equal phase and amplitude to the four symmetric feed points. The water bolus was optimized for uniform distribution of water. The PCB antenna array with the water bolus was implemented as a stretchable vest to adapt to the contoured anatomy and secure the applicator during the treatment. The effective treatment area of the CMA applicator is between 375 and 500 cm².

6.5.3 Multielement spiral antenna

Shown in Fig. 6.3C, the Pyrexar SA248 (Salt Lake City, UT, USA) is a flexible applicator with 24 heating elements that operates at 915 MHz. The unitary elements are Archimedean spirals in shape. The spirals are mounted inside a flexible silicone frame that also contains the water bolus. The silicon frame provides flexibility to adapt the applicator to curved surfaces of a body while keeping the water bolus in a constant thickness for the entire treatment area. The spiral antennas are connected in groups of three elements to be fed by one of the eight RF power amplifiers of the Pyrexar BSD-500 system. Each of the eight RF power amplifiers can be individually controlled in amplitude and phase to control energy deposition.

6.5.4 Breast array thermotherapy

A conformal array of phased antennas (Fig. 6.3D) has been proposed for the treatment of tumors located in an intact breast. The applicator was designed with a single patch antenna element operating at 915 MHz, [66]. Later design has been evolved into multiple antenna elements to develop controllable power deposition profiles for treating lesions at diverse locations within the intact breast [74]. In principle the initial design was wearable and considered antenna integration within one cup of a bra. Configurations of 2, 4, 8, 12, 16, and 20 antennas were evaluated. Target volumes of 10-mm edge length ($1 \, cm^3$) and 30-mm edge length ($27 \, cm^3$) positioned at the center of the breast and located 15 mm from the chest wall were evaluated. When excited with constant phase, applicators with 8 and 12 antennas yielded the highest average power absorption at centrally located and deep-seated targets.

A similar conformal microwave antenna applicator operating at 1.8 GHz (Fig. 6.3E) was proposed for the treatment of superficial tumors in the breast [77]. Their applicator included nine patch antennas in 3×3 array, but there was no water bolus involved within the system. This system yielded up to 3°C temperature increase at 10-mm depth within 10 min, but the temperature increase was reduced below 1°C at the deeper locations such as 25 and 40 mm.

6.5.5 Current sheet applicators

The current sheet applicator (CSA) has a very compact design that allows easy combination of antennas in a flat array to heat large tumor areas with a high spatial resolution (Fig. 6.3F). Since EM energy is inductively coupled to the tissue [78], direct contact between the antenna and the tissue is not required, which helps to improve patient comfort. It is shown that the effective field produced by pairs of these elements is continuous regardless of whether the common edges of the elements are perpendicular or parallel to the direction of impressed current [79]. Still, the temperature needs to be controlled by a water bolus to avoid overheating.

Systems incorporating single and multiple antennas have been used in thermotherapy. Single antenna applicators offer the advantage of simplified practical implementation, but they are limited in the size of treatment area and spatial control of energy deposition patterns [74]. Systems incorporating multiple antenna elements can potentially treat larger areas and facilitate electronic steering of power deposition within the treatment volume. The focusing effect may be achieved through simultaneous operations of multiple antenna applicators through a phased array [80–84], or by sequentially activating individual antennas [24]. When operated in a phased array, the amplitude and relative phase of the signal supplied to each antenna can be adjusted to yield constructive interference in a desired region (target), and destructive interference elsewhere (nontarget tissues). In general, constructive interference of multiple antenna applicators in a flat array is not perceived as beneficial over simple incoherent addition of single antenna fields [61]. When multiple antenna elements are combined in a single applicator, it improves flexibility of the device and interface to handle multiple power connections. It also helps to control water bolus and monitor temperature [24].

6.6 Other design considerations

Precise delivery of thermal energy to heterogeneous human tissues is a complex and challenging task. The type, size, and proximity of an applicator, operation frequency, applied-field polarization, and the nonuniformity of patient anatomies are critical factors that need to be considered when designing a wearable device for thermotherapy [59, 85]. The close presence of human tissues and consequently near E-field interaction is a challenging environment for an applicator. A human body presents a variety of complex impedances which makes it difficult to deliver power systematically from an external device. Modeling the complexity of the human body requires powerful computational resources and the required length of time is proportional to the model accuracy. Sufficient resources needed to be dedicated for accurate simulation [59].

The device has to be able to deliver a safe and effective treatment and allow an exact placement for the different sessions of the treatment [73]. Therefore, wearable devices should adapt to the patient anatomy. To enhance physical comfort, the device should be light and small in volume. The device requires feedback to guide and adapt the treatment to individual patient's responses and complaints, such as thermometry sensors. Magnetic resonance imaging (MRI) would be able to monitor 3D volumetric temperature as well as other morphologic and physiologic parameters during treatments.

When designing a device for thermotherapy, it is fundamental to consider the involvement of clinical personnel and patient advocacy groups from the design phase. To acquire clinical acceptability and facilitate its integration into clinical routines, the device should be seamlessly integrated into day to day clinical operations and ideally not increase the treatment time and cost of current practices.

6.6.1 Water bolus

A water bolus, which consists of a bag filled with circulating water, is usually placed between the device and skin of a patient with the purposes of cooling the skin and the superficial tissues off, improving the energy coupling into the tissue and reducing the physical size of antennas. Water is usually selected as a coupling medium due to its high dielectric constant and availability; however, other coupling media could also be considered.

The temperature of the water can be controlled to adjust potential unintended temperature elevation during the treatment and to optimize the energy delivery from superficial to deeper tissues. Combined with microwave power level adjustment, modification of the water bolus temperature has great potential to shift the depth of maximum temperature from the surface to deeper locations or more [86, 87].

Water boluses have been optimized for different applicators and systems operating at different frequencies. In order to have uniform energy deposition, the required thickness of a water bolus was found to be 9.5–12 mm when the system was operating at 433 MHz with a DCC applicator. However, for the same type of applicators, when operated at 915 MHz, optimum thickness of the water bolus was 5–10 mm [76]. While current clinical treatments employ a constant water bolus thickness during the entire treatment session, recent studies showed the possibility to improve the uniformity of the thermal dose delivered to superficial targets by cyclical variations of multiple water bolus thickness [87]. Different water bolus topologies have been implemented: the single input-single output (SISO) [88, 89] and the dual input-dual output (DIDO) [90]. The DIDO water bolus topology offers uniform distribution of water flow, but it also presents a more complex topology and added weight.

6.6.2 *Numerical and tissue-equivalent numerical phantoms*

Numerical models and tissue-equivalent experimental phantoms have been extensively used to optimize the applicator design and to evaluate their interaction with nearby human bodies [91]. Numerical phantoms are excellent tools to evaluate the applicator performance with the wide range of electrical and thermal characteristics of human tissues. Electrical and thermal characteristics of human tissues vary with the operation frequency, type of tissue, temperature, water content, disease status, etc. Numerical phantoms evolved from homogeneously layered flat phantoms [92] into more realistic human representations [93]. Recent numerical models aim to include accurate complex biophysical effects such as sweating, skin blood flow, or shivering [94].

Current treatment planning strategies employ computed tomography (CT) and MRI to develop patient-specific plans. CT or MRIs are segmented into a 3D representation of the patient and then electrical and thermal properties are assigned to each tissue. After the applicator and patient models are combined, electromagnetic, and thermal simulations are computed. Different optimizations can be performed to establish the best applicator settings for a specific treatment [95].

Tissue-equivalent experimental phantoms can facilitate measurements of the developed devices. Phantoms of different shapes have been used for different applications to head, abdomen, and torso, and they can be broadly classified as liquid, gel, semihard, or solid phantoms [91]. Different ingredient and concentrations have been proposed to achieve specific tissue characteristics. A simplified phantom, comprising chicken breast tissues in a 1.5-mm thick fixture of PTFE, was used with a wearable phased array applicator [74]. Another simple type of phantom was proposed to be a mixture of deionized water, diethylene glycol butyl ether, polyethylene glycol mono phenyl ether, and sodium chloride in gel form [96]. These homogeneous phantoms evolved into more realistic ones that imitate actual body components. For example, a human head phantom comprises brain, muscle, and eye, and different dielectric material was fabricated for each [97]. Other examples are highly detailed breast phantoms with realistic composition of fibroglandular and adipose tissues developed by Mashal et al. [98].

References

[1] Y. Khan, A. Ostfeld, C. Lochner, A. Pierre, A. Arias, Monitoring of vital signs with flexible and wearable medical devices, Adv. Mater. 28 (22) (2016) 4373–4395.

[2] A. Tabing, T. Harrell, S. Romero, G. Francisco, Supraventricular tachycardia diagnosed by smartphone ECG, BMJ Case Rep. 2017 (9) (2017).

[3] P. Pandian, K. Mohanavelu, K. Safeer, T. Kotresh, D. Shakunthala, P. Gopal, V. Padaki, Smart vest: wearable multi-parameter remote physiological monitoring system, Med. Eng. Phys. 30 (4) (2008) 466–477.

[4] A. Crema, N. Malesevic, I. Furfaro, F. Raschella, A. Pedrocchi, S. Micera, A wearable multi-site system for NMES-based hand function restoration, IEEE Trans. Neural Syst. Rehabil. Eng. 26 (2) (2017) 428–440.

[5] A. Giombini, V. Giobannini, A. Cesare, P. Pacetti, N. Ichinoseki-Sekine, M. Shiraishi, H. Naito, N. Maffulli, Hyperthermia induced by microwave diathermy in the management of muscle and tendon injuries, Br. Med. Bull. 83 (1) (2007) 379–396.

[6] N. Tempel, M. Horsman, R. Kanaar, Improving efficacy of hyperthermia in oncology by exploiting biological mechanisms, Int. J. Hyperth. 32 (4) (2016) 446–454.

[6a] M.W. Dewhirst, Z. Vujaskovic, E. Jones, D. Thrall, Re-setting the biologic rationale for thermal therapy, Int. J. Hyperth. 21 (8) (2005) 779–790.

[7] M. Greef, P. Kok, D. Correia, P. Borsboom, A. Bel, J. Crezee, Uncertainty in hyperthermia treatment planning: the need for robust system design, Phys. Med. Biol. 56 (11) (2011) 3233–3250.

[8] S. Nadler, K. eingand, R. Kruse, The physiologic basis and clinical applications of cryotherapy and thermotherapy for the pain practitioner, Pain Physician 7 (3) (2004) 395–399.

[9] D. Giansanti, G. Maccioni, Development and testing of a wearable integrated thermometer sensor for skin contact thermography, Med. Eng. Phys. 29 (5) (2007) 556–565.

[10] G. Mattana, T. Kinkeldei, D. Leuenberger, C. Ataman, J. Ruan, F. Molina-Lopez, A. Quintero, G. Nisato, G. Troster, D. Briand, N. Rooij, Woven temperature and humidity sensors on flexible plastic substrates for e-textile applications, IEEE Sensors J. 10 (10) (2013) 3901–3909.

[11] Textile Institute, in: H. Mattila (Ed.), Intelligent textiles and clothing, CRC Press, Boca Raton, FL, 2006.

[12] J. Tong, L. Li, Thermal regulation of electrically conducting fabrics, in: X. Tao (Ed.), Handbook of Smart Textiles, Singapore, Springer Singapore, 2015.

[13] Y. Cheng, H. Zhang, R. Wang, X. Wang, H. Zhai, T. Wang, Q. Jin, J. Sun, Highly stretchable and conductive copper nanowire based fibers with hierarchical structure for wearable heaters, Appl. Mater. Interfaces 8 (48) (2016) 32925–32933.

[14] X. He, R. He, Q. Lan, W. Wu, F. Duan, J. Xiao, M. Zhang, Q. Zeng, J. Wu, J. Liu, Screen-printed fabrication of PEDOT:PSS/silver nanowire composite films for transparent heaters, Materials 10 (3) (2017) 220–229.

[15] I. Kim, K. Woo, Z. Zhong, E. Lee, D. Kang, S. Jeong, Y. Choi, Y. Jang, S. Kwon, J. Moon, Selective light-induced pattering of carbon nanotube/silver nanoparticle composite to produce extremely flexible conductive electrodes, Appl. Mater. Interfaces 9 (7) (2017) 6163–6170.

[16] G. Lewis, M. Langer, C. Henderson, R. Ortiz, Design and evaluation of a wearable self-applied therapeutic ultrasound device for chronic myofascial pain, Ultrasound Med. Biol. 39 (8) (2013) 1429–1439.

[17] B. An, E. Gwak, K. Kim, Y. Kim, J. Jang, J. Kim, J. Park, Stretchable, transparent electrodes as wearable heaters using nanotrough networks of metallic glasses with superior mechanical properties and thermal stability, Nano Lett. 16 (1) (2016) 471–478.

[18] S. Choi, J. Park, W. Hyun, J. Kim, J. Kim, Y. Lee, C. Song, H. Hwang, J. Kim, T. Hyeon, D. Kim, Stretchable heater using ligand-exchanged silver nanowire nanocomposite for wearable articular thermotherapy, ACS Nano 9 (6) (2015) 6626–6633.

[19] W. Lan, Y. Chen, Z. Yang, W. Han, J. Zhou, Y. Zhang, J. Wang, G. Tang, Y. Wei, W. Dou, Q. Su, E. Xie, Ultraflexible transparent film heater made of Ag nanowire/PVA composite for rapid-response thermotherapy pads, Appl. Mater. Interfaces 9 (7) (2017) 6644–6651.

[20] D. Kennedy, T. Lee, D. Seely, A comparative review of thermography as a breast cancer screening technique, Integr. Cancer Therap. 8 (1) (2009) 9–16.

[21] D. Giansanti, G. Maccioni, G. Gigante, A comparative study for the development of a thermal odoscope for the wearable dynamic thermography monitoring, Med. Eng. Phys. 28 (4) (2006) 363–371.

[22] L. Wang, D. Yin, M. Li, L. Li, Microstrip near-field focusing for microwave non-invasive breast cancer thermotherapy, in: IEEE Proceedings of 31st URSI General Assembly and Scientific Symposium, August 16–23, Beijing, China, 2014.

[23] K. Ahmed, S. Zaidi, Treating cancer with heat: hyperthermia as promising strategy to enhance apoptosis, J. Pakistan Med. Assoc. 63 (4) (2013) 504–508.

[24] P. Stauffer, P. Maccarini, K. Arunachalam, O. Craciunescu, C. Diederich, T. Juang, F. Rossetto, J. Schlorff, A. Milligan, J. Hsu, P. Sneed, Z. Vujaskovic, Conformal microwave array (CMA) applicators for hyperthermia of diffuse chest wall recurrence, Int. J. Hyperth. 26 (7) (2010) 686–698. https://doi.org/10.3109/02656736.2010.501511.

[25] M. Stoppa, A. Chiolerio, Wearable electronics and smart textiles: a critical review, Sensors 14 (7) (2014) 11957–11992.

[26] D. Meoli, T. May-Plumlee, Interactive electronic textile development: review of technologies, J. Text. Apparel Technol. Manag. 2 (2) (2002) 1–10.

[27] D. Cottet, J. Grzyb, T. Kirstein, G. Troster, Electrical characterization of textile transmission lines, IEEE Trans. Adv. Packag. 26 (2) (2003) 182–190.

[28] G. Gonzalez, A. Chiappone, I. Roppolo, E. Fantino, V. Bertana, F. Perrucci, L. Scaltrito, F. Pirri, M. Sangermano, Development of 3D printable formulations containing CNT with enhanced electrical properties, Polymer 109 (2) (2017) 246–253.

[29] G. Postiglione, G. Natale, G. Griffini, M. Levi, S. Lurri, Conductive 3D microstructures by direct 3D printing of polymer/carbon nanotube nanocomposites via liquid deposition modeling, Composites 76 (1) (2015) 110–114.

[30] S. Faraji, K. Stano, C. Rost, J. Maria, Y. Zhu, P. Bradford, Structural annealing of carbon coated aligned multi-walled carbon nanotube sheets, Carbon 79 (2) (2014) 113–122.

[31] T. Blythe, D. Bloor, Electrical properties of polymers, Cambridge University Press, Cambridge, United Kingdom, 2005.

[32] A. Sihvola, Electromagnetic Mixing Formulas and Applications, Institution of Electrical Engineers, London, United Kingdom, 1999.

[33] K. Blattenberger, Dielectric Constant, Strength, and Loss Tangent, Retrieved from, http://www.rfcafe.com/references/electrical/dielectric-constants-strengths.htm, 2016. (February 2017).

[34] Genesys, Element Catalog: Substrate Parameter Tables, Retrieved from, http://edadocs.software.keysight.com/download/attachments/6942536/element.pdf?version=1&modificationDate=1477168187000&api=v2, 2008. (February 2017).

[35] C. Ku, R. Liepins, Electrical Properties of Polymers: Chemical Principles, Hanser Publishers, Munich/New York, 1987. New York: Distributed in the U.S.A. by Macmillan.

[36] R. Popielarz, C.K. Chiang, R. Nozaki, J. Obrzut, Dielectric properties of polymer/ferroelectric ceramic composites from 100 Hz to 10 GHz, Macromolecules 34 (17) (2001) 5910–5915.

[37] V. Komarov, Handbook of Dielectric and Thermal Properties of Materials at Microwave Frequencies, Artech House Publishers, Norwood, USA, 2012.

[38] K. Bal, V.K. Kothari, Measurement of dielectric properties of textile materials and their applications, Indian J. Fiber Text. Res. 34 (2009) 191–199.

[39] I. Locher, G. Tröster, Screen-printed textile transmission lines, Text. Res. J. 77 (11) (2007) 837–842.

[40] C. Zysset, T. Kinkeldei, L. Munzenrieder, L. Petti, G. Salvatore, G. Troster, Combining electronics on flexible plastic strips with textiles, Text. Res. J. 83 (11) (2013) 1130–1142.

[41] S. Liu, J. Tong, C. Yang, L. Li, Smart E-textile: resistance properties of conductive knitted fabric—single pique, Text. Res. J. 87 (14) (2017) 1669–1684.

[42] P. Gorder, Computers in Your Clothes? A Milestone for Wearable Electronics, Retrieved from Ohio State News, https://news.osu.edu/news/2016/04/13/computers-in-your-clothes-a-milestone-for-wearable-electronics/, 2016. (21 November 2017).

[43] E. Post, M. Orth, P. Russo, N. Gershenfeld, E-broidery: design and fabrication of textile-based computing, IBM Syst. J. 39 (3) (2000) 840–860.

[44] V. Camarchia, A. Chiolerio, M. Cotto, J. Fang, G. Ghione, P. Pandolfi, M. Pirola, M. Pirola, R. Quaglia, C. Ramella, Demonstration of inkjet-printed silver nanoparticle microstrip lines on alumina for RF power modules, Org. Electron. 15 (1) (2014) 91–98.

[45] M. Ahmadloo, P. Mousavi, A novel integrated dielectric-and-conductive ink 3d printing technique for fabrication of microwave devices, in: IEEE Proceedings of Microwave Symposium Digest, June 2–7, Seattle, WA, USA, 2013.

[46] B. Karaguzel, C. Merritt, T. Kang, J. Wilson, H. Nagle, E. Grant, B. Pourdeyhimi, Utility of nonwovens in the production of integrated electrical circuits via printing conductive inks, J. Text. Inst. 99 (1) (2008) 37–45.

[47] I. Locher, T. Kirstein, G. Tröster, Routing Methods Adapted to e-Textiles, Retrieved from, http://www.fibre2fashion.com/industry-article/1383/routing-methods-adapted-to-etextiles, 2004. (11 January 2018).

[48] Y. Guo, K. Li, C. Hou, Y. Li, Q. Zhang, H. Wang, Fluoroalkylsilane-modified textile-based personal energy management device for multifunctional wearable applications, Appl. Mater. Interfaces 8 (7) (2016) 4676–4683.

[49] E. Meletis, X. Nie, F. Wang, J. Jiang, Electrolytic plasma processing for cleaning and metal-coating of steel surfaces, Surf. Coat. Technol. 150 (2) (2002) 246–256.

[50] A. Reina, X. Jia, J. Ho, D. Nezich, H. Son, V. Bulovic, M. Dresselhaus, J. Kong, Large area, few-layer graphene films on arbitrary substrates by chemical vapor deposition, Nano Lett. 9 (1) (2009) 30–35.

[51] A. Dhawan, A. Seyam, T. Ghosh, Woven fabric-based electrical circuits; part I: evaluating interconnect methods, Text. Res. J. 74 (10) (2004) 913–919.

[52] L. Castano, A. Flatau, Smart fabric sensors and e-textile technologies: a review, Smart Mater. Struct. 23 (1) (2014) 1–27.

[53] L. Rattfalt, M. Linden, P. Hault, L. Berglin, P. Ask, Electrical characteristics of conductive yarns and textile electrodes for medical applications, Med. Biol. Eng. Comput. 45 (12) (2007) 1251–1257.

[54] F. Ceken, O. Kayacan, K. Ozkurt, S. Ugurlu, The electromagnetic shielding properties of copper and stainless steel knitted fabrics, Tekstil 60 (7) (2011) 321–328.

[55] R. Perumalraj, B.S. Dasaradan, Electromagnetic shielding Fabric, Asian Text. J. 17 (10) (2008) 62–68.

[56] L. Li, W. Au, K. Wan, S. Wan, W. Chung, K. Wong, A resistive network model for conductive knitting stitches, Text. Res. J. 80 (10) (2010) 935–947.

[57] Z. Wang, L. Lee, D. Psychoudakis, J. Volakis, Embroidered multiband body-worn antenna for GSM/PCS/WLAN communications, IEEE Trans. Antennas Propag. 62 (6) (2014) 3321–3329.

[58] C.H. Durney, Antennas and other electromagnetic applicators in biology and medicine, Proc. IEEE 80 (1) (1992) 194–199.

[59] S. Curto, Antenna Development for Radio Frequency Hyperthermia Applications (Doctoral thesis), 2010, Dublin Institute of Technology, Dublin, 2010.

[60] A. Rosen, M. Stuchly, A. Vorst, Applications of RF/microwaves in medicine, IEEE Trans. Microw. Theory Techn. 50 (3) (2002) 963–974.

[61] J. Hand, Biophysics and technology of electromagnetic hyperthermia, in: M. Gautherie (Ed.), Methods of External Hyperthermic Heating, Springer, Berlin, Heidelberg, 1990.

[62] P. Nilsson, Physics and Technique of Microwave Induced Hyperthermia in the Treatment of Malignant Tumours (Doctoral thesis), University of Lund, Sweden, 1984.

[63] M. Paulides, J. Bakker, N. Chavannes, G. van Rhoon, A patch antenna design for application in a phased-array head and neck hyperthermia applicator, IEEE Trans. Biomed. Eng. 54 (11) (2007) 2057–2063.

[64] G. Rhoon, P. Rietveld, J. Zee, A 433 MHz Lucite cone waveguide applicator for superficial hyperthermia, Int. J. Hyperth. 14 (1) (1998) 13–27.

[65] E. Gelvich, V. Mazokhin, Contact flexible microstrip applicators (CFMA) in a range from microwaves up to short waves, IEEE Trans. Biomed. Eng. 49 (9) (2002) 1015–1023.

[66] S. Curto, P. Prakash, Design of a compact antenna with flared groundplane for a wearable breast hyperthermia system, Int. J. Hyperth. 31 (7) (2015) 726–736.

[67] J. Johnson, D. Neuman, P. Maccarini, T. Juang, P. Stauffer, P. Turner, Evaluation of a dual-arm Archimedean spiral array for microwave hyperthermia, Int. J. Hyperth. 22 (6) (2006) 475–490.

[68] J. Chen, O. Gandhi, Numerical simulation of annular-phased arrays of dipoles for hyperthermia of deep-seated tumors, IEEE Trans. Biomed. Eng. 39 (3) (1992) 209–216.

[69] P. Wust, B. Hildebrandt, G. Sreenivasa, B. Rau, J. Gellermann, H. Riess, R. Felix, P. Schlag, Hyperthermia in combined treatment of cancer, Lancet Oncol. 3 (8) (2002) 487–497.

[70] M. Paulides, J. Bakker, M. Linthorst, J. Zee, Z. Rijnen, E. Neufeld, P. Pattynama, P. Jansen, P. Levendag, G. Rhoon, The clinical feasibility of deep hyperthermia treatment in the head and neck: new challenges for positioning and temperature measurement, Phys. Med. Biol. 55 (9) (2010) 2465–2480.

[71] M. Paulides, J. Bakker, E. Neufeld, J. Zee, P. Jansen, P. Levendag, G. Rhoon, The HYPERcollar: a novel applicator for hyperthermia in the head and neck, Int. J. Hyperth. 23 (7) (2007) 567–576.

[72] P. Kok, D. Correia, M. Greef, G. Stam, A. Bel, J. Crezee, SAR deposition by curved CFMA-434 applicators for superficial hyperthermia: measurements and simulations, Int. J. Hyperth. 26 (2) (2010) 171–184.

[73] G. Rhoon, External electromagnetic methods and devices, in: E. Moros (Ed.), Physics of Thermal Therapy: Fundamentals and Clinical Applications, CRC Press, Boca Raton, FL, 2013.

[74] S. Curto, A. Garcia-Miquel, M. Suh, N. Vidal, J. Lopez-Villegas, P. Prakash, Design and characterization of a phased antenna array for intact breast hyperthermia, Int. J. Hyperth. 6 (6) (2017) 1–11.

[75] W. Lee, E. Gelvich, P. Baan, V. Mazokhin, E. Rhoo, Assessment of the performance characteristics of a prototype 12-element capacitive contact flexible microstrip applicator (CFMA-12) for superficial hyperthermia, Int. J. Hyperth. 20 (6) (2004) 607–624.

[76] F. Rossetto, P. Stauffer, Theoretical characterization of dual concentric conductor microwave applicators for hyperthermia at 433 MHz, Int. J. Hyperth. 17 (3) (2001) 258–270.

[77] M. Asili, P. Chen, A. Hood, A. Purser, R. Hulsey, L. Johnson, A. Ganesan, U. Demirci, E. Topsakal, Flexible microwave antenna applicator for chemo-thermotherapy of the breast, IEEE Antennas Wireless Propag. Lett. 14 (April) (2015) 1778–1781.

[78] M. Gopal, J. Hand, M. Lumori, S. Alkhairi, K. Paulsen, T. Cetas, Current sheet applicator arrays for superficial hyperthermia of chestwall lesions, Int. J. Hyperth. 8 (2) (1992) 227–240.

[79] P. Rietveld, M. Lumori, J. Stakenborg, G. Rhoon, Theoretical comparison of the SAR distributions from arrays of modified current sheet applicators with that of Lucite cone applicators using Gaussian beam modelling, Int. J. Hyperth. 17 (1) (2001) 82–96.

[80] A.J. Fenn, G.A. King, Adaptive radiofrequency hyperthermia-phased array system for improved cancer therapy: phantom target measurements, Int. J. Hyperth. 10 (2) (1994) 189–208.

[81] G. Shi, W.T. Joines, Design and analysis of annular antenna arrays with different reflectors, Int. J. Hyperth. 20 (6) (2004) 625–636.

[82] D. Shimm, T. Cetas, J. Oleson, E. Gross, D. Buechler, A. Fletcher, S. Dean, Regional hyperthermia for deep-seated malignancies using the BSD annular array, Int. J. Hyperth. 4 (2) (1988) 159–170.

[83] J. Stang, M. Haynes, P. Carson, M. Moghaddam, A preclinical system prototype for focused microwave thermal therapy of the breast, IEEE Trans. Biomed. Eng. 59 (9) (2012) 2431–2438.

[84] R. Verhaart, G. Verduijn, V. Fortunati, Z. Rijnen, T. Walsum, J. Veenland, M. Paulides, Accurate 3D temperature dosimetry during hyperthermia therapy by combining invasive measurements and patient-specific simulations, Int. J. Hyperthermia 31 (6) (2015) 686–692.

[85] C. Chou, Evaluation of microwave hyperthermia applicators, Bioelectromagnetics 13 (6) (1992) 581–597.

[86] K. Arunachalam, P. Maccarini, O. Craciunescu, J. Schlorff, P. Stauffer, thermal characteristics of thermobrachy therapy surface applicators for treating chest wall recurrence, Phys. Med. Biol. 55 (7) (2010) 1949–1969.

[87] P. Stauffer, D. Rodrigues, R. Sinahon, L. Sbarro, V. Beckhoff, M. Hurwitz, Using a conformal water bolus to adjust heating patterns of microwave waveguide applicators, in: Department of Radiation Oncology Faculty Papers, Paper 90, 2017. Retrieved from, http://jdc.jefferson.edu/radoncfp/90.

[88] Y. Birkelund, O. Klemetsen, S. Jacobsen, K. Arunachalam, P. Maccarini, P. Stauffer, Vesicoureteral reflux in children: a phantom study of microwave heating and radiometric thermometry of pediatric bladder, IEEE Trans. Biomed. Eng. 58 (11) (2011) 3269–3278.

[89] Y. Birkelund, S. Jacobsen, K. Arunachalam, P. Maccarini, P. Stauffer, Flow patterns and heat convection in a rectangular water bolus for use in superficial hyperthermia, Phys. Med. Biol. 54 (13) (2009) 3937–3953.

[90] K. Arunachalam, P. Maccarini, J. Schlorff, Y. Birkelund, S. Jacobsen, P. Stauffer, Design of a water coupling bolus with improved flow distribution for multi-element superficial hyperthermia applicators, Int. J. Hyperth. 25 (7) (2009) 554–565.

[91] K. Ito, Human body phantoms for evaluation of wearable and implantable antennas, in: Second European Conference on Antennas and Propagation, November 11–16, Edinburgh, UK, 2007.

[92] R. Tell, Microwave Energy Absorption in Tissue, Office of Research and Monitoring, United States Environmental Protection Agency, 1972.

[93] A. Christ, W. Kainz, E. Hahn, K. Honegger, M. Zefferer, E. Neufeld, W. Rascher, The virtual family—development of surface-based anatomical models of two adults and two children for dosimetric simulations, Phys. Med. Biol. 55 (2) (2010) 23–38.

[94] K. Katić, R. Li, W. Zeiler, Thermophysiological models and their applications: a review, Build. Environ. 106 (9) (2016) 286–300.

[95] M. Paulides, P. Stauffer, E. Neufeld, P. Maccarini, A. Kyriakou, R. Canters, C. Diederich, J. Bakker, G. Rhoon, Simulation techniques in hyperthermia treatment planning, Int. J. Hyperth. 29 (4) (2013) 346–357.

[96] T. Karacolak, E. Topsakal, Electrical properties of nude rat skin and design of implantable antennas for wireless data telemetry, in: IEEE Proceedings of Microwave Symposium Digest, June 15–20, Atlanta, GA, USA, 2008.

[97] N. Graedel, J. Polimeni, B. Guerin, B. Gagoski, L. Wald, An anatomically realistic temperature phantom for radiofrequency heating measurements: realistic temperature phantom for radiofrequency heating measurements, Magn. Reson. Med. 73 (1) (2015) 442–450.

[98] A. Mashal, F. Gao, S. Hagness, Heterogeneous anthropomorphic phantoms with realistic dielectric properties for microwave breast imaging experiments, Microw. Opt. Technol. Lett. 53 (8) (2011) 1896–1902.

Soft actuator materials for textile muscles and wearable bioelectronics

Edwin W.H. Jager[a], Jose G. Martinez[a], Yong Zhong[a], Nils-Krister Persson[b]
[a]*Division of Sensor and Actuator Systems, Department of Physics, Chemistry and Biology (IFM), Linköping University, Linköping, Sweden* [b]*Smart Textiles, Swedish School of Textiles (THS), University of Borås, Borås, Sweden*

7.1 Introduction

The fabrication of textiles is one of humankind's oldest technologies and has, in principle, remained the same for centuries. Inventions like the flying shuttle in 1733 by John Kay [1] and the "Spinning Jenny" [2] in 1764 by James Hargreaves can be seen as the first steps to automate the production. The industrial revolution led to a real automation of textile production and larger-scale industrial manufacturing for instance in England from around 1790. Nowadays, yarns and fabrics can be produced at high speed, high volume, with high repeatability, accuracy, and quality at low costs. For instance, current weaving speed is over 1000 m per minute at a full-width of over 2 m [3].

Textiles are a ubiquitous technology. We are almost constantly in contact with different fabrics. This includes garments and items of clothing; textiles for interior use (e.g., bed

Wearable Bioelectronics. https://doi.org/10.1016/B978-0-08-102407-2.00008-4

linen, carpets, curtains, and table cloths); and so-called technical textiles (e.g., fluid filtration membranes, geotextiles, airbags, safety belts, reinforcements for composites, and many types of medical implants).

In the first fabrics, basic functionality was dominant. Fabrics were predominantly used to protect from weather conditions or to transport goods (bags, pockets, sacks). Later, the appearance of fabrics became important and for instance clothing was used to indicate one's status or as a fashion statement. During the last century, added functionality has become an important factor driving the development of specialized fabrics, for instance flame-resistant fabrics, moist transporting fabrics ("GoreTex"), and stain-repelling fabrics. However, all of these functionalities are passive. More recently, active functionalization is becoming important resulting in smart textiles: that is textiles that can conduct electricity, measure strain, or even provide actuation.

7.2 Advantages of textiles for actuators

As per definition, textiles always consist of long flexible units, fibers, or yarns, with very high length-to-diameter ratios. Textiles can roughly be divided in weaves and knits on one side and nonwoven fabrics on the other. Somewhat simplifying nonwoven fabrics are built by a random network of fibers, kept together by melted crossing points, glue, and/or mechanical fiber entanglement. Textiles that are not nonwoven are perhaps most well-known types and embrace several techniques: weaving, weft knitting, warp knitting, braiding, twinning, etc. Common is that the fibers here are to be regarded as ordered. For weaves, there are two perpendicular sets of fibers, the warp and the weft which are interlaced in different manners, by thus keeping the fabric together. There are thousands of different, what is called, weave patterns for doing this, creating not only different appearance but also different mechanical properties, impacting openness of the fabric, porosity, area density, stiffness, drapability, strength, and smoothness. For knitting, the fabric is kept together by fibers forming loops and by locking these loops inside another loop side-by. In principle, one system of fiber could be used. In practice, a set of fibers fed into the process is used. It should be emphasized that not only the material used for the fibers, but also the textile construction highly influences the fabric properties.

Textile processes are not limited to these fabric-forming methods. In addition, fiber melt spinning, fiber yarn spinning, cord and rope making, net manufacture as well as wadding, embroidery, tufting and sewing as well as dying, sizing, lamination, and coating are within the repertoire of textile production. This makes textile processing a very versatile technology with many degrees of freedom and numerous possibilities.

Textile production can be seen upon as an additive manufacturing method. Thread by thread the fabric is built. Furthermore, functions can be integrated while manufacturing. For instance, instead of weaving with threads having different colors, one can weave with threads having different technical properties, such as weaving conducting yarns into the

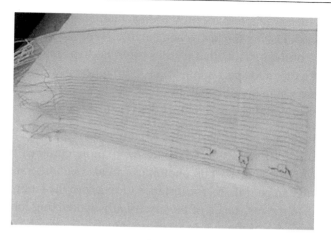

Fig. 7.1

A weave with metal yarns. Note that soldering as in normal electronics is possible (lower right part of the fabric) even if nonmetallic yarns are forming part of the weave. By this textile electronic sensor circuitries could be made. *Photo: Swedish School of Textiles, University of Borås.*

fabric (Fig. 7.1). In this way, two-dimensional (2D) surfaces with addressable properties or periodic patterns can be created. It could be noticed that a weave is in principle a discrete x (weft direction, i.e., number of warp threads)-y (warp direction, i.e., number of weft threads) coordinate system. Textiles also have several other highly interesting properties. Textile process enables materials with high tensile strength to be made, in the form of wires, ropes but also as reinforcement in composites. Still textiles are lightweight materials, once more due to the fact they are constructed out of fibers avoiding unnecessary extra material.

For biomedical applications, it is notable that no man-made class of material offers such a proximity to the body and as such ever-presence in human life as textiles. Part of this is due to textiles having the rather unique property of drapability and pliability which is used in clothing. Finally, textiles can be biocompatible, recyclable, disposable, or (bio)degradable depending on the material choice and construction, also this of importance for biomedical applications were sometimes due to spread of infections materials should be burned, sometimes should be implanted in the body and either exist in vivo for a longer time or degrade controlled, or be reused thus withstanding washing, wear, and autoclaving.

In this chapter, we will only address yarns and the weaves and knits. Nonwoven materials will be omitted.

7.3 Smart textiles

Smart textiles [4, 5], (more or less) synonymously electronic textiles, e-textiles, intelligent textiles, and alike is a class of materials, where textiles play a vital role but where functionalities from other disciplines are added [6]. The smart textiles may comprise conducting, sensing, measuring, and recently even actuating elements embedded in the otherwise passive fabric. During the last years, smart textiles have grown to be an area of its own taking advantage of the benefits that textiles offer. Perhaps most emphasized are smart textiles for medical, health, and sport applications both in terms of research carried out and market potential. There are many dimensions of smart textiles. They could act as sensors taking stimulus and they could act as actuators delivering a response.

While electrically conductive textile structures [7] are often regarded as the fundamental starting point for creating "smartness" and devices with more complex functionalities, other technologies such as chemistry and photonics can also be integrated. Still, conductive structures by their own can be utilized for instance to measure the strain of a fabric by measuring the change in the resistance of the electrically conducting fabric due to mechanical deformation of a certain part of the textile construction. These stretch sensing fabrics have been embedded in a knee sleeve to measure the bending angle of a knee in sport medicine [8], mounted on gloves to measure the bending of fingers [9], and for monitoring breath rate [10, 11]. Besides resistive [12], also capacitive sensors [13] are also possible as well as piezoresistive sensors [14]. A broad spectrum of physiological signals are possible to capture such as textile electrocardiography (ECG) [13, 15] and electromyography (EMG) [16]. The key component here is textile electrodes. These are most often knitted using electrically conductive yarns. Knit enables a stretch which is important for a close positioning to the skin. A critical factor is to be able to measure without using the electrolytic gels that otherwise is common in this context to provide good electrical contact. Problems with measurement artifacts could be handled by electrode redundancy and signal processing. Various textile biosensors have been developed [17], also covering textile microfluidics filters [18], with chemical sensing [19] and integration of fiber optics [17] as well as fluidic filters [20].

Most the smart textiles comprise "passive" functionalities where the textiles only transport (currents or liquids) or measure an external property (bending of a knee or muscle electric potentials). Recently, smart textiles also provide active functions, that is, that they can actively influence their surrounding for instance as textile actuators.

7.4 Yarn actuators

When it comes to textile actuators, most work has been focused on the elemental components of textiles that are actuating yarns or fibers, using various physical principles to provide the actuation, such as thermal expansion, electrochemistry, and solvent, or vapor swelling.

Nylon for instance, when highly oriented along its length, has an anisotropic thermal expansion behavior and this can be utilized to build actuators. Thus, when the temperature of the yarn is changed by external or electrical heating, it is possible to get linear movements [21, 22]. By twisting the nylon yarns, it is possible to get fast, scalable, tensile actuators with low hysteresis, and a long cycle lifetime. The nylon muscles achieved linear strain variations up to 49%, were 100 times stronger than human muscles and had an output mechanical work of 5.3 kW per kg of muscle weight [23]. The same actuation principle has also been applied to develop both bending [24] and torsional [25] actuators with satisfactory results. They have been used in different applications such as in a robotic human-like hand [26]. Next, 32 coiled nylon-based actuators were braided together and a glass tube containing nichrome as heating element was inserted into the braid. This enabled driving the actuators by internal resistive heating, instead of using an external heat source. Using weaving, the coiled nylon actuators were incorporated into actuating fabrics. The coiled nylon actuators were assembled in the vertical (warp) direction and polyester, cotton, and silver-plated nylon yarns were woven in the horizontal (weft) direction. The conductive silver coated yarns were used as heating elements to actuate the fabric. The woven structure could change its porosity after heating. Also, the combination of weaving resulted in a better cycle rate capability than the single yarns, as the heat could be dissipated over a much larger area than for a single large-diameter actuator of similar strength [23]. Uses of this technology have been proposed as fabrics that automatically change porosity with temperature, offering the wearer a more comfortable experience as bigger porosity can be achieved in the fabric when the temperature raises [23]. However, effort is still needed to look for materials and systems that have a better performance in the temperature range similar to that of the human body.

It is also possible to achieve bending movement from such nylon yarns. The nylon filaments have been flattened into beams and resistive heating elements deposited on both sides, resulting in 180 degrees of bending for a 115 mm long beam [27]. Later the same concept was extended to bending nylon actuators that move in multiple directions. The nylon filaments were now formed into beams with a squared cross section and resistive heating elements were applied on all four sides [24].

Order change materials or shape memory alloys (SMA) are alloys that after deformation recover their initial shape when proper energy is applied. Thus, they can be used to build actuators in the form of fibers or yarns that actuate when the temperature is altered [28–30]. Up to 500% strain variations can be achieved when a SMA fiber obtained by extrusion is heated over a wide range of temperatures. There are also yarn actuators that instead of using thermal energy to recover the initial shape use light excitation [31, 32]. In this case, they can reach similar stresses to those of the human muscles under UV light excitation [32].

Different materials respond in different ways in the presence of different vapors or solvents. This effect can also be used to make actuating fibers or yarns [33]. Yarns were made of helical assembled, aligned carbon nanotubes (CNTs) with nanometer- and micrometer-sized gaps in the fibers and thereafter twisted. Exposing the yarns to polar solvents, for example, ethanol, acetone, toluene, and dichloromethane caused the yarns to contract and rotate within 0.5 s.

Electrochemical yarn actuators have also been developed, both based on capacitive charging or Faradaic reactions. In a capacitive actuator, the yarns are immersed in an electrolyte (it can be both solid or liquid) and an electrical stimulus is applied, causing the charges to reallocate due to the electrostatic forces that appear on the yarn, promoting the reallocation of the ions in the surrounding electrolyte and the subsequent movement of the yarn without changing the composition of the material. On the other hand, in Faradaic actuators, the electrical stimulus promotes also an electrochemical reaction. The electrochemical reaction causes a change in the material composition and ions and solvent are incorporated in or expelled from the material, thus resulting in a swelling or shrinking movement. In some of the developed actuators (mainly those based on CNTs or graphene), the prevalent effect that takes place is still debated, but most probably both effects influence at the same time [34]. CNT linear actuators have been developed reaching up to 16.5% tensile contraction [35]. They have been modified such as using PVA to cross-link the CNT to increase their tensile strength and avoid undesired effects such as relaxation, which make the control of the movement hard [36, 37]. CNT yarns can also function as torsional actuators that can rotate up to 15,000° [38]. At the same time as they rotate, they also present linear actuation and by coiling the CNT yarns, a higher strain can be achieved. Conducting polymers (CPs) which show bulk swelling/shrinking (see Section 7.5.2) have been used too as linear actuators, typically as electroactive coatings on passive yarns or fibers. For instance, chitosan/polypyrrole (Cs/PPy) were fabricated by an in situ chemical polymerization of pyrrole on and in the chistosan fibers [39]. The Cs/PPy hybrid microfibers had a better performance than pure PPy films. For instance, the Young's modulus increased from 1.7 GPa for PPy films to 5.2 GPa for the hybrid fibers. The fibers exerted 0.5% strain. Another example is commercial cellulose-based yarns (Lyocell) that have been coated with the CP PPy and used as linear actuators [40]. Both single and twisted yarns were modified and actuated, giving strains of 0.075% and 0.14%, respectively. While the cellulose yarns were passive, nonconductive, conductive yarns have also been used as the core of PPy-based yarn actuators. Various commercial, off-the-shelf conductive yarns were coated with PPy and the strain and force were measured [41]. It showed that all yarns could actuate but that the mechanical properties of the yarn (e.g., Young's modulus) were of higher importance than the electrical conductivity. Even graphene fiber/CP bimorph fiber actuators have been demonstrated [42]. By coating PPy on only one side of the graphene fibers, simple bending fiber actuators were fabricated. The fibers were also intertwined in a net shape that could bend.

7.5 Textile actuators

Textile actuators have also been developed following the same actuation principles as for the single yarn or fiber actuators. For instance, SMA wires have been knitted and incorporated into fabrics. Important aspects for the fabric's behavior are the friction between the single SMA yarns or their elasticity, which both have been considered and modeled [43]. Using a so-called Garter stitch, they could be actuated between the martensite extended and austenite contracted states with a strain of 50%. Next, they have been structured into different knitted patterns (e.g., forward and reverse stockinette; vertical striped rib pattern) that can accomplish different kinds of movements with high actuation forces such as folding structures, rolling fabrics, and even rotational actuation [44]. Commercial Ni-Ti SMA yarns and polyurethane shape memory polymer yarns were fabricated and thereafter successfully incorporated, woven, as part of passive fabrics [45]. The activation of the SMA and shape memory polymer yarns could alter the three-dimensional (3D) structure of the fabrics as well as open and close the fabrics. SMA yarns incorporated into passive fabrics have been used in a wide number of applications such as fabrics that become wrinkle free at body temperature [46], in T-shirts that do not need ironing [47], in a flat fabric to emulate peristaltic movement [48], in geometrically morphing fabrics for dynamic light filters [49], prosed for compression garments [50], or as cantilevered actuators for robots able to perform simple tasks as curving a surface, lifting masses, or mimicking finger-like movements [51].

Thermal expansion as the driving mechanism has also been used in textiles. Stretchable, conductive textiles have been formed by wrapping spandex fibers with CNT aerogel sheet and knitting the CNT/spandex yarns into a fabric [52]. The fabric, pre-stretched by 100% strain, could generate 25% strain when heated to 70 °C by resistive heating using the CNT as the resistive heating element.

Fabrics have also been used as important passive components in actuators, that is, not strictly used as the active actuation providing textile. For instance, a textile comprising ionic polymer metal composite (IPMC) actuator has been developed by sandwiching the ion-containing Nafion film between two conducting fabrics that function as the electrodes of IPMC actuator [53]. By applying a potential between the two textile electrodes, the charges inside the IPMC Nafion membrane are redistributed causing the IPMC to bend. Another example is the use of a fiber glass fabric as the central reinforcement grid in an IPMC like actuator based on carbide-derived carbon (CDC) electrodes [54]. The ion-containing PVDF layer was spray coated on both sides or the fiber glass fabric, where after the CDC electrodes were spray coated on both sides of the PVDF/fabric membrane. Bending was achieved by applying a potential difference of the two CDC electrodes. When working at a constant temperature, the SMA is able to return to its original shape after a mechanical strain as the SMA presents superelasticity or pseudoelasticity [55]. This property has been tested combined with textiles in different fields as ballistics to improve high impact resistance [56].

A separated category is the so-called McKibben muscle that is an interesting actuation technology for soft robotics. A McKibben muscle comprises a soft, expanding tube, or bladder surrounded by braided mesh. When pressuring the internal tube using hydraulics or pneumatics, the tube expands in the radial direction and the braided mesh pattern converts this movement into a contractile motion of the actuator. Similar to a mammalian muscle the actuator becomes thicker and shorter. Although the braided structure that encases the internal bladder is made using textile processing, McKibben muscles per se are not regarded as textile actuators. Suzumori and coworkers have developed small McKibben actuators having an external diameter ranging as small as 18 mm [57]. Like normal muscles they bundled 10 or 30 small McKibben actuators into a multifilament muscle and achieved forces up to 9.3 N. They have woven the McKibben tubes into a "fabric" with the tubes in the warp (linear direction) and using ordinary wool in the weft (vertical or perpendicular direction) direction [58]. The "McKibben fabrics" have thereafter been integrated into a sort of exoskeleton suit that supports the lower back and should augment lifting heavy objects [58].

Thermally actuated and electrochemically actuated textiles will be described in more detail in the following two sections.

7.5.1 Thermally activated textile actuators

As mentioned, thermal energy can be used to actuate yarns and textiles. This energy can either be supplied in a controlled way, such as electrical resistive heating, or taken from the ambient. In the latter case, the surrounding heat can be used and this opens up to fabricate automatic systems, where a temperature change can create a movement.

Lamination is a widely used textile processing method. It is employed in industry both for garments such as breathable jackets and in technical textiles such as airbags and textile car interiors. A lamination in the textile field is defined [59] as "A material combined of two or more layers, at least one of which is a textile fabric, bonded closely together by means of an added adhesive, or by the adhesive properties of one or more of the component layers." So, by lamination two solid materials are combined, typically in a face-to face manner with a large interfacial area. The layers could be textile fabrics, thinner webs, or solid or perforated plastic films. The adhesion could be achieved by melting a thermoplastic (hot treatment) or gluing (cold treatment). Applied heat and/or pressure thereafter bonds the layers. By using different kinds of materials with different properties, such as layer A with uniaxial property in one direction and layer B with uniaxial property in the other direction, anisotropy is created. An example of such material properties is different (linear) expansion coefficients, c, which can be used to create thermally actuated textiles. As a proof of concept of such an actuator, we have chosen and glued together, that is, using cold treatment, two low weight materials (so that the device can handle its own weight), polyester (PES) and polyethene (PE) (Fig. 7.2). We call the device a thermally activated textile actuator (TATA). When the surrounding temperature raise above room temperature, there is a continuous reshaping of the structure due to the difference in thermal expansion of the PES and PE layers (Fig. 7.2A and B).

There are numerous applications of the TATA system. For instance, they can be used in valves for fluidics. Fig. 7.3 shows a structure with multiple laser-cut "fingers" that can open or close, thus fluids can be redirected. It is found that the actuating mechanism is fully

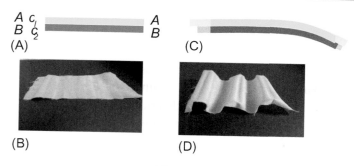

Fig. 7.2

(A) Two different materials, A, deep yellow and, B, dark blue, having thermal expansion coefficients C1 and C2, respectively, are laminated resulting in a thermally activated textile actuator (TATA). (B) At room temperature (23°C), the TATA is flat and (C) at high temperature due to the two different thermal expansion coefficients and the fact that the layers are mechanically coupled a bending movement is created. (D) By using different relative orientation of the two layers and patterning thereof, more complex movements are possible when the structure is exposed to a higher temperature. System developed at the Swedish School of Textiles, University of Borås. *Figure reproduced from Ref. N.-K. Persson, et al., Actuating textiles—next generation of smart textiles, Adv. Mater. Technol. (2018) 1700397.*

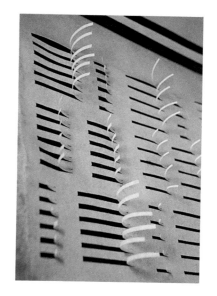

Fig. 7.3

Fluidic application of the thermally activated textile actuator. Fingers with different sizes were formed using laser cutting. Although, the heat from the laser somewhat impacted the layers due to some melting at the edges, the method turned out well. Despite having different lengths—thus different (thermal) masses of the fingers—the actuation upon heating was similar. *Photo Swedish School of Textiles, University of Borås.*

reversible; when lowering the temperature, the shape returns to the low-temperature form. This can be repeated for many cycles. By altering the construction, it is also possible to switch the behavior so that at low temperature the structure is open and at high temperatures it is closed. Furthermore, as seen in Fig. 7.3, it is possible to make many actuators at a time, that is, achieving up-scaling. In this case, a laser cutter was used. It is possible to integrate the fabrication of such devices in a continuous, industrial production line. Likewise, lamination is compatible with large-scale manufacturing of textiles and textile processes are important tools for opening up for large-scale production of cost-effective actuators.

7.5.2 CP textile actuators

Electroactive polymers (EAPs) have been proposed as the active material in soft actuators for soft robotics and wearables due to their inherent properties. EAPs are silent, lightweight, and being polymeric material, they can be potentially produced at large-scale and low costs. EAPs are generally divided into two categories: electronic EAPs and ionic EAPs. *Electronic EAPs* are driven by an electric field which causes the materials to deform. This group includes dielectric elastomers (DEs), electrostrictive polymers, and liquid crystal elastomers [60]. DE is the most commonly used electronic EAP. It consists of a soft dielectric material sandwiched between two compliant electrodes and is based on the principle of Maxwell stress [61, 62]. When a potential is applied to the two electrodes the columbic forces attract the electrodes, deforming the soft dielectric material, resulting in a lateral movement. These DE actuators are capable of exerting large forces, have a high bandwidth and have been demonstrated in a variety of actuators designs. A major drawback, especially for use in wearables, is the high voltages needed to drive these DE actuators, typically a few kVs, although recent work has demonstrated actuation at a few hundred volt.

The actuation principle of *ionic EAPs* is based on the motion of ions and solvent to induce volume changes. Ionic EAPs comprise CPs [63, 64], IPMCs [65], CNTs [66], and gels [67]. For wearables and textile actuators, CPs are particularly interesting. CP can be electrochemically oxidized and reduced in a reversible way for many cycles. This redox reaction of CPs is accompanied with a flow of ions into or out of the CP depending on the ion (called a dopant) and the redox reaction. In principle, there are two reactions that we can generalize as follows [68, 69]: a CP that has been synthesized with small, mobile anions (a^-), such as ClO_4^-, and is operated in an electrolyte containing both mobile cations and anions the redox reaction will be

$$CP^+\left(a^-\right)+e^- \leftrightarrow CP^0 +a^-\left(aq\right) \tag{7.1}$$

that is, when we reduce the CP, the anions a^- leave the material and when we oxidize the CP, the anions enter the CP to compensate for the charge imbalance. Instead, for a CP synthesized with large, immobile anions A⁻, such as dodecylbenzene sulfonate (DBS⁻) and operated in an electrolyte containing small mobile cations M⁺ the redox reaction will be

$$CP^+\left(A^-\right) + M^+\left(aq\right) + e^- \leftrightarrow CP^0\left(A^-M^+\right) \tag{7.2}$$

that is, when we reduce the CP, cations M⁺ enter the CP and when we oxidize the CP the cations leave the CP. So, depending on the dopant size, we either have cation or anion motion. In reaction (7.1), the volume expands in the *oxidized* state, that is, when we apply a positive potential and in reaction (7.2) the volume expands in the *reduced* state, that is, when we apply a negative potential. In addition to the ion motion osmotic swelling also contributes to the volume change [70, 71]. The main advantage of CPs as actuator materials is that they require a low operating potential, typically only 1–2 V. A drawback is that, since the principle is based on ion motion, an ion source is needed. This has typically been a liquid electrolyte, but currently solid polymer electrolytes are gaining interest thus enabling in-air actuation of these materials. The CP exert larges stress, typically 1–5 MPa (compared to 0.35 MPa for a mammalian muscle [72]), moderate strains (1%–10%) [73] and the materials can be coated on a wide variety of materials and shapes.

The latter property is particularly interesting for wearables and soft robotics as yarns and fabrics can be coated with CP and thus functionalized into electromechanically active materials [74] and fiber/yarn actuators [39–42]. Recently, we have developed such textile actuators from standard textile materials exploiting some of the advantages of textile fabrication to boost the performance of CP actuators while enabling wearable actuators [40]. Starting with commercial cellulose-based yarns, Lyocell, we have coated these in a two-step process. In the first step, we coated the yarns with a thin PEDOT layer using vapor-phase polymerization to make the passive yarns, and fabrics, electrically conducting. The electrical conductivity is required to be able to electropolymerize the CP PPy, which has good actuation properties, on the yarn and fabric. Next, the PPy was electrochemically synthesized on these PEDOT-coated yarns. Hereafter, the yarns were clamped in a lever arm system to measure the force and strain. This first generation of textile actuators was still operated in a liquid electrolyte. Fig. 7.4 shows the strain of a single yarn (S-yarn) a single twisted yarn (T-yarn). A clear movement of the yarn could be measured although the strain (~0.1%) is much lower than for pure PPy films. We attribute this to the fact that we have a thin PPy layer coated on a relatively stiff Lyocell yarn core, generating significant mechanical impedance. For instance, the strain using a softer, elastane yarn core gave 0.3% strain. Calculated stress of 0.5 MPa shows that the PPy layer does actuate as normal. As mentioned, the actuation mechanism of CP actuators is the insertion (and ejection) of ions into the CP. Therefore, to achieve fast actuation, thin CP layers are required, resulting in low output forces. To overcome this and achieve high forces, the thin actuators have been bundled into larger devices, which can be cumbersome to achieve practically [75, 76]. Here, the first advantage of textile fabrication comes in. Textile fabrication is a perfect means of assembling many yarns or fibers in parallel,

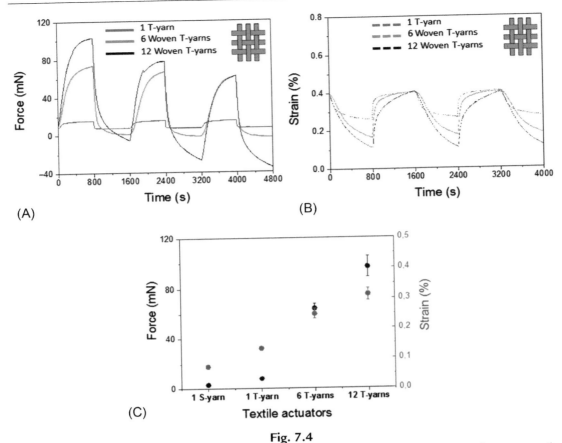

Fig. 7.4

Force (A) and strain (B) of a single yarn (S-yarn), a single twisted yarn (T-yarn), and woven textile actuator that are 6 or 12 yarns wide. (C) Peak force and strain of the single yarns and woven textile actuators. *Reproduced from Ref. A. Maziz, et al., Knitting and weaving artificial muscles, Sci. Adv. 3 (1) (2017) e1600327.*

for example, weaving. We exploited this principle in the textile actuators. Lyocell yarns were woven into a fabric, coated and characterized following the same procedures as for the single yarns. Fig. 7.4 shows the measured strain and force. As can be seen, the output force scales with the number of parallel yarns in the fabric demonstrating that indeed parallel assembly using textile processing can amplify the output force.

Another advantage of textile fabrication is that it can be used to make very different textile constructions, such as stretchable fabrics. We utilized this principle too in the textile actuators. The Lyocell yarns were knitted into a stretchable fabric, and again coated and characterized following the same procedures as for the single yarns. Fig. 7.5 shows the

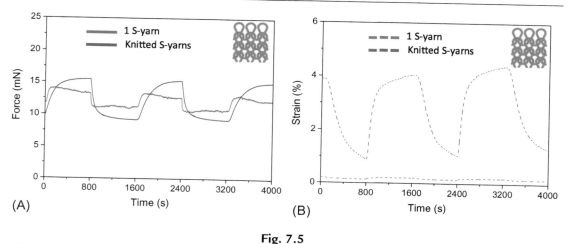

Fig. 7.5

The force and strain of a PPy coated Lyocel single yarn and knitted fabric. *Reproduced from Ref. A. Maziz, et al., Knitting and weaving artificial muscles, Sci. Adv. 3 (1) (2017) e1600327.*

measured strain and force for these knitted fabrics compared to a single yarn. The measured strain increased from 0.075% to 3% for a fabric made of the same materials and actuated in the same way. It demonstrates that one can tune the strain and force by employing different textile constructions, such as weaving to amplify the strain of PPy-based actuators.

To illustrate the possibilities of the textile actuators, we made the fabrics into actuator units, "textuators" (Fig. 7.6A) and mounted it in a LEGO setup to drive a lever arm (Fig. 7.6B–D). The textile actuator was able to move the arm up and down, while lifting a small weight. This work shows that combined with EAPs, such as CPs, conventional textiles can be turned into electromechanically active fabrics. We are currently optimizing the textile actuators to enhance the performance and simplify the production [41].

7.6 Application areas

In the same way that fabrics can be produced that have multiple colors such as lines or checkered fabrics, multiple materials can be integrated into the fabrics during productions. These can be plain electrically conducting metallic yarns (Fig. 7.1), sensing yarns, such as PEDOT-coated yarns (Fig. 7.7A) [10], actuating yarns as presented in this chapter, or optical fibers resulting in multifunctional fabrics that can be used in smart textiles. Application areas for such smart textiles can be found in broad spectrum of applications. They could be integrated into garments and used to drive a soft, textile-based exoskeleton-like suit. Such soft exoskeletons might be able to replace the stiff, hard, and noisy robotic exoskeletons [77], with a more comfortable equivalent that is soft, pliable, lightweight, and silent. Likewise, such exoskeletons could be used to active support to some part of the body. Fig. 7.7B shows

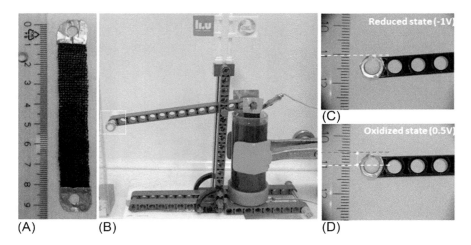

Fig. 7.6

(A) A "textuator," a textile actuator with electrical and mechanical contacts and (B) a textile actuator driving a LEGO robot arm or lever. (C) and (D) show the movement of the lever arm tip with an attached weight. *Reproduced from Ref. A. Maziz, et al., Knitting and weaving artificial muscles, Sci. Adv. 3 (1) (2017) e1600327.*

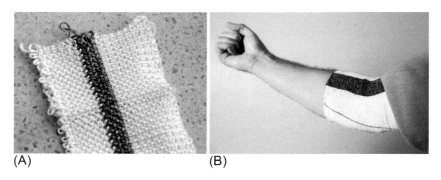

Fig. 7.7

(A) A knitted fabric with integrated PEDOT-coated yarns (black yarn) used for respiratory monitoring with normal (white) yarn. (B) A conceptual photo of an arm sleeve with integrated textile actuators as under development by Linköping University and University of Borås. *(A) Photo Swedish School of Textiles, University of Borås. (B) Photo Thor Balkhed, Linköping University.*

a concept elbow exoskeleton as being developed in a collaboration project by the Linköping University and University of Borås. Exoskeleton suits and active orthoses could augment patients with no or limited ability, assist in rehabilitation, or augment craftsmen working with heavy loads or caretakers and nurses lifting patients.

In technical textile applications, there is a broad spectrum of applications such as adaptive surfaces and haptic devices for fields ranging from medical devices and tools to the automotive industry.

7.7 Conclusions

During the last years, active smart textiles have been demonstrated using various actuation principles and much interesting work has been done. These works have already inspired others. For instance, Zakharov and Pismen devised new, complex actuation patterns by exploiting the *x-y* grid pattern that can be easily made using weaving and integrating "Janus-fibers" [78]. The works presented in this chapter demonstrate that smart textiles are no longer only a "passive" technology, for example, used to create wearable sensors, but also can be an active technology enabling actuators to be integrated in wide variety of textiles used in everyday objects such as items of clothing and technical textiles. This will hopefully generate a new class of devices and tools augmenting the users in novel ways beyond our current imagination.

Acknowledgments

The authors thank Vinnova (VinnVäxt—Smart Textiles), the Carl Tryggers Stifelsen (Grant no. CTS16:207), Swedish Research Council (Grant no. VR-2014-3079), the Erling-Persson Family Foundation (Project 2017-10-09—Textile Actuators for Wearable Assistive Devices), and Promobilia Foundation (grant no F17603) for their financial support.

References

[1] Y.E. El-Mogahzy, Engineering Textiles: Integrating the Design and Manufacture of Textile Products (Woodhead Publishing wSeries in Textiles), Woodhead Publishing, 2009.
[2] B. Wulfhorst, T. Gries, D. Veit, Textile Technology (English ed.), Hanser Publishers Distributed in the USA and in Canada by Hanser Gardner Publications, Munich Cincinnati Ohio, 2006. viii, 320.
[3] C. Sartorius, The Fastest Weaving Machine in the World, in Sulzer Technical Review, 1999. Sulzer.
[4] L. Guo, et al., Electro-conductive textiles and textile-based electro-mechanical sensors—integration in as an approach for smart textiles, in: V. Koncar (Ed.), Smart Textiles and their Applications, Elsevier, 2015.
[5] G. Cho, S. Lee, J. Cho, Review and reappraisal of smart clothing, Int. J. Human-Computer Interact. 25 (6) (2009) 582–617.
[6] L. Guo, et al., Electro-conductive textiles and textile-based electro-mechanical sensors—integration in as an approach for smart textiles, in: V. Koncar (Ed.), Smart Textiles and their Applications, Woodhead Publishing, 2016.
[7] T. Bashir, M. Skrifvars, N.K. Persson, Production of highly conductive textile viscose yarns by chemical vapor deposition technique: a route to continuous process, Polym. Adv. Technol. 22 (12) (2011) 2214–2221.
[8] B.J. Munro, et al., The intelligent knee sleeve: a wearable biofeedback device, Sens. Actuators B: Chem. 131 (2) (2008) 541–547.
[9] G.M. Spinks, et al., Conducting polymers electromechanical actuators and strain sensors, Macromol. Symp. 192 (2003) 161–169.
[10] T. Bashir, et al., Stretch sensing properties of conductive knitted structures of PEDOT-coated viscose and polyester yarns, Text. Res. J. 84 (3) (2014) 323–334.
[11] L. Guo, et al., Design of a garment-based sensing system for breathing monitoring, Text. Res. J. 83 (5) (2012) 499–509.
[12] L. Capineri, Resistive sensors with smart textiles for wearable technology: from fabrication processes to integration with electronics, Proc. Eng. 87 (2014) 724–727.

[13] B. Chamadiya, et al., Textile capacitive electrocardiography for an automotive environment, Biodevices 2011 (2011) 422–425.

[14] C.-T. Huang, et al., Parametric design of yarn-based piezoresistive sensors for smart textiles, Sens. Actuators A: Phys. 148 (1) (2008) 10–15.

[15] R. Paradiso, et al., Knitted bioclothes for cardiopulmonary monitoring, in: Proceedings of the 25th Annual International Conference of the Ieee Engineering in Medicine and Biology Society, vols. 1–4 (25), 2003, pp. 3720–3723.

[16] E.P. Scilingo, et al., Performance evaluation of sensing fabrics for monitoring physiological and biomechanical variables, IEEE Trans. Inform. Technol. Biomed. 9 (3) (2005) 345–352.

[17] S. Pasche, et al., Smart textiles with biosensing capabilities, Smart Interact. Text. 80 (2013) 129–135.

[18] G.O.F. Parikesit, et al., Textile-based microfluidics: modulated wetting, mixing, sorting, and energy harvesting, J. Text. Inst. 103 (10) (2012) 1077–1087.

[19] W. Guan, M. Liu, C. Zhang, Electrochemiluminescence detection in microfluidic cloth-based analytical devices, Biosens. Bioelectr. 75 (2016) 247–253.

[20] J. Bu, et al., Lab on a fabric: mass producible and low-cost fabric filters for the high-throughput viable isolation of circulating tumor cells, Biosens. Bioelectr. 91 (2017) 747–755.

[21] M. Suzuki, N. Kamamichi, Displacement control of an antagonistic-type twisted and coiled polymer actuator, Smart Mater. Struct. 27 (3) (2018) 035003.

[22] A. Cherubini, et al., Experimental characterization of thermally-activated artificial muscles based on coiled nylon fishing lines, AIP Adv. 5 (6) (2015) 067158.

[23] C.S. Haines, et al., Artificial muscles from fishing line and sewing thread, Science 343 (6173) (2014) 868–872.

[24] S.M. Mirvakili, I.W. Hunter, Multidirectional artificial muscles from nylon, Adv. Mater. 29 (4) (2017).

[25] S. Aziz, et al., Thermomechanical effects in the torsional actuation of twisted nylon 6 fiber, J. Appl. Polym. Sci. 134 (47) (2017) 45529.

[26] L. Wu, et al., Compact and low-cost humanoid hand powered by nylon artificial muscles, Bioinspir. Biomim. 12 (2) (2017) 026004.

[27] S.M. Mirvakili, I.W. Hunter, Bending artificial muscle from nylon filaments, in: Y. BarCohen, F. Vidal (Eds.), Electroactive Polymer Actuators and Devices (EAPAD), SPIE-Int Soc Optical Engineering, Bellingham, 2016, p. 979811. ISBN 978-1-5106-0039-3.

[28] J. Naciri, et al., Nematic elastomer fiber actuator, Macromolecules 36 (22) (2003) 8499–8505.

[29] E.-K. Fleischmann, F.R. Forst, R. Zentel, Liquid-crystalline elastomer fibers prepared in a microfluidic device, Macromol. Chem. Phys. 215 (10) (2014) 1004–1011.

[30] S.V. Ahir, A.R. Tajbakhsh, E.M. Terentjev, Self-assembled shape-memory fibers of triblock liquid-crystal polymers, Adv. Funct. Mater. 16 (4) (2006) 556–560.

[31] W. Deng, et al., Light-responsive wires from side-on liquid crystalline azo polymers, Liquid Crystals 36 (10–11) (2009) 1023–1029.

[32] L. Fang, et al., Synthesis of reactive azobenzene main-chain liquid crystalline polymers via Michael addition polymerization and photomechanical effects of their supramolecular hydrogen-bonded fibers, Macromolecules 46 (19) (2013) 7650–7660.

[33] P. Chen, et al., Hierarchically arranged helical fibre actuators driven by solvents and vapours, Nat. Nanotechnol. 10 (12) (2015) 1077–1083.

[34] T.F. Otero, J.G. Martinez, K. Asaka, Faradaic and capacitive components of the CNT electrochemical responses, Front. Mater. 3 (3) (2016).

[35] J.A. Lee, et al., Electrochemically powered, energy-conserving carbon nanotube artificial muscles, Adv. Mater. 29 (31) (2017) 1700870.

[36] T. Mirfakhrai, et al., Carbon nanotube yarn actuators: an electrochemical impedance model, J. Electrochem. Soc. 156 (6) (2009) K97–K103.

[37] A.-S. Michardiere, et al., Carbon nanotube microfiber actuators with reduced stress relaxation, J. Phys. Chem. C 120 (12) (2016) 6851–6858.

[38] J. Foroughi, et al., Torsional carbon nanotube artificial muscles, Science 334 (6055) (2011) 494–497.

[39] Y.A. Ismail, et al., Sensing characteristics of a conducting polymer/hydrogel hybrid microfiber artificial muscle, Sens. Actuators B: Chem. 160 (1) (2011) 1180–1190.

[40] A. Maziz, et al., Knitting and weaving artificial muscles, Sci. Adv. 3 (1) (2017) e1600327.

[41] J.G. Martinez, et al., Investigation of electrically conducting yarns for use in textile actuators, Smart Mater. Struct. 27 (7) (2018) 074004.

[42] Y. Wang, et al., Flexible and wearable graphene/polypyrrole fibers towards multifunctional actuator applications, Electrochem. Commun. 35 (2013) 49–52.

[43] J. Abel, J. Luntz, D. Brei, A two-dimensional analytical model and experimental validation of garter stitch knitted shape memory alloy actuator architecture, Smart Mater. Struct. 21 (8) (2012) 085011.

[44] J. Abel, J. Luntz, D. Brei, Hierarchical architecture of active knits, Smart Mater. Struct. 22 (12) (2013). 125001.

[45] Y.Y.F.C. Vili, Investigating smart textiles based on shape memory materials, Text. Res. J. 77 (5) (2007) 290–300.

[46] S. Vasile, et al., Analysis of hybrid woven fabrics with shape memory alloys wires embedded, Fibres Text. East. Eur. 18 (1) (2010) 64–69.

[47] B. Quinn, Textile Futures: Fashion, Bloomsbury Academic, Design and Technology, 2010.

[48] S. Guney, I. Ucgul, A. Koyun, Designing the medical textile material providing peristaltic motion and its computerized control, J. Text. Inst. 107 (5) (2016) 547–552.

[49] I. Cabral, et al., Exploring geometric morphology in shape memory textiles: design of dynamic light filters, Text. Res. J. 85 (18) (2015) 1919–1933.

[50] B. Holschuh, D. Newman, Two-spring model for active compression textiles with integrated NiTi coil actuators, Smart Mater. Struct. 24 (3) (2015) 035011.

[51] M.C. Yuen, R.A. Bilodeau, R.K. Kramer, Active variable stiffness fibers for multifunctional robotic fabrics, IEEE Robot. Autom. Lett. 1 (2) (2016) 708–715.

[52] J. Foroughi, et al., Knitted carbon-nanotube-sheath/spandex-core elastomeric yarns for artificial muscles and strain sensing, ACS Nano 10 (10) (2016) 9129–9135.

[53] E. Shoji, S. Takagi, H. Araie, Novel conducting fabric polymer composites as stretchable electrodes: one-step fabrication of chemical actuators, Polym. Adv. Technol. 20 (4) (2009) 423–426.

[54] F. Kaasik, et al., Scalable fabrication of ionic and capacitive laminate actuators for soft robotics, Sens. Actuators B: Chem. 246 (2017) 154–163.

[55] K. Otsuka, C.M. Wayman, Shape Memory Materials, Cambridge University Press, 1999. ISBN 978-0-521-66384-7.

[56] F. Boussu, J.I. Petitniot, Development of shape memory alloy fabrics for composite structures, in: H.R. Mattila (Ed.), Intelligent Textiles and Clothing, Woodhead Publishing, 2006, pp. 124–142.

[57] S. Kurumaya, et al., Design of thin McKibben muscle and multifilament structure, Sens. Actuators, A: Phys. 261 (2017) 66–74.

[58] A. Ohno, K. Suzumori, A. Sadic, Fabrication of active textile woven and wearable suit using thin pneumatic artificial muscle, in: JSME Conference on Robotics and Mechatronis, Robomec 2015, Kyoto, Japan, 2015.

[59] M.J. Denton, P.N. Daniels, Textile Terms and Definitions, 11 ed., The Textile Institute, Manchester, 2002.

[60] F. Carpi, et al., Electroactive polymer actuators as artificial muscles: are they ready for bioinspired applications? Bioinspir. Biomim. 6 (4) (2011) 045006.

[61] R. Pelrine, et al., High-speed electrically actuated elastomers with strain greater than 100%, Science 287 (2000) 836–839.

[62] F. Carpi, et al., Standards for dielectric elastomer transducers, Smart Mater. Struct. 24 (10) (2015) 105025.

[63] Q. Pei, O. Inganäs, Conjugated polymers and the bending cantilever method: electrical muscles and smart devices, Adv. Mater. 4 (4) (1992) 277–278.

[64] T.F. Otero, et al., Electrochemomechanical properties from a bilayer: polypyrrole/non-conducting and flexible material—artificial muscle, J. Electroanal. Chem. 341 (1–2) (1992) 369–375.

[65] M. Shahinpoor, et al., Ionic polymer-metal composites (IPMCs) as biomimetic sensors, actuators and artificial muscles—a review, Smart Mater. Struct. 7 (1998) R15–R30.

[66] R.H. Baughman, et al., Carbon nanotube actuators, Science 284 (5418) (1999) 1340–1344.

[67] Y. Osada, H. Okuzaki, H. Hori, A polymer gel with electrically driven motility, Nature 355 (6357) (1992) 242–244.

[68] Q. Pei, O. Inganäs, Electrochemical applications of the bending beam method. 1. Mass transport and volume changes in polypyrrole during redox, J. Phys. Chem. 96 (25) (1992) 10507–10514.

[69] E.W.H. Jager, E. Smela, O. Inganäs, Microfabricating conjugated polymer actuators, Science 290 (5496) (2000) 1540–1545.

[70] K.P. Vidanapathirana, et al., Ion movement in polypyrrole-dodecylbenzenesulphonate films in aqueous and non-aqueous electrolytes, Solid State Ionics 154–155 (2002) 331–335.

[71] M.J.M. Jafeen, M.A. Careem, S. Skaarup, Speed and strain of polypyrrole actuators: dependence on cation hydration number, Ionics 16 (1) (2010) 1–6.

[72] J.D. Madden, et al., Fast contracting polypyrrole actuators, Synthetic Metals 113 (1–2) (2000) 185–192.

[73] T. Mirfakhrai, J.D.W. Madden, R.H. Baughman, Polymer artificial muscles, Mater. Today 10 (4) (2007) 30–38.

[74] A. Gelmi, et al., Direct mechanical stimulation of stem cells: a beating electro-mechanically active scaffold for cardiac tissue engineering, Adv. Healthc. Mater. 5 (12) (2016) 1471–1480.

[75] A.S. Hutchison, et al., Development of polypyrrole-based electromechanical actuators, Synthetic Metals 113 (1–2) (2000) 121–127.

[76] G.M. Spinks, T.E. Campbell, G.G. Wallace, Force generation from polypyrrole actuators, Smart Mater. Struct. 14 (2) (2005) 406–412.

[77] Sarcos Corp, e.g., http://www.sarcos.com/ and Ekso Bionics, http://eksobionics.com/.

[78] A.P. Zakharov, L.M. Pismen, Active textiles with Janus fibres, Soft Matter 14 (5) (2018) 676–680.

Further reading

[79] N.-K. Persson, et al., Actuating textiles—next generation of smart textiles, Adv. Mater. Technol. (2018) 1700397.

Index

Note: Page numbers followed by *f* indicate figures and *t* indicate tables.

U

Ultra-large-scale integration
(ULSI), 140–141
Ultrathin chips (UTCs), 140–141,
146

V

Vapor-phase polymerization,
211–212

W

Water bolus, 194–195
Wearable biomarker analysis,
practical design, 58–59
Wearable biosensors
bodily fluids, 66
physical sensing, 66
point-of-care diagnostics, 65–66
saliva-based, 66, 68–70

subcutaneous and implantable,
74–77
sweat-based, 72–74
tear-based, 66–68
Wearable enzyme-based biosensors,
32–33
Wearable/implantable systems,
150–151
Wearable ion-selective chemical
sensor, 54t
Wearable technology, 90, 179–180
Wearable temperature sensors,
28–29
Weaving, 188, 204–205
Wireless communication, 94
Wireless power transfer (WPT), 90
capacitive power transfer, 121f
electromagnetic waves, 119
far-field power transfer
techniques power, 120

inductive coupling mechanism,
120
inductive power transfer, 121f
limitation, 125
power LEDs, 120
RF power transfer mechanism,
120
systems based on non-radiative
methods, 119–120
systems based on radiative
methods, 119–120
ultraminiaturized flexible device,
122f
World Health Organization (WHO),
153–154

Y

Yarn actuators, 204–206
Young's modulus, 136–139, 159,
206